Chinese Medicine: Ancient Healing Traditions

Chinese Medicine: Ancient Healing Traditions

Edited by Trinity Harper

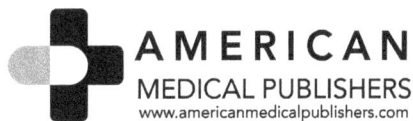

AMERICAN
MEDICAL PUBLISHERS
www.americanmedicalpublishers.com

American Medical Publishers,
41 Flatbush Avenue,
1st Floor, New York,
NY 11217, USA

Visit us on the World Wide Web at:
www.americanmedicalpublishers.com

This book contains information obtained from authentic and highly regarded sources. Copyright for all individual chapters remain with the respective authors as indicated. All chapters are published with permission under the Creative Commons Attribution License or equivalent. A wide variety of references are listed. Permission and sources are indicated; for detailed attributions, please refer to the permissions page and list of contributors. Reasonable efforts have been made to publish reliable data and information, but the authors, editors and publisher cannot assume any responsibility for the validity of all materials or the consequences of their use.

ISBN: 978-1-63927-045-3

Trademark Notice: Registered trademark of products or corporate names are used only for explanation and identification without intent to infringe.

Cataloging-in-Publication Data

Chinese medicine : ancient healing traditions / edited by Trinity Harper.
   p. cm.
Includes bibliographical references and index.
ISBN 978-1-63927-045-3
1. Medicine, Chinese. 2. Medicine, Ancient. 3. Alternative medicine--China. I. Harper, Trinity.
R601 .C45 2022
610.951--dc23

Table of Contents

Preface

The world is advancing at a fast pace like never before. Therefore, the need is to keep up with the latest developments. This book was an idea that came to fruition when the specialists in the area realized the need to coordinate together and document essential themes in the subject. That's when I was requested to be the editor. Editing this book has been an honour as it brings together diverse authors researching on different streams of the field. The book collates essential materials contributed by veterans in the area which can be utilized by students and researchers alike.

Traditional Chinese medicine is based on the ancient Chinese medical practice that involves various forms of cupping therapy, herbal medicine, bonesetter, exercise, gua sha, massage, acupuncture and dietary therapy. The Chinese herbal medicine uses both biotic and non-biotic substances including human, animal and mineral products. Chinese medicine is based on the belief that the vital energy of the body circulates through the channels known as meridians. These meridians have branches connected to body organs and functions. The primary focus of Chinese medicine is on the functions of the body such as breathing, digestion and temperature maintenance. Disease is seen as a disharmony and imbalance in the interactions and functions of yin, yang, meridians and qi along with the interaction between the human body and the environment. Diagnosis in Chinese medicine focuses on tracing symptoms in order to determine a pattern of an underlying disharmony. This book is compiled in such a manner, that it will provide an in-depth knowledge about the theory and practice of Chinese medicine. Students, researchers, experts and all associated with this field will benefit alike from this book.

Each chapter is a sole-standing publication that reflects each author's interpretation. Thus, the book displays a multi-facetted picture of our current understanding of application, resources and aspects of the field. I would like to thank the contributors of this book and my family for their endless support.

Editor

Comparison of chemical profiles and effectiveness between Erxian decoction and mixtures of decoctions of its individual herbs: a novel approach for identification of the standard chemicals

H. P. Cheung[1], S. W. Wang[1], T. B. Ng[2], Y. B. Zhang[1], L. X. Lao[1], Z. J. Zhang[1], Y. Tong[1], F. W. S. Chung[1] and S. C. W. Sze[1]*

Abstract

Background: Identification of bioactive standard chemicals is a major challenge in the study of the Chinese medicinal formula. In particular, the chemical components may interact differently depending on the preparative methods, therefore affecting the amounts of bioactive components and their pharmacological properties in the medicinal formula. With the use of Erxian decoction (EXD) as a study model—a well-known Chinese medicinal formula for treating menopausal symptoms, a novel and rapid approach in seeking standard chemicals has been established by differentially comparing the HPLC profiles and the menopause-related biochemical parameters of combined decoction of EXD (EXD-C) and mixtures of the decoctions of its individual herbs (EXD-S).

Methods: The levels of six chemicals, which exerted actions on the HPO axis, have been measured in EXD-C and EXD-S by HPLC. Twelve-month-old female Sprague-Dawley rats were employed and treated with EXD-C and EXD-S. Their endocrine functions after treatment were evaluated by determining the ovarian mRNA levels of aromatase, a key enzyme for estradiol biosynthesis. The effect of the antioxidant regimen was determined by the hepatic superoxide dismutase-1 (SOD), catalase (CAT) and glutathione peroxidase (GPx-1) mRNA levels.

Results: The amounts of mangiferine, ferulic acid, jatrorrhizine and palmatine in EXD-S were twofold higher than those in EXD-C. EXD-S was more effective in stimulating ovarian aromatase and the expression of the antioxidant enzymes compared with EXD-C.

Conclusion: Mangiferine, ferulic acid, jatrorrhizine and palmatine are suitable for use as standard chemicals for quality evaluation of EXD according to our approach. EXD-S could be more effective than EXD-C.

Keywords: Standard chemicals, Chinese medicine formula, Erxian decoction, Menopause, Novel approach

Background

The clinical use of Chinese medicine (CM) formulas for treating chronic diseases and aging-related disorders has been gaining momentum in recent years. The multiple pharmacological properties of CM formula are proved to be contributed by the multiple bioactive chemicals in a CM formula through multiple mechanisms [1]. Thus, seeking bioactive and standard chemical is crucial for quality control evaluation of CM formulas. While the contemporary analytic techniques allow us to isolate and detect multiples chemical components from CM

*Correspondence: stephens@hku.hk
[1] School of Chinese Medicine, Li Ka Shing Faculty of Medicine,
The University of Hong Kong, 10 Sassoon Road, Pokfulam,
Hong Kong, SAR, China
Full list of author information is available at the end of the article

formulas simultaneously, identification of bioactive and standard chemicals remains a tedious task.

Due to the complexity of the chemicals in a CM formula, the potential interaction and the subsequent changes in the pharmacological properties have drawn the attention of many researchers in the field [1]. Interactions leading to changes in the chemical components of TCM may arise during the processing of herbal materials or during the decoction procedures [2]. Conventionally, different herbal materials in a Chinese medicinal formula are decocted together to yield the medicinal extract, which can be regarded as a "combined decoction". To the contrary, individual herbs can be decocted separately and mixed together to compose a medicinal formula. This is particularly common in the recent development of herbal formulations, extracts of individual herbal material can be concentrated in the form of granules, and the medicinal formula can be reconstituted by mixing the corresponding amounts of granules [3]. The resulting decoction is thus regarded as a mixture of decoctions of separated individual herbs (separated decoction)". However, due to the difference in their decoction processes, there will be variations in the chemical components of the "combined decoction" and "separated decoction". It is known that during the decoction process, the chemicals from different herbs may interact to affect the solubility, conversion of chemical structures, or may lead to generation of new chemicals or precipitation [3]. For example, results obtained from a previous study revealed that the component of 1,5-dicaffeoylquinic acid in the Tibetan herb (*Saussurea laniceps*) was transesterificated into 1,3-dicaffeoylquinic acid during boiling in water [4]. These interactions may affect the amounts of bioactive components in the medicinal formula, and thus the pharmacological properties. On the one hand, the discrepancy between the chemical components and the pharmacological properties between "combined decoction" and "separated decoction" has raised concerns about the variation in quality and therapeutic efficacy of decoctions prepared using different methods. On the other hand, such discrepancy may hint the bioactive components contributing to the pharmacological properties, thus opening up the possibility of a novel and rapid approach for identification of the chemical standards of CM formulas for quality control purpose.

In this study, Erxian decoction (EXD), an anti-menopausal Chinese medicine formula, was selected as a study model to demonstrate the feasibility of our approach for identification of the chemical standards of CM formulas. Erxian decoction (EXD) is a popular TCM formula that has been clinically used for relieving menopausal syndrome for more than 60 years [5]. Our previous EXD studies have used a LC-DAD-ESI-MS/MS method in

characterising the key chemical constitutents of EXD absorbed or metabolised in vivo during the treatment of menopausal syndromes [6]. Knowing that the causes of menopausal syndromes involves the hypothalamus-pituitary-ovary (HPO) axis, target compounds of this study were identified and differentiated by their presence in the major organs of the HPO axis (i.e. brain and ovary) and serum. Six chemicals from EXD that may contribute to relief of menopausal syndrome were selected: mangiferine, ferulic acid, icariin, jatrorrhizine, palmatine and berberine [6]. Therefore, the levels of mangiferine, ferulic acid, icariin, jatrorrhizine, palmatine and berberine in both EXD-C and EXD-S were determined and compared by HPLC profiles. Besides chemical analysis, it has been found in human that during menopause, the expression of aromatase, a key enzyme for ovarian estradiol production, and the activities of some antioxidant enzymes, including superoxide dismutase-1 (SOD1), and glutathione peroxidase (GPx-1), underwent a decrease leading to a decline of ovarian estrogen production and serum estrogen level [7]. In addition, our previous study also demonstrated that EXD relieved menopausal syndrome via up-regulation of the mRNA levels of ovarian aromatase and hepatic antioxidant enzymes catalase (CAT) in twelve-month-old naturally aging SD-rats with lower serum estradiol levels compared with those of 3-month-old young SD-rat [5]. Therefore, we evaluated and compared the pharmacological properties of EXD-C and EXD-S for alleviating menopause by measurement of their mRNA levels of ovarian aromatase and hepatic antioxidant enzymes SOD-1, CAT, and GPx-1 after drug treatment. Results and approach obtained from this study could be applied in quality control studies of other existing CM formulas, which ensure the use of high-quality CM formulas clinically. The following shows our approach for selecting the standard markers for quality control of CM formulas: (i) the standard markers should be present at target sites/organs in vivo; (ii) the standard markers should be associated with pharmacological and clinical effects of CM formulas; (iii) the amounts of standard markers should have twofold differences for different decoction processing (EXD-S: separate decoction of EXD vs EXD-C: combined decoction of EXD).

Methods
Herbal materials and preparation of different decoctions of EXD
One kilogram of the six component herbs of EXD namely *Herba Epimedii, Rhizoma Curculiginis, Radix Morindae officinalis, Cortex Phellodendri, Radix Anemarrhenae,* and *Radix Angelicae sinensis* (composition ratio = 12:12:10:10:9:9) were decocted together with distilled water in 10:1 (v/w) ratio at 100 °C for 1 h to prepare "combined decoction of EXD" (EXD-C), the extraction

was repeated twice. The procedures were the same as those described in our previous publication [5]. For preparation of "mixtures of EXD individual herbs decoction" (EXD-S), the component herbs in the amounts according to above composition ratio of EXD-C were decocted separately instead and reconstituted afterward. The extraction was also repeated twice. Both of the herbal extracts, EXD-C and EXD-S, were filtered and lyophilized in a freeze drier (Labconco, Freezone). The dried powdered extracts were stored at −80 °C before use. The herbal materials were collected from various sources and their identity was confirmed by Dr YanBo Zhang (one of the authors), School of Chinese medicine, the University of Hong Kong.

Quality control and high performance liquid chromatography (HPLC)

To evaluate the consistency of the quality of EXD-S and EXD-C extracts, three batches of 0.5 g powder of extracts were extracted with 10 ml 75% methanol in a water bath at 60 °C for 15 min, followed by ultrasonication for 30 min. The extracts were centrifuged at $15,700 \times g$ and filtered with 0.45 μm Millex® syringe filter (Millipore). Six standard chemicals namely mangiferine, ferulic acid, icariin, jatrorrhizine, palmatine and berberine which are well-known compounds in EXD [5] were employed for quantitation. The HPLC profiles of the EXD-S and EXD-C were generated using Water 600S HPLC system (Waters) with a reverse-phase column (XBridge® C18, 5 μl, 250 mm × 4.6 mm i.d., Waters, USA). The mobile phase consisted of acetonitrile (solvent A) and 0.05% SDS in 0.1% acetic acid (solvent B). A programmed gradient was used for elution with 5–30% A in 0–30 min, 30% A in 30–35 min, 30–50% A in 35–40 min, 50–55% A in 40–65 min. The injection volume was 10 μl and flow rate was 1 ml/min. The ultraviolet (UV) absorbance from 200 to 400 nm was measured with a diode array detector (DAD). Chromatograms were generated at 345 nm to observed most number of peaks. The peak integration and quantitation were analyzed with the Waters Empower 2 software (Waters), the procedures were the same as those described in our previous publication [5].

Animals

Twelve-month old female Sprague-Dawley (SD)-rats with low serum estradiol levels were employed as the animal model [5]. Animals were purchased at the age of 8 months from the Laboratory Animal Units, the University of Hong Kong and housed at an ambient temperature of 24 °C with a relative humidity of 50–65% and 12-h light–dark cycles till the required age. The rats were acclimated for four months and their serum estradiol levels were monitored before the experiment. The experiments

had been approved by the Committee on the Use of Live Animals in Teaching and Research (CULATR) of the Li Ka Shing Faculty of Medicine, the University of Hong Kong.

Drug administration and organ harvesting

Rats were arbitrarily divided into six groups with ten animals each. EXD-S and EXD-C extracts dissolved in 2 ml of water (0.76 and 1.52 g/kg) were administered via gavage tubing daily for 6 weeks. The control group received an equal volume of water instead of drug. At the end of the experiment, the rats were euthanized by an intraperitoneal injection of pentobarbital (200 mg/kg). The ovaries and livers were collected and stored at −80 °C until further experiment.

RNA extraction and quantitative real-time PCR

The RNA extraction and quantitative real-time PCR were performed according to the previous methods published by our group [5]. In brief, total RNA was isolated from the ovary and liver using the TRIZOL® reagent according to instructions of the manufacturer (Invitrogen Life Technologies). The purity and concentration of RNA were determined by the absorbance at 260/280 nm and at 260 nm, respectively. The cDNA was transcribed from 1 μg of total RNA using random hexamers (Promega) and reverse transcriptase II (Invitrogen Life Technologies) following the manufacturer's instructions. Quantitative real-time PCR was performed for the expression of aromatase (Cyp19), CAT, SOD-1, glutathione peroxidase 1 (GPx-1) genes and beta-actin (β-actin) as housekeeping control using the Platinum® quantitative PCR SuperMIX-UDG (Invitrogen Life Technologies) in a final reaction volume of 25 μl in 0.25 X SYBR green (Molecular Probes®, Invitrogen Life Technologies) according to the manufacturer's protocol. The sequences of the PCR primers are described in our previous study [5]. The target genes were amplified with the following programme: pre-incubation at 94 °C for 15 min, followed by 40 cycles of incubation at 94 °C for 20 s, 57 °C for 20 s and 72 °C for 20 s. Following the amplification process, a melting curve analysis was performed by raising the temperature from 72 to 95 °C at a rate of 1 °C/5 s to ensure the specificity of PCR products. Quantitation of PCR product was performed by comparing with the standard curve (plot of number of threshold cycle (Ct) value against log of standard amount with a series of 20-fold dilution), and the results were expressed as Ct value. Quantity of the target genes was normalized with the housekeeping gene β-actin for relative quantitation. The experiments were repeated in triplicate for analysis.

Statistical analysis

For the peaks in HPLC profiles of EXD-S and EXD-C, relative standard deviation (RSD) was calculated. For PCR experiments, data were expressed as mean ± SEM. Statistically analysis was performed using One-way ANOVA followed by Tukey's Multiple Comparison Test. A p value <0.05 in a comparison was considered statistically significant. Statistical analysis was performed with GraphPad Prism 4® software (GraphPad Software).

Results

HPLC profiles of EXD-S and EXD-C

The peaks from chromatograms generated at 345 nm show most detectable peaks were integrated. The chromatograms of EXD-S and EXD-C annotated with the six standard chemicals are shown in Fig. 1. Three batches of EXD-S and EXD-C were injected. The amounts of the six standard chemicals were determined from the standard curve and are listed in Table 1. The contents of all the six marker chemicals were found to decrease to different extents in EXD-C (Fig. 2). The content of mangiferin in EXD-S and EXD-C demonstrated a 2.09-fold difference. The decrease in content of three berberine-type alkaloids (jatrorrhizine, palmatine and berberine) in EXD-C varied from 3.44-old for jatrorrhizine, 30.17-fold for palmatine and 1.62-fold for berberine. The content of ferulic acid in EXD-C decreased by 2.46-fold and the amount of icariin showed a 1.17-fold decrease in EXD-C (Fig. 3). For all the six standard chemicals, the RSD values calculated were within 5%, indicating consistency in the quality of the sample injected and reproducibility of the HPLC profile, as well as excluding the influence of any unknown variability or instability found in the composition of the active constituents in the molecular investigation of the EXD extract.

Effects of EXD-S and EXD-C on expression of Cyp19, CAT, SOD and GPx-1 at transcriptional level

After treatment with EXD-S and EXD-C for 6 weeks, the expression of ovarian Cyp19, SOD, CAT and hepatic GPx-1 was regulated differently. From the results, both treatments with EXD-S and EXD-C at high doses significantly stimulated the expression of ovarian Cyp19 gene, which encodes the key enzyme aromatase for estrogen secretion. ($p < 0.01$ compared with control group in Tukey's Multiple Comparison Test following One-way ANOVA). The stimulatory effect on up-regulation of Cyp19 was most prominent in EXD-S at high dose, which is in line with our previous finding [5], in which the expression level of Cyp19 gene was significantly higher than that of EXD-C at high dose ($p < 0.001$ compared with control group in Tukey's Multiple Comparison Test following One-way ANOVA) (Fig. 4).

The effects of EXD-S and EXD-C were less prominent on the gene expression of hepatic antioxidant enzymes.

The relative mRNA levels of CAT after treatment of EXD were slightly higher than that of control by around 1.5-fold, without statistical significance. EXD-S treatment at both dosages displayed a trend of increase in CAT expression compared with EXD-C, but again no significant differences were detected (Fig. 5).

The mRNA levels of SOD-1 and GPx-1 in all treatment groups were comparable to that of control. However, in EXD-S (low dose) treated group, the hepatic mRNA expression of SOD-1 was significantly higher than that of EXD-C (low dose) group (Fig. 6). EXD-S at high dose also displayed a tendency of increase in the mRNA level of hepatic GPx-1 compared with that of EXD-C groups, but such tendency was devoid of statistically significant difference (Fig. 7).

Discussion

The effects of different decoction methods on chemical profiles of anti-menopausal EXD formula have been demonstrated by HPLC, with the six selected chemicals that have been present at HPO-axis in vivo revealed from our previous publication [6]. Results obtained from HPLC profile revealed that all the six chemicals including mangiferin, ferulic acid, icariin, jatrorrhizine, palmatine and berberine were higher in content in EXD-S than that in EXD-C (Figs. 2, 3), the HPLC profile of EXD-S is the same as that in our previous publication [5]. Such changes in chemical profiles may be due to the interaction of different components during the decoction process. For instance, the chemical components may enhanced the solubility of each other when decocted together thus increasing the final content of chemicals in the extract [8]. On the contrary, they may precipitate with each other forming insoluble complex leading to loss of bioactive components [8]. It is known that alkaloids like berberine, palmatine and jatrorrhizine would form precipitate with the flavone baicalin [9]. Alkaloids may also precipitate with organic acids forming insoluble salts [8]. It is possible that the alkaloids species in combined decoction of EXD (EXD-C) may precipitate with organic acid from its different ingredient herbs like ferulic acid, flavonoid compounds such as icariin or other undetected flavone species and are lost from EXD-C. Also, bioactive components can be converted by chemical reactions like hydrolysis of glycosides. In the combined decoction of EXD (EXD-C), hydrolysis may be facilitated to remove the sugar units from the flavonoids glycoside icariin, leading to decrease in its content [2].

Mangiferine, ferulic acid, jatrorrhizine and palmatine were confirmed as the key chemical markers for quality control of anti-menopausal EXD according to our proposed approach. Because (i) they have been present at HPO axis, revealed by our previous study; (ii) their pharmacological effects are related to menopause. As it has

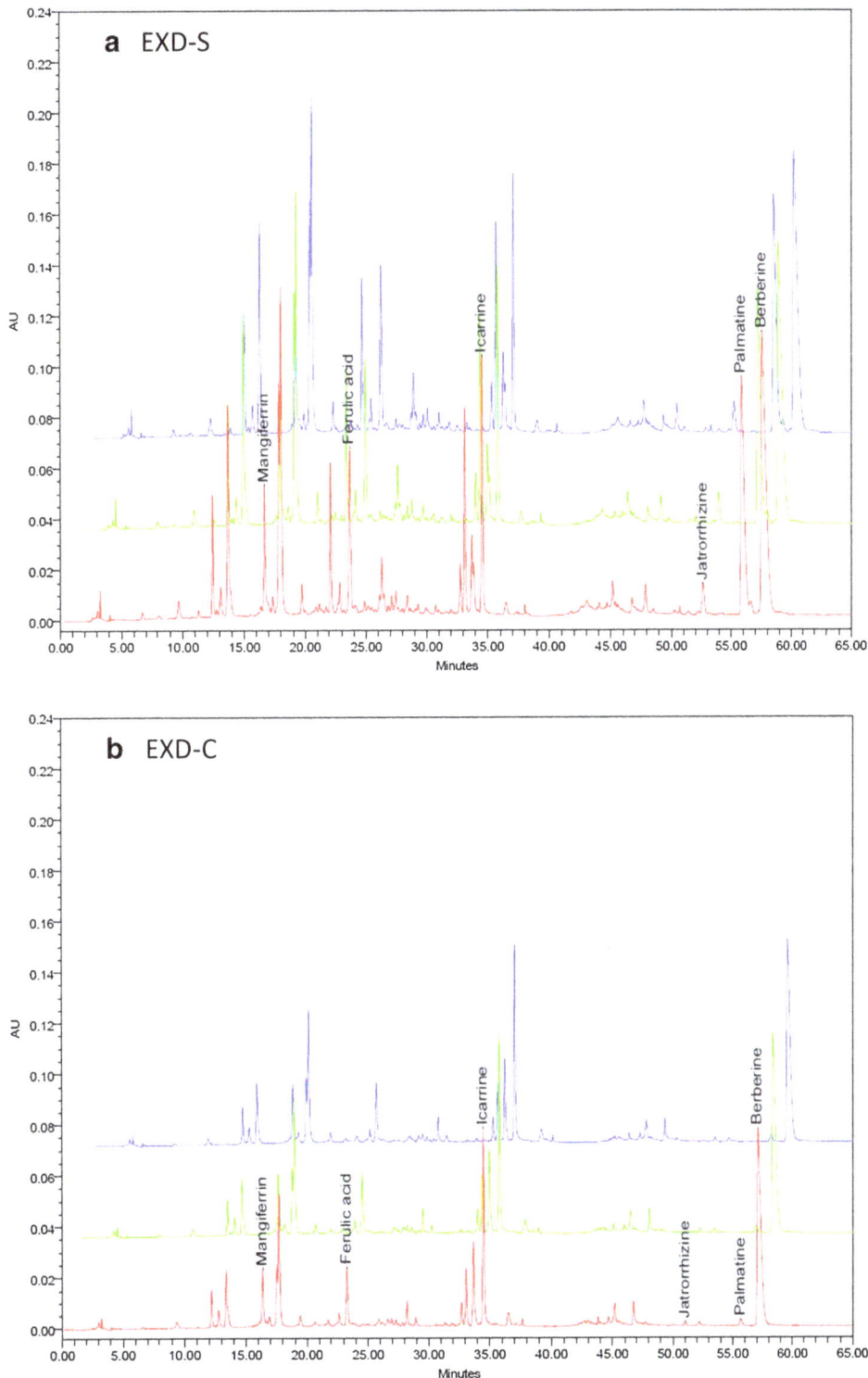

Fig. 1 Overlaid HPLC chromatograms of **a** EXD-S [4] and **b** EXD-C from three repeated injections extracted at 345 nm. The peaks of six standard chemicals were annotated as mangiferine, ferulic acid, icariin, jatrorrhizine, palmatine and berberine, in a chorological order of retention time

been reported that along with aging and menopause, the antioxidant enzymes is down-regulated, and the estrogen secretion through aromatase is hampered [6]. These four chemical markers possess antioxidant activities [10–13]. Besides, ferulic acid were also reported to have estrogenic properties, its treatment increases the bone mineral

Table 1 The contents of six standard chemicals of EXD in three injections of EXD-S and EXD-C

Injection	Mangiferin (mg/g)	Ferulic acid (mg/g)	Icariin (mg/g)	Jatrorrhizine (mg/g)	Palmatine (mg/g)	Berberine (mg/g)
EXD-S1	1.368	0.4871	1.731	0.1004	1.083	1.615
EXD-S2	1.371	0.4896	1.744	0.1010	1.090	1.617
EXD-S3	1.382	0.4996	1.745	0.1014	1.092	1.628
Mean	1.374	0.4921	1.740	0.1010	1.089	1.620
RSD (%)	0.57	1.34	0.46	0.48	0.46	0.43
EXD-C1	0.6581	0.1983	1.498	0.02865	0.03577	1.000
EXD-C2	0.6610	0.1980	1.493	0.03009	0.03661	1.001
EXD-C3	0.6583	0.2034	1.479	0.02947	0.03592	1.003
Mean	0.6591	0.1999	1.490	0.02940	0.03610	1.001
RSD (%)	0.24	1.53	0.65	2.45	1.23	0.17
Mean ratio	2.085	2.462	1.168	3.435	30.17	1.618

The results are expressed as mg or chemicals per g of EXD extract. RSD values were calculated for each chemical from three injections and the mean ratio represents the ratio of amount of chemicals in EXD-S to that of EXD-C

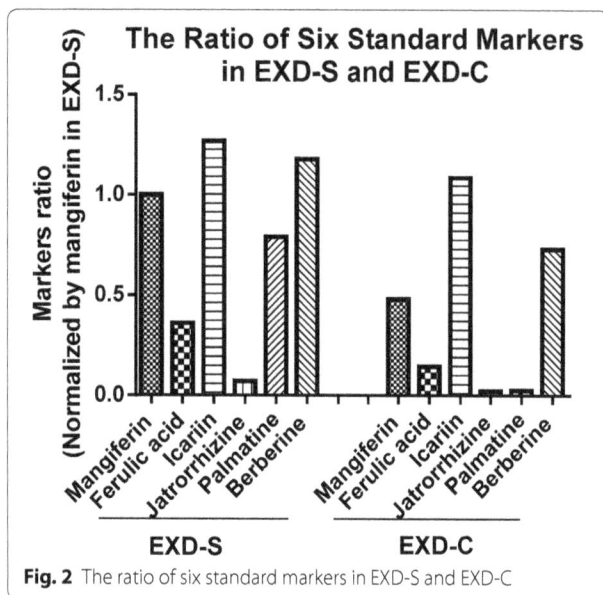

Fig. 2 The ratio of six standard markers in EXD-S and EXD-C

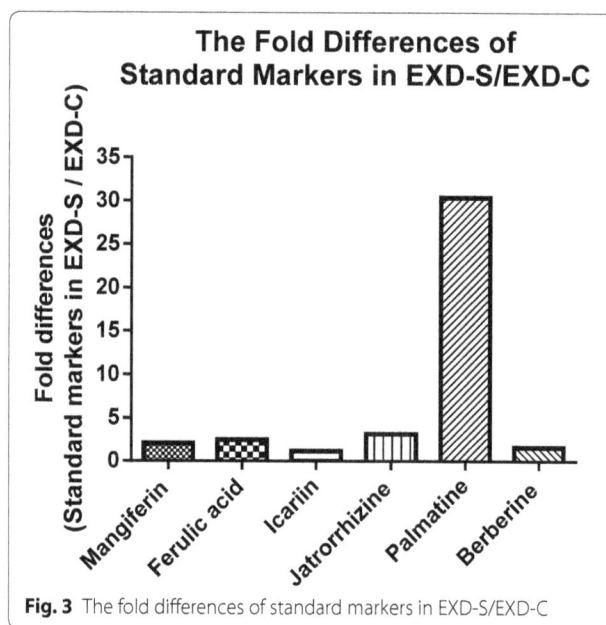

Fig. 3 The fold differences of standard markers in EXD-S/EXD-C

density in ovariectomized female rats of the Sprague-Dawley strain with slightly increasing the serum levels of estrogen [14]. In addition, it has been shown to be effective in treating hot flashes in menopausal women [15]; (iii) the amounts of these four chemical markers in EXD-S are twofold higher than those in EXD-C, thus different decoction methods could be easily revealed by different amounts of these four markers in HPLC profile (Fig. 3). In particular, palmatine is almost 30.38-fold higher in EXD-S compared with EXD-C (Fig. 3), which will be further biologically characterized in our further experiment.

Besides chemical analysis, the effects of EXD-S and EXD-C on ovarian aromatase mRNA expression and hepatic antioxidant enzymes were evaluated, which has also been proven as the targets of EXD by our group previously [5]. As anticipated, EXD stimulated ovarian aromatase (Cyp19) expression the transcriptional level at high dose (1.76 g/kg). The up-regulation of Cyp19 mRNA level in EXD-S-treated rats was significantly almost twofold higher than that of EXD-C, which may have been due to the overall increase in bioactive components in EXD-S as revealed from the HPLC profiles. It is known that the bioactive components in EXD such as mangiferin, berberine, palmatine and jatrorrhizine possess antioxidant activities [10–13]. Besides, icariin and ferulic acid were also reported to have estrogenic properties [14, 16]. The lower amounts of these bioactive compounds in EXD-C may explain the decreased bioactivity of EXD-C

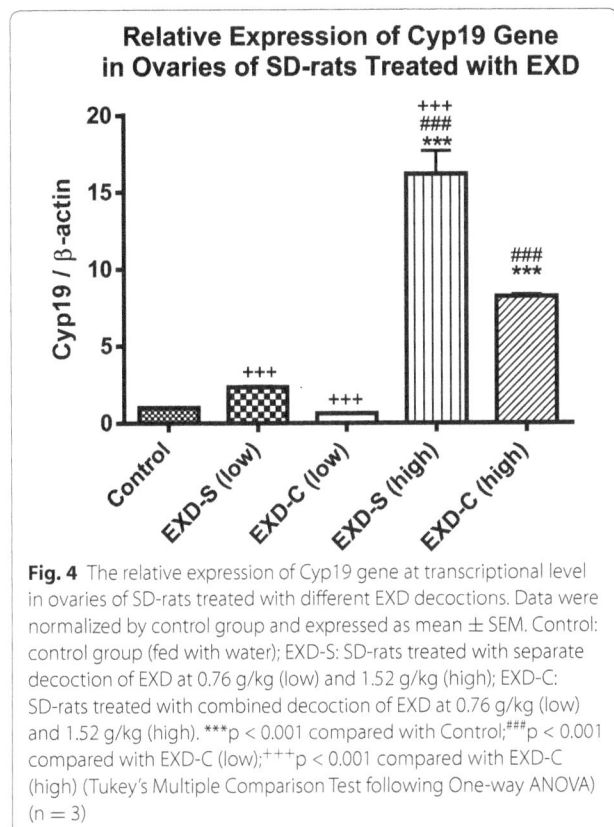

Fig. 4 The relative expression of Cyp19 gene at transcriptional level in ovaries of SD-rats treated with different EXD decoctions. Data were normalized by control group and expressed as mean ± SEM. Control: control group (fed with water); EXD-S: SD-rats treated with separate decoction of EXD at 0.76 g/kg (low) and 1.52 g/kg (high); EXD-C: SD-rats treated with combined decoction of EXD at 0.76 g/kg (low) and 1.52 g/kg (high). ***p < 0.001 compared with Control; ###p < 0.001 compared with EXD-C (low); +++p < 0.001 compared with EXD-C (high) (Tukey's Multiple Comparison Test following One-way ANOVA) (n = 3)

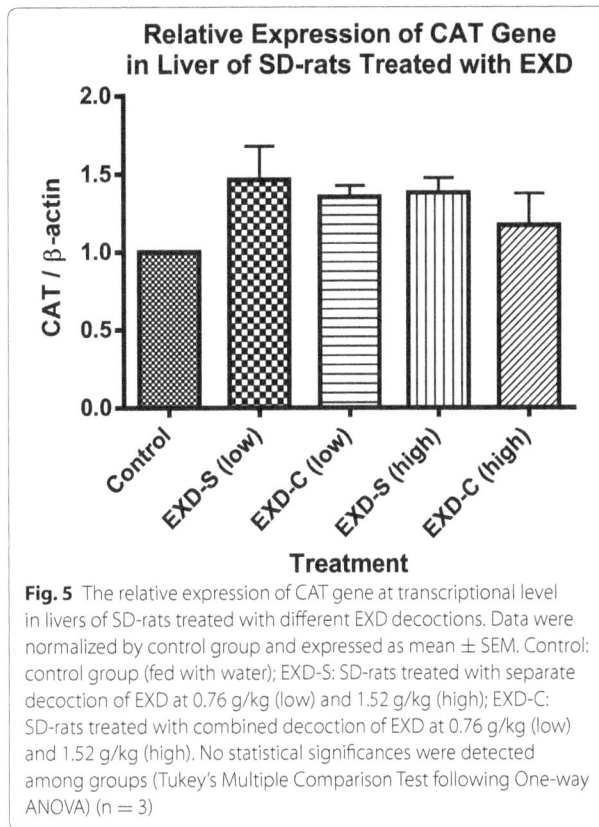

Fig. 5 The relative expression of CAT gene at transcriptional level in livers of SD-rats treated with different EXD decoctions. Data were normalized by control group and expressed as mean ± SEM. Control: control group (fed with water); EXD-S: SD-rats treated with separate decoction of EXD at 0.76 g/kg (low) and 1.52 g/kg (high); EXD-C: SD-rats treated with combined decoction of EXD at 0.76 g/kg (low) and 1.52 g/kg (high). No statistical significances were detected among groups (Tukey's Multiple Comparison Test following One-way ANOVA) (n = 3)

in vivo. The effects of EXD-S on mRNA level of hepatic antioxidants are in line with our previous findings [5]. In our previous study, EXD could significantly up-regulate CAT expression at the transcriptional level [5]. In this study, both EXD-S and EXD-C elicited around 1.5-fold of increase in the mRNA level of CAT, although no statistical significance was detected. Consistent with the results of Cyp19 expression, EXD-S showed a stronger tendency of stimulation of CAT and GPx-1 than EXD-C. The mRNA level of SOD-1 in EXD-S-treated group was significantly higher than that of the group treated with low dosages of EXD-C. These again support the better pharmacological properties of EXD-S than EXD-C.

In a TCM formula, the complexity of chemical components imposes difficulties in the identification of standard chemicals for quality control. The observation of differences in the chemical profiles of EXD-S and EXD-C in relation to their bioactivity has opened up the possibility of a novel and rapid approach to identify the standard chemicals in CM formulas. Since the pharmacological properties of a medicinal formula are conferred by the chemical components, which may change as a result of different decoction conditions. By comparing the HPLC profiles of the decoctions, the differentially extracted components would be those responsible for the observed

discrepancy in bioactivity. This would facilitate the identification and selection of bioactive components as standard chemicals out of the complex herbal mixture. In a study on Radix *Scutellariae* (Huangqin) decoction, an increase in the amount of the bioactive compound baicalin was observed in the combined decoction [17]. In another study on Tangkuei Liu Huang Decoction, the amount of baicalin was higher in separate decoctions than that of combined decoction [18]. These findings suggest that the bioactive components in a herbal extract can be affected by the decoction method as well as the herbal interaction between different herbs. The decoction methods would also affect the pharmacological properties. In some studies, the combined decoction may have better therapeutic efficacy and vice versa [19, 20]. Whether the component herbs of a Chinese medicinal formula should be decocted separately or in combination together depends on different individual formulas, but the decoction of herbal materials is often an inevitable process for the preparation of most of the CM prescriptions. The evaluation of chemical profiles as well as the pharmacological properties of different processing methods may indicate a novel approach for identifying the standard chemicals of the CM formula. In this study, the feasibility of such approach is evaluated by differential comparison

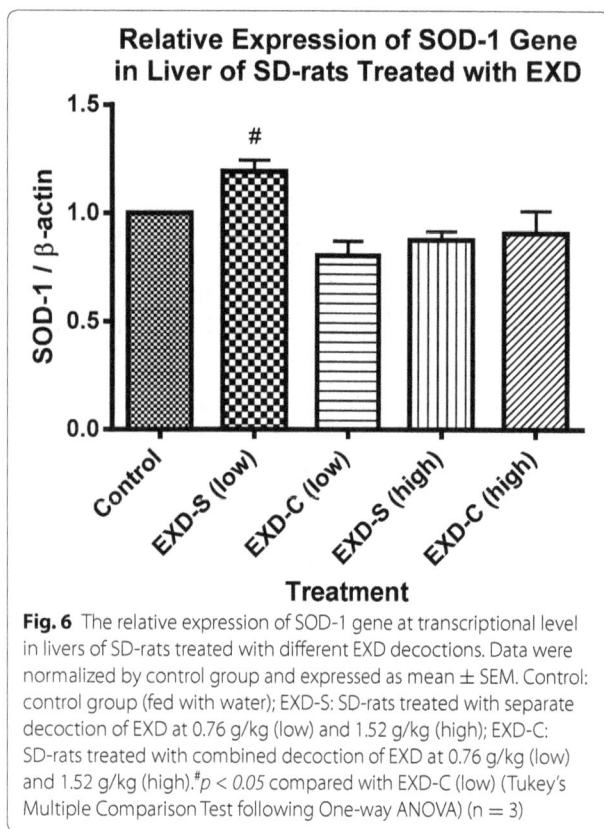

Fig. 6 The relative expression of SOD-1 gene at transcriptional level in livers of SD-rats treated with different EXD decoctions. Data were normalized by control group and expressed as mean ± SEM. Control: control group (fed with water); EXD-S: SD-rats treated with separate decoction of EXD at 0.76 g/kg (low) and 1.52 g/kg (high); EXD-C: SD-rats treated with combined decoction of EXD at 0.76 g/kg (low) and 1.52 g/kg (high).[#]$p < 0.05$ compared with EXD-C (low) (Tukey's Multiple Comparison Test following One-way ANOVA) (n = 3)

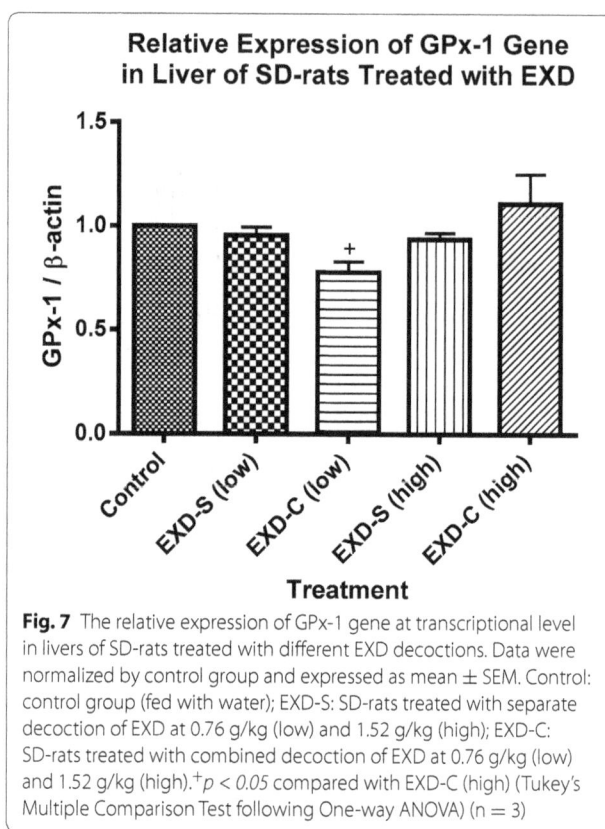

Fig. 7 The relative expression of GPx-1 gene at transcriptional level in livers of SD-rats treated with different EXD decoctions. Data were normalized by control group and expressed as mean ± SEM. Control: control group (fed with water); EXD-S: SD-rats treated with separate decoction of EXD at 0.76 g/kg (low) and 1.52 g/kg (high); EXD-C: SD-rats treated with combined decoction of EXD at 0.76 g/kg (low) and 1.52 g/kg (high).[+]$p < 0.05$ compared with EXD-C (high) (Tukey's Multiple Comparison Test following One-way ANOVA) (n = 3)

of the HPLC profile of EXD-S and EXD-C in relation to the pharmacological properties. Eventually, this approach can be coupled with analytic techniques to identify the differentially extracted components obtained by different decoction methods.

In future developments, such approach may be polished by further validations with a more comprehensive pharmacological screening platform, and further evaluation of the feasibility of this approach can be conducted with other Chinese medicinal formulas. The four key chemicals, including mangiferine, ferulic acid, jatrorrhizine and palmatine, found in EXD could be further investigated in vitro and in vitro to identify their combined effects as a mixture of four in treating menopausal syndromes.

Conclusions

In this study, the HPLC profiles of EXD-S and EXD-C have been evaluated with six known marker chemicals, which exerted actions on the HPO axis. All six chemicals were present at a higher level in EXD-S than in EXD-C. Four of them, including mangiferine, ferulic acid, jatrorrhizine and palmatine, were demonstrated to be suitable standard chemicals for quality control of EXD according

to our novel and rapid approach. Both EXD-S and EXD-C displayed stimulatory effects on the expression of ovarian aromatase and hepatic SOD-1, with the effect of EXD-S being more potent. The changes of pharmacological activity in relation to the changes in chemical profiles of EXD decoction demonstrated the feasibility of a novel and rapid approach for identification of bioactive standard compounds from TCM formulas.

Abbreviations
TCM: traditional Chinese medicine; EXD: Erxian decoction; EXD-S: mixtures of EXD individual herbs decoction; EXD-C: combined decoction of EXD; SD-rat: Sprague Dawley-rat; CAT: catalase; SOD-1: superoxide dismutase 1; GPx-1: glutathione peroxidase; Ct: threshold cycle; RSD: relative standard deviation; HPLC: high performance liquid chromatography; HPO: hypothalamus-pituitary-ovary.

Authors' contributions
SCWS, YBZ, ZJZ and YT conceived and designed the study. HPC and SWW conducted the experiment and analyses. HPC, FWSC and SCWS wrote the manuscript. LXL and ZJZ provided invaluable comments. SCWS and TBN revised the manuscript. All authors read and approved the final manuscript.

Author details
[1] School of Chinese Medicine, Li Ka Shing Faculty of Medicine, The University of Hong Kong, 10 Sassoon Road, Pokfulam, Hong Kong, SAR, China. [2] School of Biomedical Science, Faculty of Medicine, The Chinese University of Hong Kong, Shatin, N.T., Hong Kong, SAR, China.

Acknowledgements

This study was partially supported by grants from the Seed Funding Programme for Basic Research (Project Number 201211159146 and 201411159213), the University of Hong Kong. We thank Mr Keith Wong and Ms Cindy Lee for their technical assistances.

Competing interests

The authors declare that they have no competing interests.

References

1. Zhang LH. Studies of active ingredients of Chinese traditional compound medicine (CTCM) (我對中藥複方有效成分研究的一些看法). Prog Chem (化學進展). 1999;2(11):186–8.
2. Cai BC, Qin KM, Wu H, Cai H, Lu TL, Zhang XD. Chemical mechanism during Chinese medicine processing (中藥炮制過程化學機理研究). Prog Chem (化學進展). 2012;24(4):637–49.
3. Deng YY, Gao WY, Chen HX, Wu SS. 中藥複方合煎與分煎的差異性研究進展. Chin Tradit Herb Drugs (中草藥). 2005;36(12):1909–11.
4. Yi T, Lo H, Zhao Z, Yu Z, Yang Z, Chen H. Comparison of the chemical composition and pharmacological effects of the aqueous and ethanolic extracts from a Tibetan "Snow Lotus" (Saussurea laniceps) herb. Molecules. 2012;17(6):7183–94.
5. Sze SCW, Tong Y, Zhang YB, Zhang ZJ, Lau AS, Wong HK, Tsang KW, Ng TB. A novel mechanism: Erxian decoction, a Chinese medicine formula, for relieving menopausal syndrome. J Ethnopharmacol. 2009;123(1):27–33.
6. Hu YM, Wang YT, Sze SCW, Tsang KW, Wong HK, Liu Q, Zhong LD, Tong Y. Identification of the major chemical constituents and their metabolites in rat plasma and various organs after oral administration of effective Erxian decoction (EXD) fraction by liquid chromatography-mass spectrometry. Biomed Chromatogr. 2010;24(5):479–89.
7. Okatani Y, Morioka N, Wakatsuki A, Nakano Y, Sagara Y. Role of the free radical-scavenger system in aromatase activity of the human ovary. Horm Res. 1993;39(Suppl 1):22–7.
8. Yuan ST, Du HY, Xia C. Effect of separated and combined decoction of Chinese medicinal formula on solubility of components (中藥複方湯劑分煎合煎對溶出效果的影響). Chin J Inf Tradit Chin Med (中國中醫藥訊息雜誌). 1999;6(7):29–32.
9. Yi L, Xu X. Study on the precipitation reaction between baicalin and berberine by HPLC. J Chromatogr B. 2004;810(1):165–8.
10. Sato T, Kawamoto A, Tamura A, Tatsumi Y, Fujii T. Mechanism of antioxidant action of pueraria glycoside (PG)-1 (an isoflavonoid) and mangiferin (a xanthonoid). Chem Pharm Bull (Tokyo). 1992;40(3):721–4.
11. Kaewpradub N, Dej-adisai S, Yuenyongsadwad S. Antioxidant and cytotoxic activities of Thai medicinal plants named Khaminkhruea: Arcangelisia flava, Coscinium blumeanum and Fibraurea tinctoria. Songklanakarin J Sci Technol. 2005;27(Suppl. 2):455–67.
12. Yokozawa T, Ishida A, Kashiwada Y, Cho EJ, Kim HY, Ikeshiro Y. Coptidis Rhizoma: protective effects against peroxynitrite-induced oxidative damage and elucidation of its active components. J Pharm Pharmacol. 2004;56(4):547–56.
13. Rackova L, Majekova M, Kost'alova D, Stefek M. Antiradical and antioxidant activities of alkaloids isolated from Mahonia aquifolium. Structural aspects. Bioorg Med Chem. 2004;12(17):4709–15.
14. Sassa S, Kikuchi T, Shinoda H, Suzuki S, Kudo H, Sakamoto S. Preventive effect of ferulic acid on bone loss in ovariectomized rats. In Vivo. 2003;17(3):277–80.
15. Philp HA. Hot flashes–a review of the literature on alternative and complementary treatment approaches. Altern Med Rev. 2003;8(3):284–302.
16. Ye HY, Lou YJ. Estrogenic effects of two derivatives of icariin on human breast cancer MCF-7 cells. Phytomedicine. 2005;12(10):735–41.
17. Chen JZ, Lu GY, Luo XM, Ye L, Chen JM. Comparison of baicalin, paeoniflorin and glycyrrhetic acid in different decoctions of Huangqin decoction (黃芩湯分煎液與合煎液中黃芩苷，芍藥苷和甘草酸含量的比較). Chin Tradit Patent Drugs (中成藥). 2008;30(9):1330–3.
18. Jin FY, Zhong ZL, Zhang LY, Liang GY, Cao PX, Yang YQ. Comparison of the content of baicalin in the different decoctions of TangKuei six yellow decoction (當歸六黃湯分煎樣品與合煎樣品中黃芩苷含量的比較). Lishizhen Med Materia Medica Res (時珍國醫國藥). 2009;20(3):681–2.
19. Gao L, Xie M, Sun MY. Experimental research on the anti-febrile effect of mingled decoction and separated decoction of Bupleurium roots and Scutellaria root on the fever induced by LPS in rats (柴芩合煎液與分煎液對LPS 誘導的大鼠發熱模型的影響). Chin J Exp Tradit Med Formulae (中國實驗方劑學雜誌). 2003;9(6):22–5.
20. Wang XT, Lu Y, Hu YL, Hou SK. Effect of separated and combined decoction of Chinese medicinal extract on mastitis in dairy cattle (分煎和合煎對中藥乳康灌注液治療奶牛乳腺炎效果的影響). Anim Husb Vet Med (畜牧與獸醫). 2008;40(3):69–71.

2

Comparing the antidiabetic effects and chemical profiles of raw and fermented Chinese Ge-Gen-Qin-Lian decoction by integrating untargeted metabolomics and targeted analysis

Yan Yan[1†], Chenhui Du[2†], Zhenyu Li[1], Min Zhang[1,3], Jin Li[2], Jinping Jia[1], Aiping Li[1], Xuemei Qin[1*] and Qiang Song[2*] [iD]

Abstract

Background: Microbial fermentation has been widely applied in traditional Chinese medicine (TCM) for thousands of years in China. Various beneficial effects of fermentation for applications in TCM or herbals have been reported, such as enhanced anti-ovarian cancer, antioxidative activity, and neuroprotective effects. Ge-Gen-Qin-Lian decoction (GQD), a classic TCM formula, has been used to treat type 2 diabetes mellitus in China. In this study, GQD was fermented with *Saccharomyces cerevisiae*, and the antidiabetic activities and overall chemical profiles of raw and fermented GQD (FGQD) were systematically compared.

Methods: First, the antidiabetic effects of GQD and FGQD on high-fat diet and streptozotocin (STZ)-induced diabetic rats were compared. Then, high-performance liquid chromatography Q Exactive MS was applied for rapid characterization of the chemical components of GQD. Additionally, we proposed an integrated chromatographic technique based untargeted metabolomics identifying differential chemical markers between GQD and FGQD and targeted analysis determining the fermenting-induced quantitative variation tendencies of chemical marker strategy for overall chemical profiling of raw and fermented GQD.

Results: Both GQD and FGQD displayed effects against HFD and STZ-induced diabetes, and FGQD showed a better recovery trend associated with profound changes in the serum lipoprotein profile and body weight gain. In addition, 133 compounds were characterized from GQD. It was demonstrated that the integrated strategy holistically illuminated 30 chemical markers contributed to the separation of GQD and FGQD, and further elucidated the fermenting-induced chemical transformation mechanisms and inherent chemical connections of secondary metabolites. Although there were no new secondary metabolites in FGQD compared with GQD, the amounts of secondary metabolites, which were mostly deglycosylated, were redistributed in FGQD.

*Correspondence: qinxm@sxu.edu.cn; sxhpe@163.com
†Yan Yan and Chenhui Du contributed equally to this work
[1] Modern Research Center for Traditional Chinese Medicine of Shanxi University, No. 92, Wucheng Road, Taiyuan 030006, Shanxi, China
[2] School of Traditional Chinese Materia Medica, Shanxi University of Chinese Medicine, No. 121, Daxue Street, Taiyuan 030619, Shanxi, China
Full list of author information is available at the end of the article

Conclusion: The anti-diabetic activities of GQD could be improved by applying fermentation technology. Moreover, the proposed strategy could serve as a powerful tool for systematically exploring the chemical profiles of raw and fermented formulas.

Keywords: Ge-Gen-Qin-Lian decoction, Fermentation, Untargeted metabolomics, Targeted analysis, Antidiabetic effects

Background

Herbal fermentation, which began approximately 4000 years ago in China, is used to produce secondary metabolites from plants in bulk by utilizing the metabolic pathways of microorganisms [1]. Fermented medicinal plants and traditional Chinese medicine (TCM) are attracting increasing attention in East Asia, especially in Taiwan and Korea. During the fermentation of TCM, certain glycosides are deglycosylated into small, hydrophobic molecules that may be more efficacious than the original herbal medicines due to increased absorption and bioavailability of the active components in the body [2–5]. Fermented medicinal plants and traditional herbal medicine have been shown to exhibit enhanced anti-ovarian cancer activity, antioxidative activity, and neuroprotective effects compared to the raw formulas [6–9]. The yeast *Saccharomyces cerevisiae* (SC) is the most widely used organism for fermentation and has been successfully used for the biotransformation of TCM formula [4, 5, 10].

Although various beneficial effects of fermentation applied to TCM or medicinal plants have been reported, systematic comparisons of the pharmacological actions and overall chemical profiles of raw and fermented TCM formulas are scarce. TCM is a complex system comprising hundreds of different compounds. Thus, the most critical difficulty is distinguishing and matching herbal biotransformed secondary metabolites in complex microorganism matrixes. Metabolomics, a novel approach for rapidly identifying the global metabolic composition of biological systems, has been widely used for the overall chemical characterization of herbal medicines [11]. Thus, metabolomics analysis could be used to study the effects of fermentation on TCM. In general, the purpose of untargeted metabolomics is to identify statistically significant differences based on unbiased differential analysis of as many signals as possible [12]. By contrast, targeted quantitative metabolomics is intended mainly to accurately determine metabolites in various samples by comparison with authentic compounds to improve the repeatability, comparability and reproducibility of data [13]. Liquid chromatography coupled with mass spectrometry (LC–MS)-based untargeted metabolomic approach can provide global profiles of abundant (up to hundreds of) secondary metabolites by determining their presence, amount and occasionally their structures [14, 15] and has been successfully used to study the effects of processing on herbal drugs, such as Rehmanniae Radix and Fructus corni [15, 16].

Ge-Gen-Qin-Lian decoction (GQD), a well-known TCM formula, was first recorded in "Treatise on Febrile Diseases" compiled by Zhong-jing Zhang of the Han Dynasty (202 BC-220 AD). GQD consists of four herbs, Pueraria Lobatae Radix, Scutellariae Radix, Coptidis Rhizoma, and Glycyrrhizae Radix et Rhizoma Praeparata cum Melle, in a weight ratio of 8:3:3:2. Extensive chemical studies have shown that flavones (free form and glycosides), flavanones, alkaloids and triterpene saponins are the major compounds in GQD [17, 18]. Modern pharmacological studies have revealed that GQD has antidiabetic effects in vivo and in vitro [19–22]. GQD is also clinically used to treat type 2 diabetes mellitus (T2DM) [23].

Since GQD and SC have a long history and extensive range of use, their safety and efficacy are demonstrated and widely accepted by the public. Here, GQD was fermented using SC, and the antidiabetic effects of GQD and fermented GQD (FGQD) on high-fat diet (HFD) and streptozotocin (STZ)-induced diabetic rats were compared. An integrated strategy based on untargeted and targeted metabolomic analysis was proposed for the overall chemical profiling of raw and fermented GQD. Finally, the correlations of the biological and chemical differences are discussed.

Methods
Information on experimental design and resources
The information regarding the experimental design, statistics, and resources used in this study is attached in the minimum standards of reporting checklist (Additional file 1).

Chemicals, materials and reagents
Acetonitrile (HPLC and MS grade) and methanol (HPLC grade) were purchased from Tedia (Fairfield, USA) and Hanbon (Nanjing, China), respectively. Formic acid (analytical grade) was provided by Aladdin Chemistry Co. Ltd (Shanghai, China). De-ionized water was prepared in-house by a Milli-Q water purification system (Millipore, MA, USA). Other chemicals and reagents were analytical grade. The chemical reference substances (purity > 98%,

HPLC–DAD) of 3′-hydroxypuerarin, puerarin, daidzin, daidzein, baicalin, wogonoside, baicalein, wogonin, coptisine, berberine, palmatine, magnoflorine, genistin, genistein, ononin and formononetin were purchased from Chengdu Wei ke-qi Bio-Technology Co., Ltd. (Chengdu, China). Liquiritin, isoliquiritin, liquiritigenin, isoliquiritigenin and glycyrrhizic acid were purchased from Chunqiu Bio-Technology Co., Ltd. (Nanjing, China). Scutellarein (purity > 98%, HPLC–DAD) was isolated, purified and identified in our lab.

Puerariae Lobatae Radix (Gegen), Scutellariae Radix (Huangqin), Coptidis Rhizoma (Huanglian) and Glycyrrhizae Radix et Rhizoma Praepapata Cum Melle (Zhigancao) were purchased from Wan Min pharmacy (Taiyuan, China) and authenticated by Associate Professor Chenhui Du, according to the standard of the Chinese Pharmacopeia (2015 edition). Voucher specimens were deposited in the Modern Research Center for Traditional Chinese Medicine of Shanxi University. SC (CICC 1205) was purchased from the China Center of Industrial Culture Collection (CICC).

Preparation of GQD and FGQD extracts

Herb pieces of 3200 g (Gegen:Huangqin:Huanglian:Gancao = 8:3:3:2) were immersed in a 10-fold volume of distilled water (w/v) for 0.5 h and then extracted by refluxing two times (40 min, 30 min). For each extract, the decoction was filtered through eight layers of gauze to remove the herbal residue. The two filtrates were combined, condensed under reduced pressure with a rotary evaporator at 70 °C and evaporated to dryness (yield: 28.6%).

Freeze-dried spores of SC were recovered in 25 mL of potato dextrose (PD) medium and then incubated at 28 °C on a rotary shaker at $180 \times g$ for 24 h. A 20-mL volume of GQD (0.5 g mL^{-1}, crude drug per g mL^{-1}) was mixed with 30 mL of distilled water in a 250-mL flask. The substrates of GQD were subjected to autoclaving at 121 °C for 20 min, then shook evenly and allowed to cool naturally. The sterilized substrates of GQD were inoculated with 2% (v/v) recovered SC and incubated at 28 °C in a shaking incubator ($180 \times g$). GQD samples were fermented for 48 h and then evaporated to dryness.

The concentrations of GQD and FGQD were approximately 2 g mL^{-1} (crude drug per g mL^{-1}) for the animal experiments. In addition, the GQD and FGQD extracts for LC and LC–MS analysis were also prepared using the same protocol mentioned above in triplicate.

Animal handing and biochemical parameters related to T2DM measurement

Male Sprague–Dawley rats (200–220 g) were purchased from Beijing Vital River Laboratories Co., Ltd. (SCXK (Jing) 2014-0013, Beijing, China). The rats were housed at a controlled room temperature of 23 ± 2 °C, $55 \pm 10\%$ humidity and a 12-h dark–light cycle for 10 days with free access to food and water. Then, 70 rats were randomly divided into two groups: the normal control group (NC, n = 10) and the diabetic rats group (n = 60). The NC group was fed a regular diet. The diabetic rats group was fed a high-sugar and HFD containing 5% sucrose, 10% lard, 5% yolk powder, 1% cholesterol, 0.1% sodium cholate and 78.9% regular diet. After 4 weeks of dietary intervention, the diabetic rats were fasted for 24 h and then received STZ (35 mg kg^{-1}) dissolved in citrate buffer (0.1 M, pH 4.5) by intraperitoneal injection. The rats in the NC group received an equivalent volume of citrate buffer vehicle. One week after injection, fasting blood glucose (FBG) levels were determined using a drop of blood from the tail vein. Rats with FBG level above 11.1 mM were randomly subdivided into four groups (n = 13 for each group): the diabetic model group (DM) and three treatment groups. The treatment groups were fed 0.67 mg kg^{-1} of metformin hydrochloride (HM), 20 g kg^{-1} of GQD, or 20 g kg^{-1} of FGQD (crude drug per g kg^{-1} of body weight) every day for 8 weeks. Body weights were recorded every week, and FBG levels were measured every 2 weeks throughout the experiment.

At the end of the experimental period, the rats were sacrificed under anaesthesia, and blood was immediately collected. Total serum cholesterol (TC), triglycerides (TG), high-density lipoprotein cholesterol (HDL-C) and low-density lipoprotein cholesterol (LDL-C) levels were measured by an ELISA kit (Nanjing jiancheng Bioengineering Institute, Nanjing, China). The fast serum insulin (FINS) concentration was measured using commercial kits (Wa Lan Biotechnology, Shanghai, China). The insulin sensitivity index (ISI) was calculated according to FBG and FINS. The following formula for ISI was used: Ln (1/FBG * FINS) [24]. Homeostasis model assessment-insulin resistance (HOMA-IR) was calculated to measure the insulin sensitivity of the rats fed the experimental diets using the following formula: [FINS × FBG] 22.5^{-1} [25].

Statistical analysis

Data are expressed as the mean ± S.D. All grouped data were statistically analysed with SPSS 13.0. Statistical significances between means were determined using one-way ANOVA followed by the LSD test of variance homogeneity and Dunnett's T3 test of variance heterogeneity after the normal distribution test. Unless otherwise specified, a value of $p < 0.05$ was selected for discriminating significant differences throughout.

Preparation of standard and sample solutions for HPLC–MS and HPLC analysis

For HPLC quantification, a mixed stock solution of ten reference substances was prepared at concentrations ranging from 1.0 to 2.5 mg mL^{-1} in 70% methanol. A standard working solution of the mixtures was obtained by diluting the stock solutions to the desired concentrations. All solutions were stored at 4 °C before use.

To obtain sufficient chemical ingredients in the GQD and FGQD extracts, dried extracts (0.1 g) were accurately weighted and separately extracted in 25 mL of 70% methanol (v/v) for 30 min by ultrasonication. After adjustment to the initial weight with methanol, 1 μL and 10 μL of the supernatant solution (obtained by centrifuging at 13,000×g for 10 min) were subjected to LC–MS and LC analysis, respectively. To validate the stability of the sample preparation and instrument, a pooled sample of all samples was prepared as quality control samples (QCs) for LC–MS. QCs were injected six times before the batch process and injected one time every 12 samples during the analysis process.

Untargeted metabolomics analysis by HPLC Q Exactive MS

An HPLC Ultimate™ 3000 instrument coupled with a Q Exactive MS (Thermo Scientific, Bremen, Germany) was used for untargeted metabolomics in this study. Chromatographic separation was performed on an Agilent Poroshell 120 EC-C$_{18}$ column (3 × 100 mm, 2.7 μm, Agilent, CA, USA). The mobile phase consisted of water containing 0.1% (v/v) formic acid (A) and acetonitrile (B). The following gradient was used: 0–10 min, 5% B to 17% B; 10–12 min, 17% B; 12–14 min, 17% B to 22% B; 14–19 min, 22% B; 19–29 min, 22% B to 32% B; 29–30 min, 32% B to 50% B; 30–34 min, 50% B to 90% B. The column was equilibrated for 5 min prior to each analysis. The flow rate was 0.3 mL min^{-1}, and the column temperature was maintained at 30 °C. The mass spectrometer was operated in both positive and negative ESI full MS–dd-MS/MS acquisition mode with the use of the following parameter settings: spray voltage, 3.5 kV; sheath gas: 35 arbitrary units; auxiliary gas: 10 arbitrary units; capillary temperature: 320 °C; S lens RF level: 55; heater temperature: 300 °C. Full scan data were recorded for ions with m/z 100–1500 at a resolution of 70,000 (FWHM defined at m/z 200) in profile format. The automatic gain control (AGC) target values were set at $1 \times e^6$ and $3 \times e^6$ ions, respectively. The injection time was set to 250 ms in ESI$^-$ mode and 100 ms in ESI$^+$ mode. The MS/MS event was triggered when the given precursor ion was detected in an isolation window of m/z 2.0. The stepped normalized collision energies (NCE) of the analytes were 10, 30 and 50.

Targeted quantification analysis by HPLC

Targeted metabolite quantification was performed on a Waters ACQUITY UPLC H-Class system (Milford, MA, USA). Samples were separated on an Agela-MP C$_{18}$ column (2.1 mm × 250 mm, 5 μm, Agela, Tianjin, China) maintained at 30 °C. The binary mobile phase consisted of water containing 0.1% formic acid (A) and acetonitrile (B) at a flow rate of 1.0 mL min^{-1}. The optimized gradient elution program was set as follows: 5–20% B (0–25 min), 20% B (25–30 min), 20–22% B (30–35 min), 22–40% B (35–55 min), 40–63% B (55–65 min), 63–80% B (65–70 min). The UV signals from two separate channels of 254 nm and 276 nm were recorded.

Data processing and analysis

Data from the HPLC Q Exactive MS acquisition and processing were used for chemical profile analysis using Xcalibur™ 2.2 (Thermo Fisher). The untargeted metabolomics analysis was conducted by using Compound Discovery (version 1.2.1, Thermo SCIEX), and the detailed workflow is shown in Additional file 2: Figure S1. The multivariate data matrix was introduced into SIMCA-P (Version 13.0, Umetrics AB, Umea, Sweden) software for "unsupervised" principal component analysis (PCA) and "supervised" orthogonal projection to latent structure-discriminant analysis (OPLS-DA). All variables were UV-scaled for PCA and Pareto-scaled for OPLS-DA.

Results

Antidiabetic effect

As shown in Fig. 1, the body weight of the diabetic rats decreased significantly compared with the NC group after STZ injection ($p < 0.01$). HM reversed the diabetes-induced body weight decrease from the 6th week ($p < 0.05$), whereas FGQD significantly reversed the body weight decrease from the 7th and 8th weeks ($p < 0.01$, $p < 0.05$). However, no significant ($p > 0.05$) effect was observed for the GQD group, suggesting that GQD had

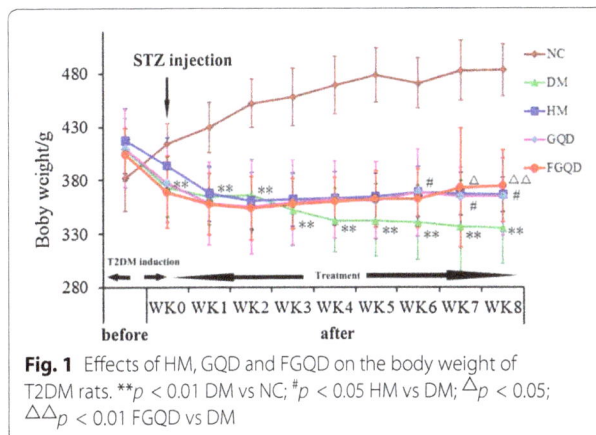

Fig. 1 Effects of HM, GQD and FGQD on the body weight of T2DM rats. **$p < 0.01$ DM vs NC; #$p < 0.05$ HM vs DM; $^\triangle p < 0.05$; $^{\triangle\triangle}p < 0.01$ FGQD vs DM

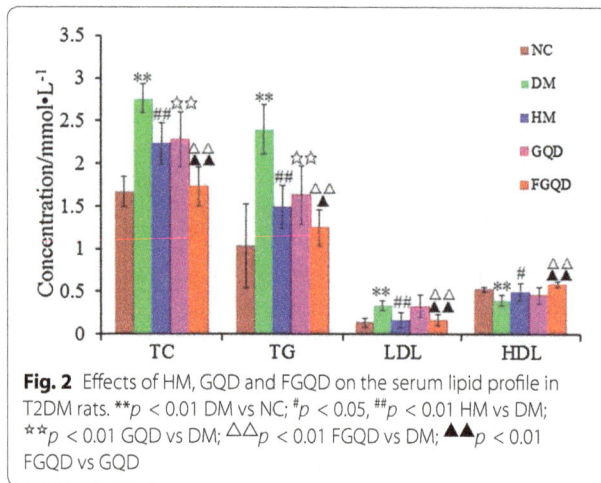

Fig. 2 Effects of HM, GQD and FGQD on the serum lipid profile in T2DM rats. $**p < 0.01$ DM vs NC; $^{\#}p < 0.05$, $^{\#\#}p < 0.01$ HM vs DM; $\star\star p < 0.01$ GQD vs DM; $^{\triangle\triangle}p < 0.01$ FGQD vs DM; $\blacktriangle\blacktriangle p < 0.01$ FGQD vs GQD

Table 1 Effects of HM, GQD and FGQD on FINS, ISI and HOMA-IR of T2DM rats

Group	FINS (mIU/L)	ISI	HOMA-IR
NC	4.92 ± 0.74	-3.38 ± 0.24	1.33 ± 0.30
DM	$9.88 \pm 0.58**$	$-5.24 \pm 0.22**$	$8.59 \pm 1.75**$
HM	$7.17 \pm 0.54^{\#\#}$	$-4.47 \pm 0.36^{\#\#}$	$3.98 \pm 1.07^{\#\#}$
GQD	$6.78 \pm 0.35^{\star\star}$	$-4.52 \pm 0.23^{\star\star}$	$4.18 \pm 0.95^{\star\star}$
FGQD	$5.86 \pm 0.55^{\triangle\triangle\blacktriangle\blacktriangle}$	$-4.26 \pm 0.18^{\triangle\triangle}$	$3.20 \pm 0.60^{\triangle}$

NC normal control, *DM* diabetic model, *HM* metformin hydrochloride, *ISI* insulin sensitivity index, *FINS* fast serum insulin, *HOMA-IR* homeostasis model assessment-insulin resistance, *T2DM* type 2 diabetes mellitus

$**p < 0.01$ DM vs NC; $^{\#}p < 0.05$, $^{\#\#}p < 0.01$ HM vs DM; $\star\star p < 0.01$ GQD vs DM; $^{\triangle\triangle}p < 0.01$ FGQD vs DM; $\blacktriangle\blacktriangle p < 0.01$ FGQD vs GQD

no significant effect on weight gain. As shown in Additional file 2: Figure S2, the FBG level was significantly increased in the diabetic rats compared to the NC group ($p < 0.01$) and was decreased in all drug-treated groups from the 4th week ($p < 0.01$, $p < 0.05$) after the injection of STZ. Although no significant difference was observed among the drug-treated groups ($p > 0.05$), the diabetic rats in FGQD showed a better trend of recovery. Rats in the model group had significantly higher levels of TC and TG ($p < 0.01$) than those in the NC group, and these levels were reduced in all drug-treatment groups ($p < 0.01$) (Fig. 2). Notably, the levels of TC and TG were significantly lower in the FGQD group than in the GQD group ($p < 0.01$) (Fig. 2). In addition, the treatments with HM and FGQD reversed the up-regulation of LDL and down-regulation of HDL in the diabetics rats group to the control level, whereas no significant ($p > 0.05$) effect was observed for GQD (Fig. 2). As shown in Table 1, the diabetic rats showed significant increases in FINS and HOMA-IR ($p < 0.01$) and a decrease in ISI ($p < 0.01$) compared with the NC group. After 8 weeks of drug

administration, the levels of FINS, ISI and HOMA-IR were reversed compared with the DM group ($p < 0.01$). In addition, a notable difference in FINS level was observed in the FGQD group ($p < 0.01$) compared with the GQD group. In short, the body weight gain and the regulation of the levels of FINS, TC, TG, LDL and HDL in the FGQD group were significantly better than those in the GQD group ($p < 0.01$), but there were no significant differences in FBG, ISI and HOMA-IR levels between GQD and FGQD. These results suggested that FGQD had better therapeutic effect against diabetes than GQD.

Characterization of the chemical constituents in the GQD extract

Since herbal medicines are generally taken as a decoction, we focused on boiled water extracts of GQD and their fermentation. The structural characterization of compounds in GQD is an essential step in identifying and matching those compounds with their secondary metabolites obtained through biotransformation. All known compounds were identified by comparison with chemical standards. For unknown compounds, structures were tentatively characterized based on retention time and MS spectra by referring to the previous literature. Finally, assignments of all compounds were further conducted by comparing the corresponding extracted ion chromatography (EIC) of GQD with those of the individual herbs. In total, 133 compounds were rapidly identified or tentatively characterized; these compounds were divided into six structural types. The detailed information, including retention times, accurate *m/z*, ppm errors, characteristic fragment ions, identified names and formulas, are summarized in Table 2, Additional file 2: Figure S3. Notably, two compounds were identified for the first time in GQD: 6-D-xylose-genistin and kuzubutenolide A.

Isoflavone glycosides

In total, 17 isoflavone *C*-glycosides and 15 isoflavone *O*-glycosides were identified as the dominant compounds from Gengen in GQD (Additional file 2: Figure S4A). P6, P11, P18, P26 and P34 were unambiguously identified by comparison with reference compounds. According to the MS/MS analysis of these authentic compounds, isoflavone *O*-glycosides (P18, P26 and P34) showed dominant aglycone ions at *m/z* 255, 271 and 269, respectively, due to the loss of a glucose group (162 Da). By contrast, isoflavone *C*-glycosides (P6 and P11) were hardly cleaved under the same conditions and shared the common principal fission pattern of successive or simultaneous losses of CO, CHO and CH_2O groups caused by cleavage of the *C*-ring. Consequently, the major fragmentation behaviours were summarized and then applied as rules to

Table 2 Retention time (t_R), and MS data for identification of 133 compounds in GQD by HPLC Q Exactive MS

Source	t_R (time)	Compound	Formula	Experimental m/z	Error ppm	Mode	MS/MS (m/z)	Structure type
P1	6.85	3'-Hydroxypuerarin-4'-O-glucoside	$C_{27}H_{30}O_{15}$	595.16559	−0.263	+	475, *433*, 415, 397, 379, 367, 337, *313*, *283*	C-glycoside-O-glu
P2	7.19	Puerarin-4'-O-glucoside	$C_{27}H_{30}O_{14}$	579.17120	0.636	+	417, 399, 381, 351, 321, *297*, *267*, 255	C-glu-O-glu
P3	7.80	3'-Methyoxy puerarin-4'-O-glucoside	$C_{28}H_{32}O_{15}$	609.18237	1.598	+	447, 429, 411, 393, 381, 365, 351, 327, *297*	C-glycoside-O-glu
P4	8.03	Mirificin-4'-O-β-D-glucoside	$C_{32}H_{38}O_{18}$	709.19830	0.859	−	457, 429	C-glycoside-O-glu
P5	8.33	Daidzein-4,7-O-glucoside	$C_{27}H_{30}O_{14}$	579.17084	0.014	+	417, *255*	O-glu
P6	8.77	3'-Hydroxypuerarin*	$C_{21}H_{20}O_{10}$	433.11276	−0.377	+	415, 397, 379, 367, 337, *313*, *283*	C-glu
P7	8.89	3'-Methoxy-4'-O-glucoside-daidzin	$C_{28}H_{32}O_{15}$	609.18262	2.008	+	447, 285	O-glu
P8	9.63	3'-Hydroxypuerarin xyloside	$C_{26}H_{28}O_{14}$	565.15509	−0.163	+	433, *415*, 397, 379, *367*, 337, *313*, *283*	C-glycoside-O-xyl
C1	10.07	Dihydro-11-Hydroxy-stepholidine-glucoside	$C_{25}H_{31}NO_{10}$	506.20200	−0.073	+	344, 326, 295, 277	alkaloid-O-glu
P9	10.30	6"-O-α-D-glucopyranosylpuerarin	$C_{27}H_{30}O_{14}$	579.17059	−0.242	+	417, 399, 381, 351, 321, *297*, 267	C-glu-O-glu
P10	10.43	3'-Hydroxydaidzin	$C_{21}H_{20}O_{10}$	433.11389	0.967	+	271	O-glu
P11	10.62	Puerarin*	$C_{21}H_{20}O_9$	417.11786	−0.356	+	399, 381, 363, 351, 321, *297*, *267*, 255	C-glu
P12	10.73	Mirificin	$C_{26}H_{28}O_{13}$	549.16016	−0.107	+	417, 399, 363, 351, 321, *297*, *267*	C-glycoside-O-api
P13	11.16	3'-Methoxypuerarin	$C_{22}H_{22}O_{10}$	447.12827	−0.678	+	429, 411, 381, 351, 327, *297*	C-glu
P14	11.22	6"-O-Xylosylpuerarin	$C_{26}H_{28}O_{13}$	549.15997	−0.541	+	417, 399, 363, 351, 321, *297*, 267	C-glycoside-O-xyl
C2	11.52	Magnoflorine*	$C_{20}H_{23}NO_4$	342.16996	−0.189	+	297, 265, 250, 237	alkaloid
P15	11.65	3'-Methoxypuerarin6"-O-D-api	$C_{27}H_{30}O_{14}$	579.17053	−0.521	+	447, 429, 411, 393, 381, 365, 351, 327, *297*	C-glu
C3	12.03	Norisocorydine	$C_{19}H_{22}NO_4$	328.15411	−0.225	+	313, 298, 282	alkaloid
S1	12.11	2',3,5,6',7-Pentahydroxyflavanone	$C_{15}H_{12}O_7$	303.05096	1.031	−	285, 275, 217, 177	flavanones aglycone
P16	12.15	3'-Methoxydaidzin 6"-O-D-api	$C_{27}H_{34}O_{11}$	579.17108	0.428	+	255	O-glu
P17	12.19	5'-Hydroxypuerarin	$C_{21}H_{20}O_{10}$	433.11328	0.824	+	415, 397, 367, *313*, *283*	C-glu
P18	12.57	Daidzin*	$C_{21}H_{20}O_9$	417.11807	0.147	+	*255*	O-glu
C4	12.75	11-Hydroxy-stepholidine-glucoside	$C_{25}H_{30}NO_{10}$	505.18610	−0.322	+	342, 324, 275	alkaloid-O-glu
P19	13.02	Genistein-8-C-xyl-glucoside	$C_{26}H_{28}O_{14}$	565.15619	1.008	+	433, *415*, 397, *367*, *313*, *283*	C-glycoside O-xyl
P20	13.40	BiochaninA-7-O-glucoside	$C_{22}H_{22}O_{10}$	447.12933	1.692	+	285, 270, 253, 225	O-glu
C5	13.61	O,O'-Dimethoxyl magnoflorine	$C_{21}H_{25}NO_5$	372.18045	−0.099	+		alkaloid
P21	13.72	Genistein-8-C-api-glucoside	$C_{26}H_{28}O_{14}$	565.15503	−0.269	+	433, *415*, *367*, 337, *313*, *283*	C-glycoside-O-api
P22	14.48	PuerosideA	$C_{29}H_{34}O_{14}$	607.20148	−0.652	+	592, 461, 299, 281, 253	O-glu
P23	14.53	Daidzein 4'-O-glucoside	$C_{21}H_{20}O_9$	417.11771	−0.229	+	*255*, 199	O-glu
G1	14.79	Liquiritengin-glucopyranoside-(1→2)-β-D-apiofuranoside	$C_{26}H_{30}O_{13}$	549.16101	1.352	−	255, 153, 135, 119	O-glu-O-api
S2	14.96	Chrysin-6-C-pen-8-C-hex	$C_{26}H_{28}O_{13}$	547.14851	2.180	−	487, 457, *427*, 367, 337, 281	C-glu
S3	15.00	Viscidulin I	$C_{15}H_{10}O_7$	301.03522	1.241	−	283, 273, 257, 229, 193, 151	flavone aglycone
C6	15.10	13-Hydroxyepiberberine	$C_{20}H_{17}NO_5$	352.11787	−0.149	+	336, 322, 294	alkaloid
S4	15.36	Chrysin-6-C-pen-8-C-hex	$C_{26}H_{28}O_{13}$	547.14600	2.527	−	487, 457, *427*, 367, 337, 281	C-glu
G2	15.38	Liquiritin apioside	$C_{26}H_{30}O_{13}$	549.16046	0.351	−	*255*, 153, 135, 119, 91	O-glu

Table 2 (continued)

Source	t_R (time)	Compound	Formula	Experimental m/z	Error ppm	Mode	MS/MS (m/z)	Structure type
G3	15.44	Liquiritin*	$C_{21}H_{22}O_9$	417.11917	2.784	–	**255**, 153, 135, 119	O-glu
S5	15.83	Chrysin 6-C-α-L-arabinoside-8-C-β-D-glucoside	$C_{26}H_{28}O_{13}$	547.14581	2.18	–	487, 457, 427, 367, 337, 281	C-glu
P24	15.90	Neopuerarin	$C_{21}H_{20}O_9$	417.11755	–1.100	+	399, 381, 363, 351, 321, **297, 267**	C-glu
P25	15.97	6-D-xylose-Genistin	$C_{26}H_{28}O_{14}$	565.15768	2.408	+	433, **271**	O-glu
S6	16.14	Scutellarein 7-β-D-glucuronoside	$C_{21}H_{18}O_{12}$	461.07266	2.619	–	285, **267**	O-gluA
S7	16.16	Chrysin 6-C-β-L-arabinoside-8-C-β-D-glucoside	$C_{26}H_{28}O_{13}$	547.14587	2.290	–	487, 457, 427, 367, 337, 281	C-glu
C7	16.28	Stecepharine	$C_{21}H_{25}NO_5$	372.18015	–0.399	+	222, 207, 189	alkaloid
S8	16.31	Viscidulin III 2'-O-glucoside	$C_{23}H_{24}O_{13}$	507.11469	2.707	–	345, 330, 315	O-glu
S9	16.43	Acteoside	$C_{29}H_{36}O_{15}$	623.19861	2.509	–	461, 161, 179	O-glu
P26	16.44	Genistin*	$C_{21}H_{20}O_{10}$	433.11334	0.417	+	**271**	O-glu
P27	16.46	Kuzubutenolide A	$C_{23}H_{24}O_{10}$	461.14017	–4.053	+	299, 281, 253, 239	O-glu
S10	16.52	Chrysin 6-C-β-D-glucoside-8-C-α-L-arabinoside	$C_{26}H_{28}O_{13}$	547.14569	1.961	–	457, 427, 367, 337, 321	C-glu
P28	16.74	Formononetin-8-C-glucoside-O-api	$C_{27}H_{30}O_{13}$	563.17694	1.023	+	431, 413, 311, 281	C-glu-O-api
C8	16.88	Groenlandicine	$C_{19}H_{15}NO_4$	322.10712	–0.821	+	307, 279	alkaloid
C9	16.99	Demethyleneberberine	$C_{19}H_{17}NO_4$	324.12283	–0.205	+	308, 266, 281	alkaloid
S11	17.02	chrysin6-hexosyl-8-C-pentosyl	$C_{26}H_{28}O_{13}$	547.14612	1.503	–	457, 427, 367, 337, 321	C-glu
P29	17.05	Formononetin-8-C-glucoside-O-xyloside	$C_{27}H_{30}O_{13}$	563.17554	–0.670	+	431, 413, 311, 281	C-glu
P30	17.10	6''-O-Malonyl daidzin	$C_{24}H_{22}O_{12}$	503.11804	–0.362	+	**255**	O-glu
S12	17.19	Chrysin 6-C-β-D-glucoside-8-C-β-L-arabinoside	$C_{26}H_{28}O_{13}$	547.14575	2.070	–	457, 427, 367, 337, 321	C-glu
P31	17.22	4'-Methoxypuerarin	$C_{22}H_{22}O_9$	431.13364	–0.043	+	413, 395, 377, 335, 311, 281	C-glu
S13	17.34	5,2',6'-Trihydroxy-7,8-dimmethoxy flavone-2'-glucoside	$C_{23}H_{24}O_{12}$	491.11948	2.194	–	329, 314, 299	O-glu
S14	17.36	Isoacteoside	$C_{29}H_{36}O_{15}$	623.19843	1.383	–	461, 161, 179	O-glu
C10	17.38	Oxyberberine	$C_{20}H_{17}NO_5$	352.11789	–0.059	+	337, 336, 322, 308, 294	alkaloid
C11	17.64	Oxidated palmatine	$C_{21}H_{21}NO_5$	368.14893	–0.314	+	352, 336	alkaloid
G4	18.06	Pyrroside B	$C_{26}H_{30}O_{14}$	565.15649	2.315	–	**271**, 151	O-glu
G5	18.59	5-Hydroxylliquiritin	$C_{21}H_{22}O_{10}$	433.11404	1.117	+	**271**, 151, 119	O-glu
S15	19.12	5,7,2',6'-Tetrahydroxyflavone	$C_{15}H_{10}O_6$	285.04050	3.984	–	241, 199, 133, 151	flavone aglycone
P32	19.21	6''-O-Acetyl daidzin	$C_{23}H_{22}O_{10}$	459.12839	–0.183	+	**255**	O-glu
C12	19.49	Columbamine	$C_{20}H_{19}NO_4$	338.13849	–0.576	+	323, **308**, 294	alkaloid
S16	19.58	5,7,2'-Trihydroxy-6-methoxyflavone 7-O-glu-curonide	$C_{22}H_{20}O_{12}$	475.08975	0.848	–	299, 284, 175, 113	O-gluA
C13	19.70	Epiberberine	$C_{20}H_{18}NO_4$	336.12274	–0.876	+	321, 320, 292	alkaloid
C14	19.98	Coptisine*	$C_{19}H_{13}NO_4$	320.09174	0.017	+	292, 262	alkaloid
C15	20.13	Jatrorrhizine	$C_{20}H_{19}NO_4$	338.13855	–0.398	+	323, **308**, 294	alkaloid

Table 2 (continued)

Source	t_R (time)	Compound	Formula	Experimental m/z	Error ppm	Mode	MS/MS (m/z)	Structure type
P33	20.81	Sophoraside A or isomer	$C_{24}H_{26}O_{10}$	473.14496	0.737	−	311, 267, 252	O-glu
G6	20.89	Isoliquiritin apioside	$C_{26}H_{30}O_{13}$	549.16150	0.191	−	255, 153, 135, 119, 91	O-glu
S17	21.68	Scutellarein*	$C_{15}H_{10}O_6$	285.04071	4.720	−	267, 239, 166, 137, 117	flavone aglycone
P34	22.04	Ononin*	$C_{22}H_{22}O_9$	431.13361	−0.101	+	269	O-glu
G7	22.13	Licuraside	$C_{26}H_{30}O_{13}$	549.16040	0.133	−	255, 153, 135, 119	O-glu
G8	22.23	Isoliquiritin*	$C_{21}H_{22}O_9$	417.11948	1.471	−	255, 153, 135, 119	O-glu
S18	22.44	Baicalein 7-β-D-glucoside	$C_{21}H_{20}O_{10}$	433.11276	−0.163	+	271	O-glu
S19	22.50	Baicalin*	$C_{21}H_{18}O_{11}$	445.09216	0.028	−	269, 241, 223, 175, 113	O-gluA
S20	22.60	Eriodictyol	$C_{15}H_{12}O_6$	287.05630	1.285	−	218, 161, 125	flavanones aglycone
C16	22.65	Worenine+CH2+2H	$C_{21}H_{21}NO_4$	352.15433	−0.285	+	334, 320	alkaloid
P35	23.45	Daidzein*	$C_{15}H_{10}O_4$	255.06509	−0.374	+	227, 199, 181, 153	flavanones aglycone
G9	23.47	Neoisoliquiritin	$C_{21}H_{22}O_9$	417.11954	1.531	−	255, 153, 119	O-glu
C17	23.56	Worenine	C20H15NO4	334.10721	−0.174	+	319, 306, 291	alkaloid
G10	23.59	Licochalcone B	$C_{16}H_{14}O_5$	285.07687	3.929	−	270, 253, 191, 150	chalcones aglycone
G11	24.13	Licorice glycosideB	$C_{35}H_{36}O_{15}$	695.19727	0.223	−	549, 531, 399, 255	O-glu
G12	24.18	Liquiritigenin*	$C_{15}H_{11}O_4$	255.06641	4.801	−	237, 153, 135, 119, 91	flavanones aglycone
P36	24.21	Isoononin	$C_{22}H_{22}O_9$	431.13461	0.951	+	269	O-glu
C18	24.53	Palmatine*	$C_{21}H_{21}NO_4$	352.15417	−0.468	+	337, 336, 322, 308, 294	alkaloid
P37	24.69	BiochaninA	$C_{16}H_{12}O_5$	283.06110	3.533	−	268, 240, 211	flavone aglycone
P38	24.82	Apigenin*	$C_{15}H_{10}O_5$	269.04568	1.230	−	241, 225, 213, 197	flavone aglycone
S21	24.88	Naringenin 7-O-β-D-glucuronide	$C_{21}H_{20}O_{11}$	447.09454	2.352	−	271, 243, 113	O-gluA
C19	24.96	Berberine*	$C_{20}H_{17}NO_4$	336.12274	−0.876	+	321, 320, 306, 292	alkaloid
C20	25.27	Demethylcoptichine	$C_{30}H_{25}NO_8$	528.16552	−0.073	+	334, 319, 304	alkaloid
S22	25.52	Norwogonin-8-Oglucuronide	$C_{21}H_{18}O_{11}$	445.07779	2.814	−	269, 251, 241	O-gluA
S23	26.15	Trihydroxymethoxyflavone-Oglucoside	$C_{22}H_{22}O_{11}$	461.10977	1.932	−	299, 284, 283, 211, 173	O-glu
S24	26.18	Hydroxyl oroxylin A-7-O-glucuronide	$C_{22}H_{20}O_{12}$	475.08813	1.028	−	299, 284	O-gluA
S25	26.40	4'-Hydroxylwogonin	$C_{16}H_{12}O_6$	299.05606	1.0455	−	271, 227, 211, 165, 133	O-gluA
S26	26.57	Norwogonin-7-Oglucuronide	$C_{21}H_{18}O_{11}$	445.07748	2.117	−	269, 251, 241	O-gluA
S27	26.98	Chrysin-7-O-glucuronide	$C_{21}H_{18}O_{10}$	431.09763	0.828	+	255	O-gluA
S28	27.00	Oroxylin A-7-O-glucuronide	$C_{22}H_{20}O_{11}$	459.09357	3.001	−	283, 268, 175, 113, 85	O-gluA
S29	27.38	Hydroxyl wogonoside	$C_{22}H_{20}O_{12}$	475.08810	0.998	−	299, 284	O-gluA
P39	27.49	Isoformononetin	$C_{16}H_{12}O_4$	267.06650	1.315	−	252, 223, 199	isoflavone aglycone
C21	27.84	13-Methylberberine	$C_{21}H_{19}NO_4$	350.13864	−0.045	+	335, 334, 320, 318, 306	alkaloid
S30	28.09	Baicalein 6-O-glucuronide	$C_{21}H_{18}O_{11}$	445.07791	3.083	−	269, 241, 225, 197	O-gluA
C22	28.16	Demethylcoptichine	$C_{30}H_{25}NO_8$	528.16595	1.244	+	334, 319, 304	alkaloid

Table 2 (continued)

Source	t_R (time)	Compound	Formula	Experimental m/z	Error ppm	Mode	MS/MS (m/z)	Structure type
S31	28.52	Wogonoside*	$C_{22}H_{20}O_{11}$	459.09348	2.815	−	*283*, *268*, 175, 113, 85	O-gluA
S32	29.11	5,7-Dihydroxy-6,8-dimethoxyflavone-7-O glucuronide	$C_{23}H_{22}O_{12}$	489.10565	2.898	−	313, 298, 283	O-gluA
P40	30.47	Genistein*	$C_{15}H_{10}O_5$	269.04572	4.721	−	241, 225, 183, 159	isoflavone aglycone
S33	30.53	5,7,4'-Trihydroxy-8-methoxyflavone	$C_{16}H_{12}O_6$	299.05637	4.532	−	*284*, *231*, 136, 94	flavone aglycone
G13	31.48	Licorice saponin A3	$C_{48}H_{72}O_{21}$	983.44867	0.435	−	821, *351*	O-gluA-gluA
S34	31.88	Norwogonin	$C_{15}H_{10}O_5$	269.04578	1.330	−	*251*, *241*, *223*	flavone aglycone
G14	32.14	22β-Acetoxylglycyrrhizic acid	$C_{44}H_{64}O_{18}$	879.40295	2.341	−	*351*	O-gluA-gluA
S35	32.20	5,7,2'-Trihydroxy-6-methoxyflavone	$C_{16}H_{12}O_6$	299.05630	1.285	−	*284*, 255	flavone aglycone
G15	32.19	Licorice saponin G2	$C_{42}H_{62}O_{17}$	837.39185	1.819	−	*351*, 193	O-gluA-gluA
S36	32.19	Trihydroxydimethoxyflavone	$C_{17}H_{14}O_7$	329.06674	3.528	−	314, 299	flavone aglycone
S37	32.40	Baicalein*	$C_{15}H_{10}O_5$	269.06000	−0.100	−	*251*, *241*, *223*, 213, 197	flavone aglycone
S38	32.64	Trihydroxy-methoxyflavone	$C_{16}H_{12}O_6$	299.05627	4.198	−	*284*, 165, 137	flavone aglycone
G16	32.73	Isoliquiritigenin*	$C_{15}H_{11}O_4$	255.06633	4.566	−	237, 153, 119, 91	chalcones aglycone
G17	32.80	Glycyrrhizic acid*	$C_{42}H_{62}O_{16}$	821.39655	1.385	−	*351*	O-gluA-gluA
P41	32.97	Formononetin*	$C_{16}H_{12}O_4$	267.06647	4.810	−	252, 223	isoflavone aglycone
G18	33.07	Glycyrrhizin isomer	$C_{42}H_{62}O_{16}$	821.39642	1.227	−	*351*	O-gluA-gluA
G19	33.39	Licorice saponin C2	$C_{42}H_{62}O_{15}$	805.40094	0.433	−	*351*, 193	O-gluA-gluA
G20	33.50	Licorice saponin B2	$C_{42}H_{64}O_{15}$	807.41724	1.093	−	*351*, 193	O-gluA-gluA
S39	33.54	Skullcapflavone	$C_{18}H_{16}O_7$	343.08255	1.321	−	328, 313, 298, 285	flavone aglycone
G21	33.72	Liconeolignan	$C_{21}H_{22}O_5$	353.13947	1.120	−	338, 321, 295, 283, 269	others
S40	33.77	Wogonin*	$C_{16}H_{12}O_5$	283.06140	4.593	−	*268*, *239*, 163	flavone aglycone
S41	33.78	Chrysin	$C_{15}H_{10}O_4$	255.06497	−0.215	+	238, 214	flavone aglycone
S42	33.90	Dihydroxy-dimethoxyflavone	$C_{17}H_{14}O_6$	315.08600	−0.315	+	300, 285	flavone aglycone
C23	33.95	Berberastine	$C_{20}H_{18}NO_5$	352.11774	−0.209	+	336, 322, 308	alkaloid
S43	34.03	Oroxylin A	$C_{16}H_{12}O_5$	283.06137	4.487	−	*268*, *239*, 163	flavone aglycone
S44	34.21	Tenaxin I	$C_{18}H_{16}O_7$	343.08252	1.321	−	268, 239, 163	flavone aglycone
G22	34.40	Licoisoflavone A	$C_{20}H_{18}O_6$	353.10330	1.335	−	284, 267, 243, 216, 201, 83	isoflavone aglycone
G23	34.45	Licochalcone A	$C_{21}H_{22}O_4$	337.14484	1.404	−	305, 281, 243, 229, 201	chalcones aglycone
G24	35.03	Glabrone	$C_{20}H_{16}O_5$	335.09271	1.310	−	305, 291, 275, 213, 199, 107	isoflavone aglycone
G25	35.03	Licoisoflavone B	$C_{20}H_{16}O_6$	351.08755	1.235	−	283, 265, 241, 199, 83	isoflavone aglycone

Major signals in MS spectra were indicated in bolditalic

t_R retention time, P Pueraria Lobatae Radix, S Scutellariae Radix, C Coptidis Rhizoma, G Glycyrrhizae Radix et Rhizoma Praeparata cum Melle, + detected in positive ion mode, − detected in negative ion mode, *confirmed with reference compounds

elucidate the structures of the other 27 unknown compounds with the same basic skeleton [18, 26, 27]. Among them, P25 showed a precursor ion with m/z 565.15509 and further fragmented into the characteristic ion at m/z 271, corresponding to [M+H–xyl/api–glu]$^{+}$. More importantly, P25 was tentatively deduced as 6-D-xylose-genistin in GQD for the first time.

Flavone glycosides

The occurrence of flavone O-glucuronides is less common in plants. Previously published studies have thoroughly summarized the fragmentation pathways of flavonoids O-glucuronides in Huangqin [28]. As characteristic components, a total of 12 flavone O-glucuronides (S6, S16, S19, S22, S24, S26, S27, S28, S29, S30, S31 and S32) all from Huangqin were identified and tentatively characterized in GQD (Additional file 2: Figure S4B) [28–33]. Moreover, S2, S4, S5, S7, S10, S11 and S12 were tentatively characterized as flavone C-glycosides. In addition, S8, S13, S18 and S23 were excluded from flavone O-glucuronides by analysing the MS/MS spectra and then were finally identified as flavone O-glycosides [33].

In addition, six flavanones glycosides and five chalcones glycosides were putatively characterized in GQD (Additional file 2: Figure S4C). Among them, G3 and G8 were identified as liquiritin and isoliquiritin, respectively, by comparison with reference standards, and the others from Gancao were characterized by analysing their MS/MS spectra [32, 34]. In addition, S21 was characterized as a flavanone glycoside from Huangqin.

Free flavones

In total, 30 free flavones were tentatively assigned and could be further divided into isoflavones (8), flavones (16), flavanones (3) and chalcones (3) in GQD (Additional file 2: Figure S4D). P35, P40 and P41 were confirmed by comparison with reference standards. P37 and P39 from Gegen and G22, G24 and G25 from Gancao were tentatively characterized as isoflavone aglycones by analysing the MS/MS spectra [2, 32]. In addition, the flavones comprised 16 compounds from Huangqin. Baicalein (S37) produced characteristic ions with m/z 251, 241 and 223 by loss of H_2O and CO. Wogonin (S40), a methoxylated flavonoid, presented a deprotonated ion [M–H]$^{-}$ at m/z 283.06140 and characteristic fragment ions with m/z 268 and 239. In addition, a low signal intensity ion with m/z 163 ($^{0,2}A^{-}$) through Retro-Diels–Alder (RDA) cleavage was observed. Thus, the other 14 flavones in the complex mixtures were characterized based on the literature [28, 33]. In negative ion mode, liquiritigenin (G12) and isoliquiritigenin (G16), a pair of isomers, showed fragmentation patterns associated with RDA cleavage at m/z 135 or 119. Thus, S1, S20, G10 and G23 were tentatively

characterized according to the above mentioned MS behaviours [28].

Alkaloids

A total of 23 alkaloids from Huanglian were characterized based on positive ion mode mass spectra (Additional file 2: Figure S4E). Three benzylisoquinoline alkaloids, i.e., coptisine, palmatine and berberine, were identified by comparison with their authentic standards and the production of one or multiple common small fragments such as H_2O, CH_3 and C_2H_6N, respectively. Based on these rules, C6, C8, C9, C10, C11, C12, C13, C15, C16, C21 and C23 were observed and further tentatively characterized by analysing characteristic ions [35, 36]. Magnoflorine, an aporphinoid alkaloid, exhibited a precursor ion at m/z 342.16996 and characteristic ions at m/z 297, 265, 250 and 237. Similarly, C4 and C5 were tentatively identified as aporphinoid alkaloids. The others (C1, C3, C7, C17, C20 and C22) were characterized by comparison to the literature [27].

Triterpene saponins

Triterpene saponins were the other characteristic constituents from Gancao. In total, six triterpene saponins were putatively identified (Additional file 2: Figure S4C). Glycyrrhizic acid (G17 or G18) presented an [M–H]$^{-}$ ion with m/z 821.39655 and characteristic fragment ions at m/z 351 and 193 [32]. G13, G14, G15, G19 and G20 showed characteristic ions similar to those of glycyrrhizic acid and were tentatively characterized according to the literature [18].

Others

In addition to the major compounds described above, atypical structures were also found in GQD (Additional file 2: Figure S4C). P22 and P33, which belong to aromatic glycosides, were identified as pueroside A and sophoroside A or their isomers [26]. P27 showed an [M+H]$^{+}$ ion at m/z 461.14017 with MS^{2} characteristic peaks at m/z 299, 281, 253 and 239 and was tentatively identified as kuzubutenolide A in GQD for the first time [37]. In addition, S9 and S14 were tentatively identified as isomers of acteoside and isoacteoside [12, 38], and P38 and G21 were also tentatively characterized by comparison with the literature [33].

Multivariate statistical analysis

To identify chemical markers distinguishing GQD and FGQD samples, the negative and positive ion mode data detected by HPLC Q Exactive MS were simultaneously used for global analysis. Visual inspection of the chromatograms for GQD and FGQD indicated that the fermentation process induced obviously different peak

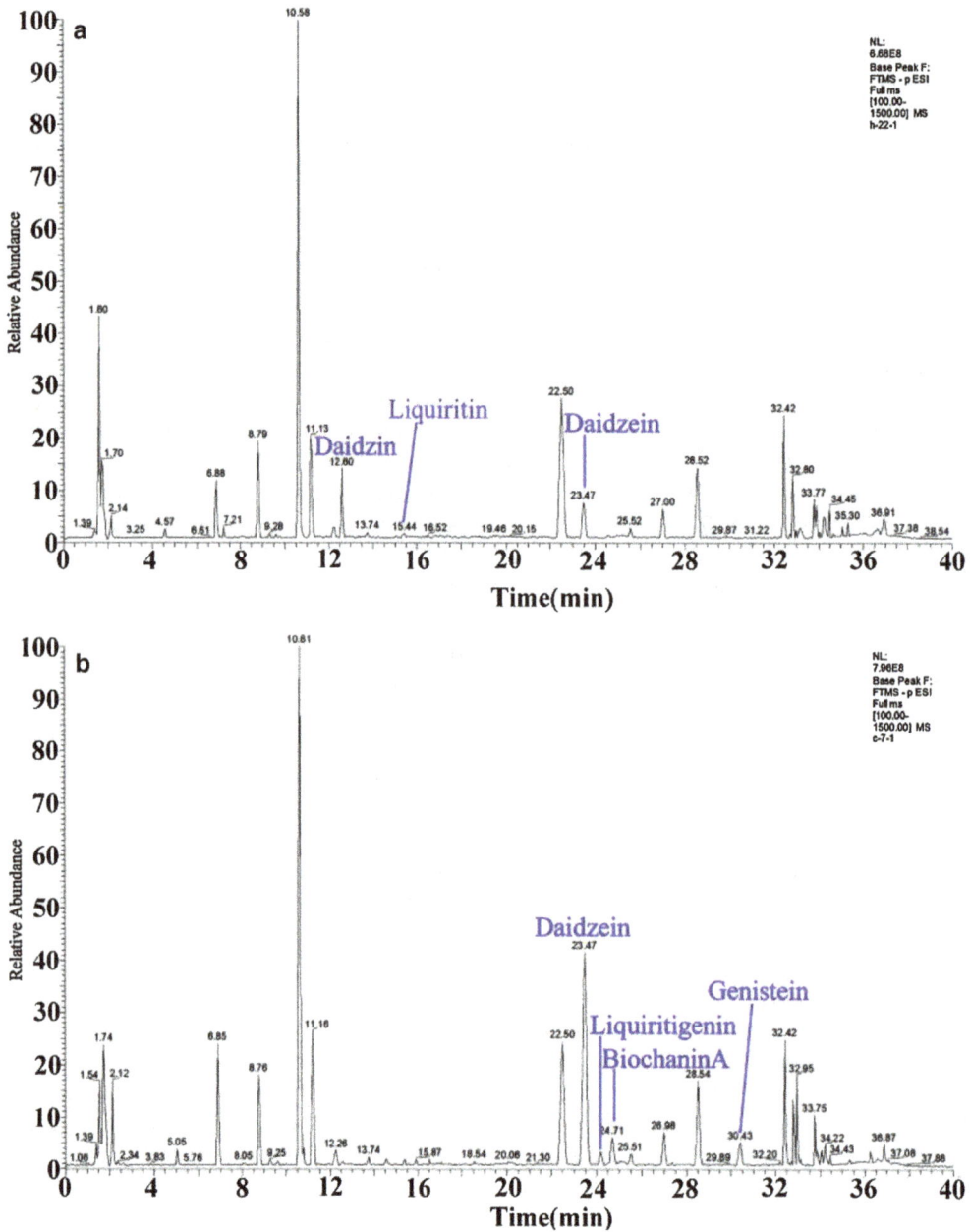

Fig. 3 Typical basic peak ion chromatograms obtained by HPLC Q Exactive MS. **a** GQD; **b** FGQD. All chromatograms were obtained in negative ion mode

intensities; that is, FGQD contained more daidzein, liquiritigenin, genistein, and biochanin A and less daidzin and liquiritin than GQD (Fig. 3). Multivariate statistical analysis was subsequently applied to further reveal the minor differences between GQD and FGQD. In the PCA score plot (Additional file 2: Figure S5A, B) generated by PC1 (46.2%) and PC2 (17.9%) for positive ion mode and PC1 (51.1%) and PC2 (17.9%) in negative ion mode, clear separation can be observed between GQD

and FGQD. Then, OPLS-DA was further performed to process the secondary metabolome data between the GQD and FGQD groups by S-plot and VIP-value analysis. The model fit parameters were 0.999 for R^2Y (cum) and 0.971 for Q^2 (cum) for positive ion mode and 0.999 for R^2Y (cum) and 0.987 for Q^2 (cum) for negative ion mode, respectively, suggesting that the OPLS-DA model exhibited good fitness and predictability. In the S-plots, each point represented an ion t_R-m/z pair, whereas the

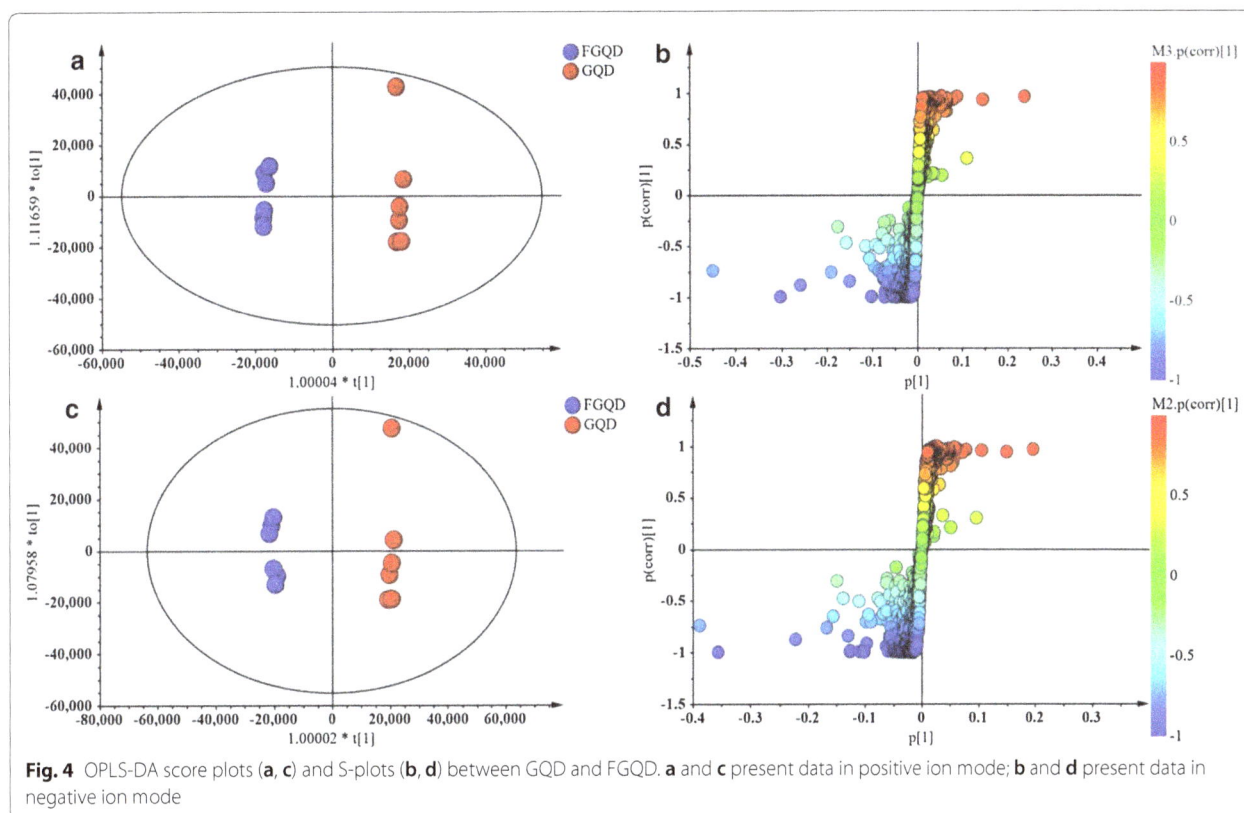

Fig. 4 OPLS-DA score plots (**a**, **c**) and S-plots (**b**, **d**) between GQD and FGQD. **a** and **c** present data in positive ion mode; **b** and **d** present data in negative ion mode

distances of the pair points from the mean centre indicate the contribution of the variables in discriminating the GQD and FGQD groups (Fig. 4a, b). The VIP-value threshold cut-off of the variables was set to one, and thus 83 and 117 variables were finally screened in LC/MS (ESI$^+$) and LC/MS (ESI$^-$), respectively. Among them, 25 variables were identified in both ion modes. Three variables and two variables were identified in negative ion mode and positive ion mode, respectively. Thus, 30 compounds that had different intensities between GQD and FGQD were detected.

To maximize the understanding of the effect of fermentation on GQD, the mean peak areas and the t-test results for the significant differences in the 30 compounds from GQD and FGQD are shown in Figs. 5, 6. As shown in Fig. 5a1, the mean peak areas of free flavones (P35, P37, P40 and G12) were larger in FGQD than in GQD ($p < 0.001$), whereas the mean peak areas of their corresponding O-glycosides (P5, P18, P20, P26, G2 and G3) were smaller in FGQD than in GQD ($p < 0.001$, $p < 0.05$), indicating that O-glycoside hydrolysis occurred during fermentation processing (Fig. 5a2). P23 could also be transformed to P35 by O-glycoside hydrolysis. In addition, P10 and P34 contained abundant hydroxyl and methyl and were deduced to possibly produce P18 by dehydroxylation or demethylation. Actually, a marked

decline in the level of P34 was also observed ($p < 0.01$) (Fig. 5a1), however, its corresponding aglycone P41 was not obviously altered in FGQD, which might be due to a dynamic equilibrium between their formation (from O-glycoside hydrolysis) and further transformation (e.g., demethylation). By contrast, C-glucosides appeared to be more difficult to transform by SC, since five C-glucosides (P6, P11, P13, P14 and P24) were detected in FGQD (Fig. 5b1). Their significant increasing trend was probably caused by the hydrolysis of low contents of puerarin C-glucoside-O-glucoside derivatives, such as P1, P2, P3, P4, P8, P12 and P15 (Fig. 5b2). O-C glycoside bonds have been reported to be the main effective target of β-glucosidase [13], in agreement with our results that puerarin (P11) and its derivatives were difficult to hydrolyse by β-glucosidase.

As shown in Fig. 6a1, the remarkable increase in the level of flavone aglycone (S43) was potentially due to hydrolysis of the corresponding flavone O-glucuronide (S28), which contains a 6-OCH$_3$ group ($p < 0.001$). S31, which contains an 8-OCH$_3$ group, was more difficult to transform by hydrolysis by SC but was easier to produce from S25 by dehydroxylation (Fig. 6a2). Although a different strain of yeast was used, the current findings are still in agreement with those in a previous study [39]. Notably, the increasing trend of S37 is likely partially

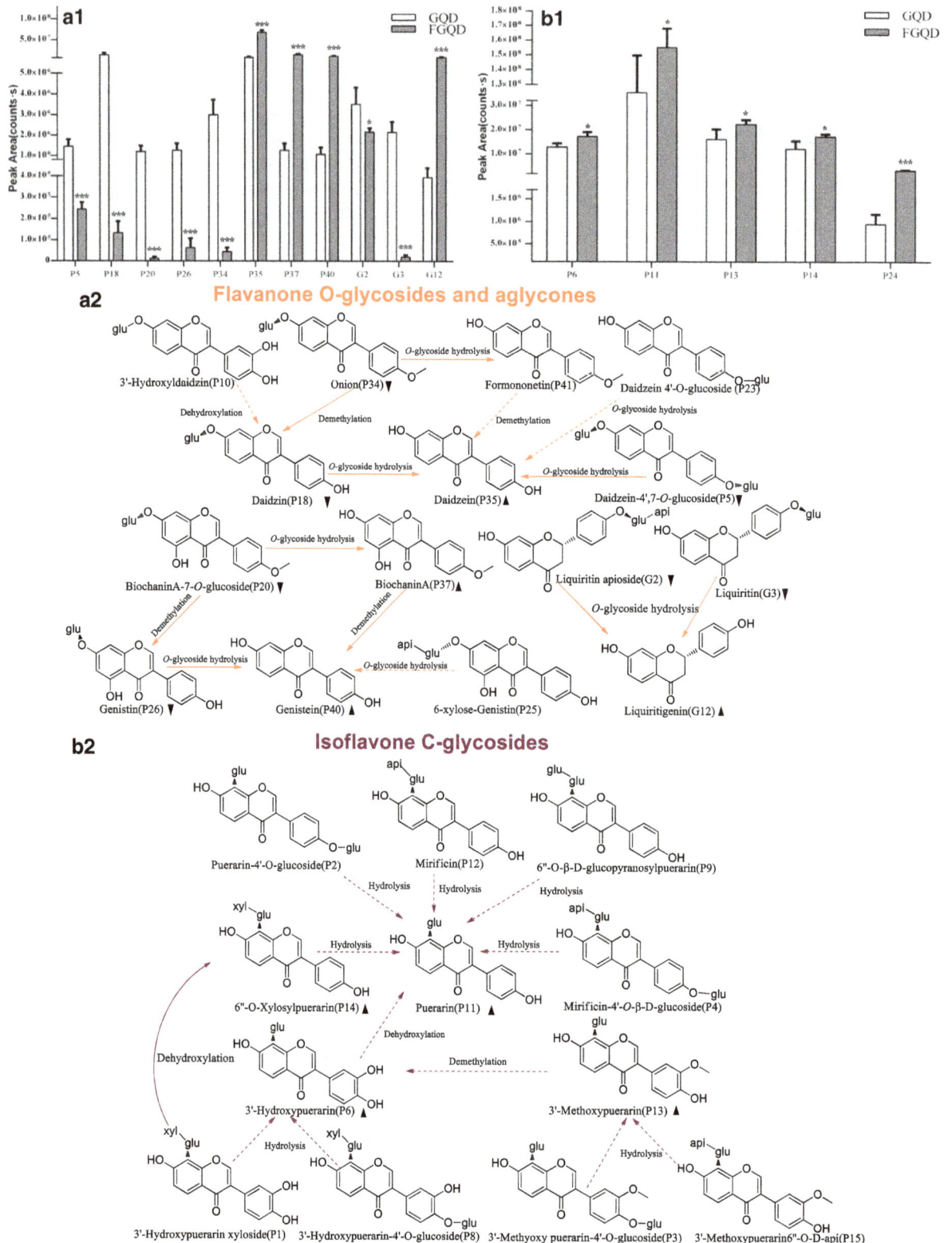

Fig. 5 Proposed fermentation-induced chemical transformation mechanisms. **a1** Flavone O-glycosides and aglycones; **b1** isoflavone C-glycosides; **a2** proposed biotransformed pathways of flavone O-glycosides and aglycones; **b2** proposed biotransformed pathways of isoflavone C-glycosides. Solid arrows: prone to happen; dotted arrows: speculated/less likely to happen. ▲ Indicates an elevation of the compound content; ▼ Indicates a decrease in the compound content (***$p < 0.001$, *$p < 0.05$ GQD vs FGQD)

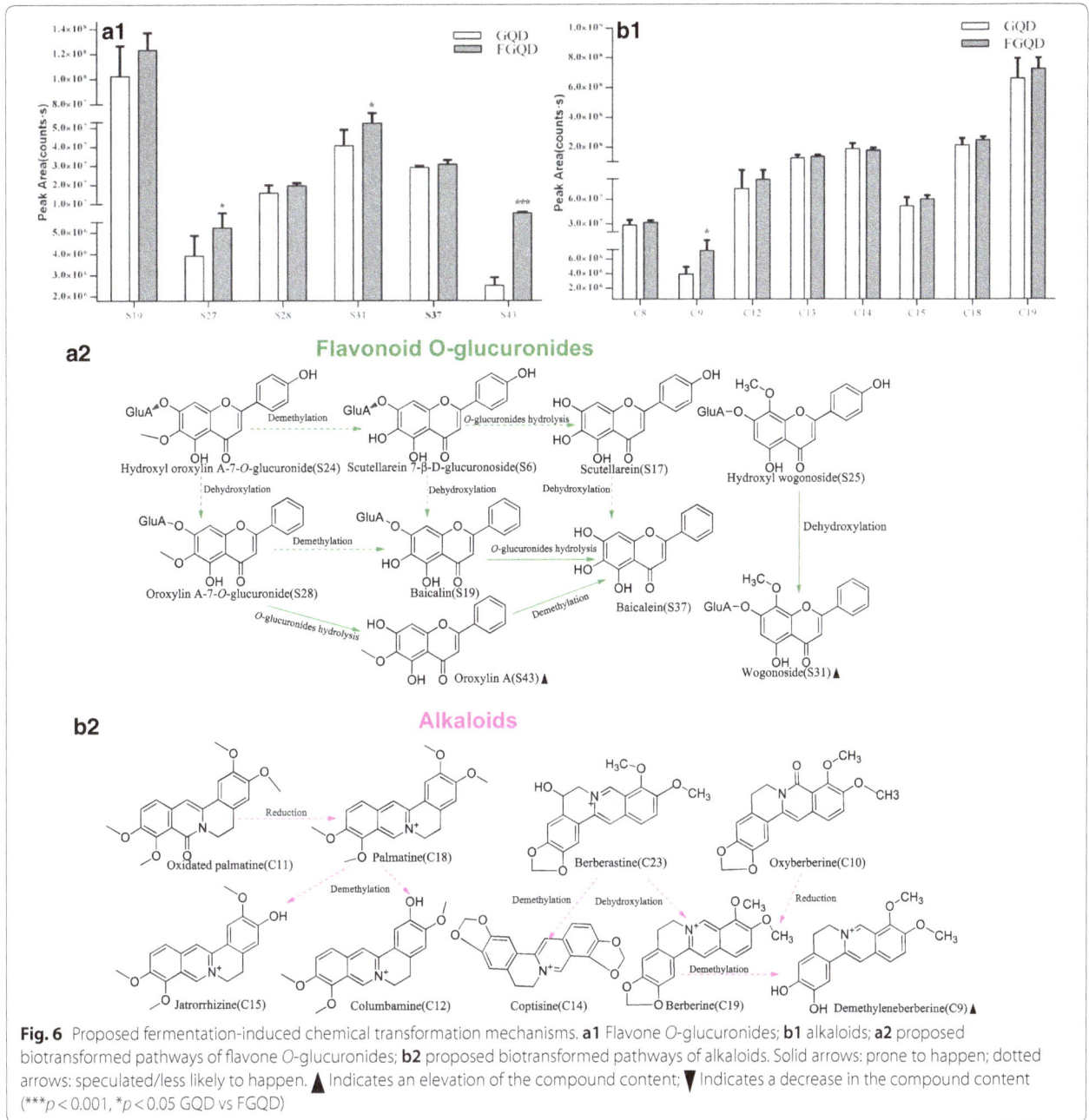

Fig. 6 Proposed fermentation-induced chemical transformation mechanisms. **a1** Flavone *O*-glucuronides; **b1** alkaloids; **a2** proposed biotransformed pathways of flavone *O*-glucuronides; **b2** proposed biotransformed pathways of alkaloids. Solid arrows: prone to happen; dotted arrows: speculated/less likely to happen. ▲ Indicates an elevation of the compound content; ▼ Indicates a decrease in the compound content (***$p < 0.001$, *$p < 0.05$ GQD vs FGQD)

responsible for the hydrolysis reactions of the corresponding compound (S19) (Fig. 6a2). A previous study demonstrated that *Escherichia* (*E.*) *coli* β-glucuronidases could hydrolyse glucuronic acid at the 7-position if the structure contains a 6-OH group [39]. Other metabolic reactions for flavone-*O*-glucuronides, including demethylation and dehydroxylation, were also deduced.

Due to the lack of a free hydroxyl group, alkaloids are demethylated to form free hydroxyl groups by SC [36]. In this study, a significant increase in demethyleneberberine (C9) was observed in FGQD compared to GQD ($p < 0.05$),

which probably contributed to the demethylation of C19 during fermentation processing (Fig. 6b1, b2). There were no significant differences in the other benzylisoquinoline alkaloids between GQD and FGQD ($p > 0.05$), thus indicating that the contents of these molecules remained stable during the fermentation process.

Targeted quantification analysis

As mentioned above, the untargeted metabolomic studies indicated that isoflavone *O*-glycosides, flavone *O*-glycosides, flavone *O*-glucuronides and alkaloids were

Table 3 Contents of 10 chemical markers in GQD and FGQD by SC (mg g^{-1}, n = 3)

Compound	0 h	48 h
Puerarin	20.30 ± 0.05	23.57 ± 0.02*
Daidzin	3.67 ± 0.08	n.d.***
Daidzein	0.50 ± 0.02	3.80 ± 0.01***
Liquiritin	0.80 ± 0.06	0.48 ± 0.02*
Liquiritigenin	0.17 ± 0.05	0.50 ± 0.01*
Coptisine	2.23 ± 0.12	2.68 ± 0.003
Palmatine	2.01 ± 0.03	2.36 ± 0.15
Berberine	7.70 ± 0.03	8.10 ± 0.02
Baicalin	10.80 ± 0.02	11.85 ± 0.01
Baicalein	1.26 ± 0.04	1.27 ± 0.03

The content is expressed in units of mg/g. n.d. indicates under the LOQ. *$p < 0.05$, ***$p < 0.001$ FGQD vs GQD

potential chemical markers for distinguishing GQD and FGQD. Thus, three *O*-glycosides (daidzin, baicalin and liquiritin), one *C*-glycoside (puerarin), three flavones (daidzein, liquiritigenin, and baicalein), and three alkaloids (coptisine, berberine and palmatine) were quantitatively determined as examples to illustrate the effects of processing (Additional file 2: Figure S3, Table S1). Their content changes in GQD and FGQD are summarized in Table 3. As expected, fermentation processing significantly depleted liquiritin (*O*-glycoside) from 0.80 ± 0.06 mg g^{-1} to 0.48 ± 0.02 mg g^{-1} ($p < 0.05$), whereas daidzin was not even detectable in FGQD ($p < 0.001$) after fermentation with SC. Interestingly, the concentrations of daidzein and liquiritigenin (free flavones) in FGQD were greatly enhanced ($p < 0.001$, $p < 0.05$, respectively). In addition, an obvious increase in the level of puerarin (isoflavone *C*-glycoside) was observed until the end of fermentation. Regarding alkaloids, the contents of coptisine, palmatine and berberine remained relatively stable ($p > 0.05$). Moreover, there was a slight increasing trend for baicalin (flavone *O*-glucuronide), whereas no significant difference was found between GQD and FGQD. Interestingly, the quantitative results revealed an increasing trend for baicalein ($p > 0.05$) did not correspond to the results of the untargeted studies, which showed a significant increase in the content of baicalein in FGQD compared with GQD ($p < 0.05$).

Discussion

GQD is a well-known TCM formula that has been reported to display anti-diabetic properties in the clinic [20]. In the present study, we investigated the efficiency of FGQD and confirmed that fermentation actually enhanced the anti-diabetic activities of GQD in vivo in diabetic rats induced by HFD and STZ. The present results suggested that GQD had no significant effect on weight gain, in agreement with a previous study [19], whereas FGQD showed a significant reversed trend. In addition, our study indicated that the level of FBG was conspicuously decreased, accompanied by decreases in serum TG, TC, LDL-C and FINS and increased HDL-C after GQD treatment, consistent with previous work [21]. FGQD exerted greater regulatory effects on the levels of TC, TG, LDL-C, HDL-C and FINS compared to GQD. Thus, both GQD and FGQD displayed effects against HFD and STZ-induced diabetes, and FGQD showed a better recovery trend associated with profound changes in the serum lipoprotein profile and body weight gain. These findings further suggest that fermentation can play a key role in the search for therapeutically useful drugs. Given the pharmacologically decisive roles of the involved ingredients, chemical transformations might significantly contribute to the therapeutic differences between GQD and FGQD. Thus, the chemical profiles of GQD and FGQD were further systematically compared using the proposed integrated strategy based on untargeted and targeted metabolomic analysis.

In this study, 133 secondary metabolites analysed using UPLC-Q Exactive MS were identified and characterized by comparison with standard references and the literature. Then, untargeted metabolomics was performed to find statistically significant differences between GQD and FGQD groups via OPLS-DA S-plot and VIP-value analysis. The OPLS method is a modification of the PLS method with a multivariate pre-processing filter called orthogonal signal correction (OSC). The OSC filter removes uncorrelated signals to provide information on the within-class variation [40]. Overall, 30 potential chemical markers contributed to the separation of GQD and FGQD, and the mechanisms of the processing-induced chemical transformation of the secondary metabolites were further elucidated. Although there were no new secondary metabolites in FGQD compared with GQD, the amounts of these secondary metabolites were redistributed in FGQD. Deglycosylation reaction by stepwise cleavage of the sugar moieties was considered the main metabolic pathway. Other chemical reactions, i.e., dehydration, demethylation and reduction, were also potentially implicated in the processing. These chemical transformations should mainly contribute to the fluctuation in the contents of isoflavone *O*-glycosides and flavone *O*-glucuronides due to processing. These results for the in vitro biotransformation of GQD by SC demonstrated that the fermentation of TCM formulas is a complex process.

Due to the lack of reference standards for quantitation and poor baseline separation, only ten representative compounds with high contents were subjected to targeted analysis to illustrate the effects of processing.

For puerarin, daidzin, daidzein, liquiritin and liquiritigenin, the results of the targeted quantification were consistent with those obtained in the untargeted studies, thus demonstrating that the hydrolysis of O-glycosides occurred due to the effect of β-glucosidase of SC [2, 41, 42] and further supporting speculation that C-glucoside is more difficult to transform via biotransformation with SC. In addition, the variation trends of coptisine, berberine, palmatine and baicalin in the targeted quantification corresponded with the results of the untargeted metabolomics, suggesting that multiple reactions might simultaneously occur, resulting in a dynamic equilibrium (Figs. 5, 6). Interestingly, the increasing trend of baicalein in the targeted analysis was highly different from the significant increase in baicalein observed in the untargeted analysis. Thus, we conclude that baicalein is altered slightly due to the dynamic equilibrium between flavone O-glucuronides and their derivatives. According to these results, our integrated strategy was useful for screening, matching and identifying the metabolites of FGQD.

Increasing evidence has indicated that the ten targeted compounds detected in raw and fermented GQD have various regulatory actions against T2DM. The antidiabetic effects of Gegen isoflavones have been demonstrated in several studies [43–46]. A previous study showed that both puerarin and daidzein from Gegen could reduce FBG and improve ISI and hyperlipidaemia in diabetic mice or rats [43–45], whereas daidzin showed an opposite effect by stimulating glucose uptake [46]. In addition, it was reported that daidzein can improve plasma TC, TG and HDL-C concentrations in db/db mice [43]. Gaur reported that liquiritigenin from Gancao could be used as a possible lead for the control of FBG levels [47]. Several studies have shown that daidzein and liquiritigenin, which are small, hydrophobic molecules, are absorbed faster and in higher amounts than their glucosides, daidzin and liquiritin, in humans [44]. Thus, the increasing trends of flavone aglycones (daidzein and liquiritigenin) and isoflavone C-glycosides (puerarin), as well as other homologous compounds, might be helpful for explaining the greater anti-diabetic effects of FGQD, which occur partially via regulation of the levels of ISI, TC, TG, and HDL. Moreover, baicalin and baicalein from Huangqin have been demonstrated to exhibit excellent anti-diabetic activities [48–50]. Berberine, palmatine and coptisine have also been reported to exert antidiabetic effects involved in improving insulin resistance and secretion and promoting glucose consumption in 3T3-L1 murine pre-adipocytes cells [51–53]. Thus, the stable contents of baicalin, baicalein, coptisine, berberine and palmatine, which showed obvious antidiabetic effects, as well as other compounds in FGQD, may contribute to the

observed anti-diabetic effects. Taken together, these findings will help enhance our understanding of the greater anti-diabetic effects of FGQD.

Conclusions
In the present study, the antidiabetic effects and chemical profiles between GQD and FGQD were systematically compared. The anti-diabetic effects of FGQD were more potent than those of GQD, suggesting that the anti-diabetic activities of TCM formulas might be improved by applying fermentation technology. Moreover, the integration of chromatographic technique-based untargeted metabolomics and targeted analysis can be considered a useful approach for systematically exploring the chemical profiles of raw and fermented formulas. The increasing activities might be ascribed to the main constituents of transformation between GQD and FGQD. To ensure the therapeutic effects and safety of FGQD, the role of fermentation in processing should be further studied.

Additional files

Additional file 1. Minimum standards of reporting checklist.

Additional file 2: Table S1. Calibration curves, LODs, LOQs, repeatability, accuracy and stability of the quantitative assays for 10 analytes in GQD. **Figure S1.** Workflow of the untargeted metabolomic analysis. **Figure S2** Effects of HM, GQD and FGQD on the FBG levels in T2DM rats. $^{**}p<0.01$ DM vs NC; $^{\#}p<0.05$, $^{\#\#}p<0.01$ HM vs DM; $^{*}p<0.05$, $^{**}p<0.01$ DM vs GQD; $^{\triangle}p<0.05$, $^{\triangle\triangle}p<0.05$ FGQD vs DM. **Figure S3.** Chemical structures of the compounds identified in GQD. P: Pueraria Lobatae Radix; S: Scutellariae Radix; C: Coptidis Rhizoma; G: Glycyrrhizae Radix et Rhizoma Praeparata cum Melle. **Figure S4.** Extracted ion chromatograms of 133 constituents from GQD. P: Pueraria Lobatae Radix; S: Scutellariae Radix; C: Coptidis Rhizoma; G: Glycyrrhizae Radix et Rhizoma Praeparata cum Melle. **Figure S5.** PCA score plots of GQD and FGQD. A: negative ion; B: positive ion. **Figure S6.** Representative HPLC chromatograms of ten marker compounds at 254 nm and 276 nm. P11: puerarin, P18: daidzin, P35: daidzein, C14: coptisine, C18: palmatine, C19: berberine, G3: liquiritin, G12: liquiritigenin, S19: baicalin, S37: baicalein.

Abbreviations
GQD: Ge-Gen-Qin-Lian decoction; FGQD: fermented Ge-Gen-Qin-Lian decoction; TCM: traditional Chinese medicine; SC: Saccharomyces cerevisiae; HPLC: high-performance liquid chromatography; MS: mass spectrometry; PD: potato dextrose; T2DM: type 2 diabetes mellitus; STZ: streptozotocin; NC: control group; HFD: high-fat diet; FBG: fasting blood glucose; HM: metformin hydrochloride; TC: total serum cholesterol; TG: triglycerides; HDL-C: high-density lipoprotein cholesterol; LDL-C: low-density lipoprotein cholesterol; FINS: fast serum insulin; HOMA-IR: homeostasis model assessment-insulin resistance; RDA: Retro-Diels–Alder; QCs: quality control samples; PCA: principal component analysis; OPLS-DA: orthogonal projection to latent structure-discriminant analysis; AGC: automatic gain control; NCE: normalized collision energies; EIC: extracted ion chromatography.

Authors' contributions
YY, CD, XQ, and QS conceived and designed the experiments. MZ, JL and JJ performed the experiments. YY wrote the manuscript. ZL and AL revised the manuscript. All authors read and approved the final manuscript.

Author details
[1] Modern Research Center for Traditional Chinese Medicine of Shanxi University, No. 92, Wucheng Road, Taiyuan 030006, Shanxi, China. [2] School of Traditional Chinese Materia Medica, Shanxi University of Chinese Medicine, No. 121, Daxue Street, Taiyuan 030619, Shanxi, China. [3] College of Chemistry and Chemical Engineering of Shanxi University, No. 92, Wucheng Road, Taiyuan 030006, Shanxi, China.

Acknowledgements
We thank the Scientific Instrument Center of Shanxi University for Q Exactive HR-MS analysis.

Competing interests
The authors declare that they have no competing interests.

Consent for publication
All authors consent to publication of this study in the journal *Chinese Medicine*.

Funding
This research was supported by the National Natural Science Foundation of China (No. 81273659).

References

1. Dong JW, Cai L, Xiong J, Chen XH, Wang WY, Shen N, Liu BL, Ding ZT. Improving the antioxidant and antibacterial activities of fermented *Bletilla striata* with *Fusarium avenaceum* and *Fusarium oxysporum*. Process Biochem. 2015;50(1):8–13.
2. Huang Q, Zhang H, Xue D. Enhancement of antioxidant activity of Radix Puerariae and red yeast rice by mixed fermentation with *Monascus purpureus*. Food Chem. 2017;226:89–94.
3. Fu Y, Yin Z, Wu L, Yin C. Fermentation of ginseng extracts by *Penicillium simplicissimum* GS33 and antiovarian cancer activity of fermented products. World J Microbiol Biotechnol. 2014;30(3):1019.
4. Tan L, Zhang X, Mei Z, Wang J, Li X, Huang W, Yang S. Fermented Chinese formula Shuan-Tong-Ling protects brain microvascular endothelial cells against oxidative stress injury. Evid Based Complement Altern Med. 2016;2016:5154290.
5. Kim DS, Um YR, Ma JY. Flavonoid content, free radical scavenging and increase in xanthine oxidase inhibitory activity in Galgeun-tang following fermentation with *Lactobacillus plantarum*. Mol Med Rep. 2014;10(5):2689–93.
6. Huang Q, Zhang H, Xue D. Enhancement of antioxidant activity of Radix Puerariae and red yeast rice by mixed fermentation with *Monascus purpureus*. Food Chem. 2017;226:89–94.
7. Fu Y, Yin Z, Wu L, Yin C. Fermentation of ginseng extracts by *Penicillium simplicissimum* GS33 and anti-ovarian cancer activity of fermented products. World J Microbiol Biotechnol. 2014;30(3):1019.
8. Kim DS, Um YR, Ma JY. Flavonoid content, free radical scavenging and increase in xanthine oxidase inhibitory activity in Galgeun-tang following fermentation with *Lactobacillus plantarum*. Mol Med Rep. 2014;10(5):2689.
9. Tan L, Zhang X, Mei Z, Wang J, Li X, Huang W, Yang S. Fermented chinese formula Shuan-Tong-Ling protects brain microvascular endothelial cells against oxidative stress injury. Evid Based Complement Altern Med. 2016;2016:5154290.
10. Limón RI, Peñas E, Torino MI, Martínez-Villaluenga C, Dueñas M, Frias J. Fermentation enhances the content of bioactive compounds in kidney bean extracts. Food Chem. 2015;172:343–52.
11. Li ZY, He P, Sun HF, Qin XM, Du GH. ^{1}H NMR based metabolomic study of antifatigue effect of Astragali Radix. Euro J Integr Med. 2014;6(6):3022–30.
12. Zhou H, Liang J, Lv D, Hu Y, Zhu Y, Si J, Wu S. Characterization of phenolics of *Sarcandra glabra* by non-targeted high-performance liquid chromatography fingerprinting and following targeted electrospray ionisation tandem mass spectrometry/time-of-flight mass spectrometry analyses. Food Chem. 2013;138(4):2390–8.
13. Chen Y, Zhou Z, Yang W, Bi N, Xu J, He J, Zhang R, Wang L, Abliz Z. Development of a data-independent targeted metabolomics method for relative quantification using liquid chromatography coupled with tandem mass spectrometry. Anal Chem. 2017;89:6954–62.
14. Naz S, Vallejo M, García A, Barbas C. Method validation strategies involved in non-targeted metabolomics. J Chromatogr A. 2014;1353:99–105.
15. Li Z, Xu JD, Zhou SS, Qian M, Ming K, Hong S, Li XY, Duan SM, Xu J, Li SL. Integrating targeted glycomics and untargeted metabolomics to investigate the processing chemistry of herbal medicines, a case study on Rehmanniae Radix. J Chromatogr A. 2016;1472:74–87.
16. Cao G, Zhang C, Zhang Y, Cong X, Cai H, Cai B, Li X, Yao J. Global detection and identification of components from crude and processed traditional Chinese medicine by liquid chromatography connected with hybrid ion trap and time-of-flight-mass spectrometry. J Sep Sci. 2011;34(15):1845–52.
17. Qi W, Wei S, Xue Q, Shuai J, Yi K, Zhang ZX, Tao B, Guo DA, Ye M. Simultaneous quantification of 50 bioactive compounds of the traditional Chinese medicine formula Gegen-Qinlian decoction using ultra-high performance liquid chromatography coupled with tandem mass spectrometry. J Chromatogr A. 2016;1454:15–25.
18. Mlao WJ, Wang Q, Bo T, Ye M, Qiao X, Yang WZ, Xiang C, Guan XY, Guo DA. Rapid characterization of chemical constituents and rats metabolites of the traditional Chinese patent medicine Gegen-Qinlian-Wan by UHPLC/DAD/qTOF-MS. J Pharm Biomed Anal. 2013;72:99–108. https://doi.org/10.1016/j.jpba.2012.09.015.
19. Zhang CH, Xu GL, Liu YH, Rao Y, Yu RY, Zhang ZW, Wang YS, Tao L. Anti-diabetic activities of Gegen Qinlian decoction in high-fat diet combined with streptozotocin-induced diabetic rats and in 3T3-L1 adipocytes. Phytomedicine. 2013;20(3–4):221–9.
20. Tong XL, Zhao LH, Lian FM, Qiang Z, Le X, Zhang J, Chen XY, Ji HY. Clinical observations on the dose-effect relationship of Gegen Qin Lian decoction on 54 out-patients with type 2 diabetes. J Tradit Chin Med. 2011;31(1):56–9.
21. Tian N, Wang J, Wang P, Song X, Yang M, Kong L. NMR-based metabonomic study of Chinese medicine Gegen Qinlian decoction as an effective treatment for type 2 diabetes in rats. Metabolomics. 2013;9(6):1228–42.
22. Chen H, Guo J, Pang B, Zhao L, Tong X. Application of herbal medicines with bitter flavor and cold property on treating diabetes mellitus. Evid Based Complement Altern Med. 2015;2015:529491.
23. Li H, Zhao L, Zhang B, Jiang Y, Wang X, Guo Y, Liu H, Li S, Tong X. A network pharmacology approach to determine active compounds and action mechanisms of ge-gen-qin-lian decoction for treatment of type 2 diabetes. Evid Based Complement Altern Med. 2014;2014:495840. https://doi.org/10.1155/2014/495840.
24. Jiang S, Du P, An L, Yuan G, Sun Z. Anti-diabetic effect of *Coptis chinensis* polysaccharide in high-fat diet with STZ-induced diabetic mice. Int J Biol Macromol. 2013;55(3):118–22.
25. Ji YJ, Lim Y, Min SM, Ji YK, Kwon O. Onion peel extracts ameliorate hyperglycemia and insulin resistance in high fat diet/streptozotocin-induced diabetic rats. Nutr Metab. 2011;8(1):18.
26. Du G, Zhao H, Zhang Q, Li GH, Yang F, Wang Y, Li Y, Wang Y. A rapid method for simultaneous determination of 14 phenolic compounds in Radix Puerariae using microwave-assisted extraction and ultra high performance liquid chromatography coupled with diode array detection and time-of-flight mass spectrometry. J Chromatogr A. 2010;1217(5):705–14.
27. Xue Q, Qi W, Wei S, Yi Q, Yao X, Rong A, Guo DA, Ye M. A chemical profiling solution for Chinese medicine formulas using comprehensive and loop-based multiple heart-cutting two-dimensional liquid chromatography coupled with quadrupole time-of-flight mass spectrometry. J Chromatogr A. 2016;1438:198–204.
28. Yang ZW, Xu F, Liu X, Cao Y, Tang Q, Chen QY, Shang MY, Liu GX, Wang X, Cai SQ. An untargeted metabolomics approach to determine component differences and variation in their in vivo distribution between Kuqin and Ziqin, two commercial specifications of Scutellaria Radix. RSC Adv. 2017;7(86):54682–95.
29. Zhang L, Zhang RW, Li Q, Lian JW, Liang J, Chen XH, Bi KS. Development

of the fingerprints for the quality evaluation of Scutellariae Radix by HPLC-DAD and LC-MS-MS. Chromatographia. 2007;66(1):13–20.

30. Islam MN, Downey F, Ng KY. Comprehensive profiling of flavonoids in *Scutellaria incana* L. using LC–Q-TOF–MS. Acta Chromatogr. 2013;25(3):555–69.

31. Han J, Ye M, Xu M, Sun J, Wang B, Guo DA. Characterization of flavonoids in the traditional Chinese herbal medicine-Huangqin by liquid chromatography coupled with electrospray ionization mass spectrometry. J Chromatogr B Analyt Technol Biomed Life Sci. 2007;848(2):355–62.

32. Montoro P, Maldini M, Russo M, Postorino S, Piacente S, Pizza C. Metabolic profiling of roots of liquorice (*Glycyrrhiza glabra*) from different geographical areas by ESI/MS/MS and determination of major metabolites by LC-ESI/MS and LC-ESI/MS/MS. J Pharm Biomed Anal. 2011;54(3):535–44.

33. Xue Q, Ru L, Wei S, Miao WJ, Jia L, Chen HB, Guo DA, Ye M. A targeted strategy to analyze untargeted mass spectral data: rapid chemical profiling of *Scutellaria baicalensis* using ultra-high performance liquid chromatography coupled with hybrid quadrupole orbitrap mass spectrometry and key ion filtering. J Chromatogr A. 2016;1441:83–95.

34. Qiao X, Song W, Ji S, Wang Q, Guo DA, Ye M. Separation and characterization of phenolic compounds and triterpenoid saponins in licorice (*Glycyrrhiza uralensis*) using mobile phase-dependent reversed-phase x reversed-phase comprehensive two-dimensional liquid chromatography coupled with mass spectrometry. J Chromatogr A. 2015;1402:36–45.

35. Wang D, Liu Z, Guo M, Liu S. Structural elucidation and identification of alkaloids in Rhizoma Coptidis by electrospray ionization tandem mass spectrometry. J Mass Spectrom. 2004;39(11):1356–65.

36. Chuang WC, Young DS, Liu LK, Sheu SJ. Liquid chromatographic-electrospray mass spectrometric analysis of Coptidis Rhizoma. J Chromatogr A. 1996;755(1):19–26.

37. Hirakura K, Morita M, Nakajima K, Sugama K, Takagi K, Niitsu K, Ikeya Y, Maruno M, Okada M. Phenolic glucosides from the root of *Pueraria lobata*. Phytochemistry. 1997;46(5):921–8.

38. Xue Q, Qi W, Shuang W, Miao W, Li Y, Cheng X, Guo DA, Ye M. Compound to extract to formulation: a knowledge-transmitting approach for metabolites identification of Gegen-Qinlian decoction, a traditional Chinese medicine formula. Sci Rep. 2016;6:39534.

39. Choi RJ, Ha IJ, Choi JS, Park YM, Kim YS. Biotransformation of flavonoid-7-O-glucuronides by β-glucuronidases. Nat Prod Sci. 2010; 16(1):1–5. http://www.koreascience.or.kr/article/ArticleFullRecord.jsp?cn=E1HSBY_2010_v16n1_1. Accepted 3 Mar 2010.

40. Wang C, Yin YH, Wei YJ, Shi ZQ, Liu JQ, Liu LF, Xin GZ. Rapid identification of herbal compounds derived metabolites using *Zebrafish larvae* as the biotransformation system. J Chromatogr A. 2017;1515:100–8.

41. Hernández LF, Espinosa JC, Fernández-González M, Briones A. β-Glucosidase activity in a *Saccharomyces cerevisiae* wine strain. Int J Food Microbiol. 2003;80(2):171–6.

42. Amor IL, Hehn A, Guedone E, Ghedira K, Engasser JM, Chekir-Ghedrira L, Ghoul M. Biotransformation of naringenin to eriodictyol by *Saccharomyces cerevisiea* functionally expressing flavonoid 3′ hydroxylase. Nat Prod Commun. 2010;5(12):1893–8.

43. Ae PS, Choi MS, Cho SY, Seo JS, Jung UJ, Kim MJ, Sung MK, Park YB, Lee MK. Genistein and daidzein modulate hepatic glucose and lipid regulating enzyme activities in C57BL/KsJ-db/db mice. Life Sci. 2006;79(12):1207–13.

44. Kwon DY, Daily JW III, Kim HJ, Park S. Antidiabetic effects of fermented soybean products on type 2 diabetes. Nutr Res. 2010;30(1):1–13.

45. Wu K, Liang T, Duan X, Xu L, Zhang K, Li R. Anti-diabetic effects of puerarin, isolated from *Pueraria lobata* (Willd), on streptozotocin-diabetogenic mice through promoting insulin expression and ameliorating metabolic function. Food Chem Toxicol. 2013;60(10):341–7.

46. Meezan E, Meezan EM, Jones K, Moore R, Barnes S, Prasain JK. Contrasting effects of puerarin and daidzin on glucose homeostasis in mice. J Agric Food Chem. 2005;53(22):8760–7.

47. Gaur R, Yadav KS, Verma RK, Yadav NP, Bhakuni RS. In vivo anti-diabetic activity of derivatives of isoliquiritigenin and liquiritigenin. Phytomedicine. 2014;21(4):415–22.

48. Hsu FL, Liu IM, Kuo DH, Chen WC, Su HC, Cheng JT. Antihyperglycemic effect of puerarin in streptozotocin-induced diabetic rats. J Nat Prod. 2003;66(6):788–92.

49. Yu F, Luo J, Jia Z, Wei Z, Zhou K, Gilbert E, Liu D. Baicalein protects against type 2 diabetes via promoting islet β-cell function in obese diabetic mice. Int J Endocrinol. 2014;2014:846742. https://doi.org/10.1155/2014/846742.

50. Ahad A, Mujeeb M, Ahsan H, Siddiqui WA. Prophylactic effect of baicalein against renal dysfunction in type 2 diabetic rats. Biochimie. 2014;106:101–10.

51. Dong Y, Chen YT, Yang YX, Zhou XJ, Dai SJ, Tong JF, Shou D, Li C. Metabolomics study of type 2 diabetes mellitus and the antidiabetic effect of berberine in zucker diabetic fatty rats using UPLC-ESI–HDMS. Phytother Res. 2016;30(5):823–8.

52. Aggarwal BB, Prasad S, Reuter S, Kannappan R, Yadev VR, Park B, Kim JH, Gupta SC, Phromnoi K, Sundaram C, Prasad S, Chaturvedi MM, Sung B. Identification of novel anti-inflammatory agents from ayurvedic medicine for prevention of chronic diseases: "reverse pharmacology" and "bedside to bench" approach. Curr Drug Targets. 2011;12(11):1595–653.

53. Jung HA, Na YY, Bae HJ, Min BS, Choi JS. Inhibitory activities of the alkaloids from Coptidis Rhizoma against aldose reductase. Arch Pharm Res. 2008;31(11):1405–12.

3

SWOT analysis and revelation in traditional Chinese medicine internationalization

Haitao Tang[1,2], Wenlong Huang[1*], Jimei Ma[2] and Li Liu[1]

Abstract

Traditional Chinese medicine (TCM) is currently the best-preserved and most influential traditional medical system with the largest number of users worldwide. In recent years, the trend of TCM adoption has increased greatly, but the process of TCM internationalization has suffered from a series of setbacks for both internal and external reasons. Thus, the process of TCM internationalization faces formidable challenges, although it also has favourable opportunities. Using SWOT analysis, this paper investigates the strengths, weaknesses, opportunities and threats for TCM. These findings can serve as references for TCM enterprises with global ambitions.

Keywords: TCM, Internationalization, SWOT analysis

Background

At present, the pace of the expansion of traditional Chinese medicine (TCM) into the overseas market continues to accelerate. Both the Chinese government and Chinese medicine enterprises are making efforts to promote TCM as it moves into the overseas market. However, particular issues associated with TCM, such as its complex composition, various effects of its actions, insufficient systematic studies during its internationalization, etc., hinder the adoption of specific TCM drugs in the internationally recognised pharmaceutical market. In this study, we use the SWOT method to analyse the current situation of TCM internationalization, and the analysis is divided into four aspects.

Strength analysis of the internationalization of traditional Chinese medicine

Strengths of traditional Chinese medicine in theory and in treating disease

There are many strengths of TCM in the treatment of diseases which are not found in Western medicine

(Table 1). First, TCM and Western medicine are two different medical theoretical systems with different modes and substantial differences in such aspects as theoretical foundations, methods of thinking, as well as diagnostic and treatment approaches. In the latter, the treatments are partial; in the former, symptoms and root causes are treated simultaneously. TCM has a unique theory as well as diagnostic and treatment techniques and methods. Compared with modern Western medicine, which focuses on detailed molecular targets, TCM thought takes an overall approach and pays attention to syndrome differentiation based on an overall analysis of the illness and the patient's condition. TCM adopts multiple levels (dimensions) and a multi-targeted method to make overall adjustments and restore the human body to achieve the goal of treating both the manifestation of the disease and its cause.

Second, TCM can be used to treat various diseases and especially has advantages for treating incurable diseases and chronic diseases [1, 2]. Berberine exhibits beneficial anti-inflammation effects for the inflammatory bowel diseases, it also differentially modulates the activities of ERK, p38 MARK, and JNK to suppress Th17 and Th1 T cell differentiation indicating that it could be a potential therapeutic drug to treat type 1 diabetes mellitus (DM) [3]. Even for a disease without an obvious clinical

*Correspondence: ydhuangwenlong@126.com
[1] China Pharmaceutical University, Longmian Road 639, Nanjing 211198, China
Full list of author information is available at the end of the article

Table 1 Comparison of TCM and Western medicine in the treatment of diseases

Subjects	Characteristics
TCM	Based on the traditional Chinese medicine theory
	Symptoms and root causes are treated simultaneously
	Only less adverse side effects
	TCM works slowly and requires a long course of treatment
Western medicine	Based on the Western medicine theory
	The treatments are partial
	Produce some adverse side effects
	Western medicine works quickly

manifestation according to Western medicine principle, TCM treatment can use its theoretical advantages of syndrome differentiation and effective timing to relieve the disease and make up for the deficiencies of modern Western medicine [4, 5]. For example, in management of metabolic syndrome, TCM is an excellent representative in alternative and complementary medicines with a complete theory system and substantial herb remedies. Ginseng, rhizoma coptidis (berberine, the major active compound) and bitter melon were discussed for their potential activities in the treatment of metabolic syndrome [6–11]. Recently, a search of active ingredient(s) from some commonly used TCM has revealed a wide variety of compounds that are biologically active with therapeutic potentials. About 62% of the 240 species were found to contain chemical compounds with pharmacological procies were found for the treatment of at least one disease and 53% of them for two or more diseases [12]. Virtual mapping between databases of Chinese herbal ingredients and molecular targets of diseases is likely to offer a new avenue for drug discovery [13].

Third, some new TCM drugs are being successfully developed based on many years of clinical practice; these drugs can generally have precise effects and have only less adverse side effects [14]. Only minimal adverse effects were reported for Chinese medicines used in treating type 2 DM indicating certain advantages in the prevention of diabetes and delay of its complications [15].

At the same time, combined traditional Chinese and Western medicine has good effect in the treatment for patients which is beneficial to improve patients' quality of life [16]. For example, TCM in combination with insulin exhibited better clinical effect in the treatment of gestational diabetes [17].

Strengths in international demand for TCM

In present-day society, the concept of healthy living has undergone tremendous changes, and people are increasingly pursuing improved health and quality of life. The unique effects of TCM are not only valued by domestic intellectuals but have also attracted the attention of the international community. Correspondingly, the demand for natural botanical medicine is also increasing.

Compared with the research and development (R&D) of TCM, there are some problems in R&D of chemical medicine. First, the process of chemical drug discovery is long and arduous that it begins from the search of a potential candidate to the development of a marketable drug. The course could be as long as more than a decade [18]. Second, the R&D cost for a new drug can be, in average, more than 800 million USD in the United States (US) [19]. Third, the development of new chemical drugs remains very a low rate of success. Among thousands chemical compounds only a few candidates could reach their first markets as new drugs in recent years. Finally, synthetic chemical drugs are often associated with undesirable side effects in patients. It is now clear that the need of therapeutic intervention in many clinical conditions cannot be satisfactorily met by synthetic chemical drugs. Since the research and development of new chemical drugs remain time-consuming, capital-intensive, safety issues, and undesired side effects, much effort has been put in the search for alternative routes for drug discovery in China [20]. TCM has a long history of use, with extensive literature and clinical applications covering thousands of years. Such as berberine, an active ingredient from Coptis chinensis Franch, is widely used for the treatment of infectious diseases in China [21]. As TCM has the advantages of treatment of special diseases safety, and so on, there are many countries and regions begin to study it. At present, more than 150 countries and regions [22] have established natural botanical institutions, and pharmaceutical companies are increasingly focusing on research and development of botanicals, paying attention to the construction of traditional botanical studies and development teams, and focusing on the search for effective natural medicines to replace chemical treatments. Furthermore, there are over 1300 medicinal plants used in Europe [23]. As safe and healthy treatments are associated with a return to nature, TCM can make up for the shortcomings of Western medicine in many areas. We can find the solutions to different kinds of diseases that are hard to cure by using the innovations and developments of TCM. TCM displays a distinctive curative effect for different diseases that are hard to cure and for technological difficulties that are recognized worldwide, such as tumours [24], chronic liver disease [25] and chronic kidney disease [26].

Strengths of natural medicine resources

China has rich natural medicine resources, with the world's largest treasure of Chinese herbal medicine, and has a unique advantage in nurturing and developing the TCM industry. According to statistical studies, there are 12,807 TCM resources in China, including 11,146 medicinal plants, 1581 medicinal animals, and 80 medicinal minerals. At present, there are more than 600 commonly used Chinese medicinal materials, in which near 400 plant and animal species are artificially cultured. In addition, a statistical analysis of 320 commonly used plant medicinal materials indicates that the total resources storage has reached approximately 8.5 million tons [27].

At present, domestic cultivation is a widely used and generally accepted practice in China. Cultivation provides the opportunity to use new techniques to solve problems encountered in the production of medicinal plants, such as toxic components, pesticide contamination, low contents of active ingredients, and the misidentification of botanical origin. Cultivation under controlled growth conditions can improve the yields of bioactive components and obtain improved yields of target products [28].

Strengths in the scale and power of TCM enterprises

China has a number of large-scale TCM enterprises with strong scientific research abilities. Chinese TCM enterprises are strengthening their research and development abilities while continuing to conduct studies of listed products and move forward with adaptions for the international market. At the same time, drug regulatory authorities continue to promote Chinese production and quality management systems in connection with international standards and to improve the good manufacturing practice (GMP) management level. Chinese TCM enterprises should achieve the GMP requirements and make efforts to connect to the international production management system. They have increased their investment in technological transformation so that the TCM production quality management level has reached a historical new height through the improvement of the production environment and conditions as well as the promotion of staff quality and production quality management.

In addition, in recent years, upstream and downstream enterprises and industries related to TCM, such as Chinese herbal planting, research and development; the manufacture and marketing of pharmaceutical equipment; TCM transportation; and many other supporting industries, have continued to grow and develop through the promotion and rapidly expanding development of the TCM industry. Thus, the development of the TCM industry can also advance the development of supporting industrial chains, forming a favourable interaction.

Weakness analysis of the internationalization of TCM

We have analyzed the strengths of the internationalization of TCM, but we should also realize that many unfavourable factors are also related to the internationalization of TCM.

Cultural diversity

Chinese medicine theory has many ancient Chinese-based terms that cannot be expressed in objective and modern scientific language and evidence, so that many Chinese medicine terms, such as yin-yang and the five elements, assistant and guide and other traditional theories and terms, are not understood and accepted by the international community [29]. TCM is a medical system developed on the basis of Taoist philosophy. The theory of TCM was first documented in an ancient Chinese book, Huangdi Neijing (Yellow Emperor's Inner classic). The book proposes that the human body contains Yin and Yang. A disease is a consequence of disbalance of Yin and Yang. Qi (air) and blood serve as mediators in communication between Yin and Yang. The primary aim in the treatment of illness is to restore the balance, and replenish Qi or blood. Herbal medicines, acupuncture, and massage are often used to restore the balance in the clinical practice in TCM [2, 30].

Eastern and Western cultures are different not only in language systems but also in values, ways of thinking, etc. Chinese medicine and pharmacy are a huge, complex system of long-term experience based practice, emphasizing an overall view that is totally different from the perspective of Western medicine and pharmacy. In the TCM theory, diabetes is considered a result of Yin deficiency with dryness-heat. The treatment of diabetes should be focused on replenishing Yin (fluid) and evacuating fire (heat) from the body [31]. However, for Western medicine, such as Metformin is commonly used in the treatment of diabetes. It acts primarily by decreasing hepatic glucose output, largely by inhibiting gluconeogenesis [32].

Chinese medicine is based on a holistic approach, while Western medicine is based on a reductionistic approach. For example, in the treatment of cancer, Western medicine often take the tumor mass reduction as the ultimate goal, regardless of normal cells; while the TCM in addition to tumor inhibition, but also intend to alleviate the symptoms, strengthen the body resistance, improve the quality of life, prolong the survival time of cancer patients for the therapeutic purpose [32, 33].

Weakness in quality control of TCM

In the cultivation of herbs, the quality of Chinese medicinal herbal products directly affects the quality of TCM.

However, most of the cultivation, harvesting and processing management procedures of Chinese herbal medicinal materials are extensive. There is a lack of relevant technological innovations, the production process is not well scientifically based, the yield per unit area is low, the quality of the herbs is uneven, and the classification of species is not strictly enforced. There are no effective means to manage and resolve the problems of pesticide residues during pest control, and heavy metal residues occur through the process of planting, leading to the existence of unwanted chemicals in the herbs [34]. There are only a few quality control indicators for most of Chinese medicinal materials, and some of them have no quantitative indicators and even no qualitative indicators. Currently, the majority of the existing Chinese medicinal materials quality control specifications are not effectively to ensure the stable quality of Chinese medicinal materials, and the medicinal ingredients in these materials, which are the most direct causes for the unstable quality of TCM and the unevenness of its clinical efficacy [34].

TCM is more complex and comprehensive than Western medicine in terms of finished product quality, whether for a single drug prescription (prescriptions consisting of a single medicinal material) or a compounded Chinese medicine (prescriptions consisting of two or more medicinal materials). There is a lack of studies on material basis, active ingredients, and mechanism of action and no scientific and reasonable quality control indicators and methods [35]. Therefore, the uniformity, safety and effectiveness of inter-assay stability for TCM products cannot be guaranteed.

The implementation periods required by Chinese good clinical practice (GCP), good laboratory practice (GLP), GMP and other specifications are shorter than the international standards for pharmacology, toxicology, standardization, GMP construction, etc. The foundation is weak, various research data have not yet gained acceptance in international communities, and there is still a long way to go before TCM can harmonize with international standards [36]. Most TCM enterprises commonly experience the following problems: there is not enough application of advanced technology, and there is a large gap between TCM practices and international advanced technologies [37]. Although the implementation of a new version of the GMP forced out some non-standard enterprises, some Chinese medicine enterprises still use outdated hardware and facilities, including outdated technologies for extraction, concentration and purification of Chinese herbal medicines; therefore, some key parameters are unclear and cannot be effectively controlled. There is a large gap between China and developed countries in terms of the extraction process and production technology of natural medicine.

Difficulty in identification of active principle from TCM composition

Regardless of specific national drug regulations there is an international consensus that all TCM drugs must meet stipulated high quality standards focusing on authentication, identification and chemical composition [38]. Chinese herbal medicine and TCM itself have complicated components that change constantly during the production of TCM, especially in the extraction process. Some components are not originally from Chinese herbal medicine itself but are transformed during the process of extraction and concentration, leading to difficulty in the identification of TCM components. In addition, TCM emphasizes mutual synergy, so it cannot simply use one or several indicators to fully represent the effect of TCM products. TCM consists of many chemical ingredients, and these ingredients play synergistic roles in human body [39], thus, the active medical ingredients are not clear. TCM adopts multi-target, multi-functional method to make overall adjustments and restore the human body to achieve the goal of treating both the manifestation of the disease and its cause. TCM is difficult to be clearly expressed by the chemical compositions in accordance with the requirements of chemical drugs, where the compositions are clearly expressed in chemical formulas.

At present, many enterprises and research institutions are committed to the pharmacology and composition of traditional Chinese medicine research. Advances in phytochemistry, high throughput screening, DNA sequencing, systems biology, and bioinformatics can reveal the chemical composition and molecular mechanisms of TCM [39–41]. In the TCM hospital Bad Kötzting, 171 TCM drugs underwent an analytical quality proof including thin layer as well as high performance liquid chromatography [38]. As from now mass spectroscopy will also be available as analytical tool. The findings are compiled and will be published one after another. The main issues of the analytical procedure in TCM drugs like authenticity, botanical nomenclature, variability of plant species, as well as medicinal parts processing are pointed out and possible ways to overcome them are sketched [38]. At present, the construction of chromatographic fingerprints plays an important role in the quality control of complex herbal medicines [42]. Many companies utilize advanced technologies to develop multi-component determination technics and chromatographic fingerprint analysis for qualitative and quantitative assessments. These assays will create a complete monitoring and evaluation system to ensure the efficacy, consistency, and inter-batch stability of the product. It is possible to clarify the role of the composition of TCM in the future.

Limited research input into TCM and challenge for technological innovation

In recent years, Europe, the US, Japan, South Korea and many other developed countries and regions have adopted modern research methods and techniques to increase the development of traditional botanical drugs, the screening and confirmation of active ingredients, the establishment of international advanced quality standards and the development of new formulations [43]. Most domestic Chinese enterprises and research institutes make relatively less investment in the R&D of TCM. Insufficient R&D investment leads to a lack of competitiveness of the enterprise products. Chemical drugs and biological products enjoy obvious competitive advantages, seriously affecting the growth rate of the market share of TCM. TCM products feature more impurity or low purity and a lack of innovation in dosage forms; traditional dosage forms still hold a dominant position. The development and application of quick-acting, long-term, efficient and convenient emergency dosage forms and other new dosage forms are still in the beginning stage. The production and application of new pharmaceutical excipients are insufficient and have a large gap with the mainstream trend of international drugs, directly affecting the competitiveness of TCM in the international market [43].

Opportunity analysis of internationalization of TCM

Continuous improvement of attention to TCM by the international community

With the progress of society and changes in the human disease spectrum, the medical model has undergone tremendous changes; people are not simply seeking disease treatment but are focusing on the comprehensive management of disease prevention, treatment and health protection [44]. People are inclined to treat disease with natural medicine due to the obvious toxic and side effects of chemical drugs, and Chinese medicine is aligned with this development tendency [45]. In addition, many national governments have gradually accepted and attached importance to TCM and natural herbal medicine because of the high bio-pharmaceutical R&D costs, medical costs, long-term costs and other issues. The international community continues to accept natural medicine, and market demand will continue to grow. More than 90 countries and regions are introducing laws and regulations for the registration of Chinese herbal medicine [46].

TCM herbal drugs are increasingly used in many countries of the EU [47]. In Europe, it is very good to know that European Pharmacopeia (Ph Eur) is working on TCM herbal drug quality monographs. The European Directorate for the Quality of Medicines (EDQM) has established two groups of experts in pharmacognosy, who elaborate monographs on herbal drugs and herbal drug preparations. Since 2007 a special working group has been established with the elaboration of monographs on traditional Chinese medicinal plants and preparations [48]. Till now, a working program, existing of 75 monographs was established by the Commission of Ph Eur, out of which almost 50 new TCM herbal drug monographs have been implemented for the Ph Eur so far [49]. The standards put forward in these monographs not only define the quality of these products, but also eliminate dangerous counterfeit, substandard, adulterated and contaminated (traditional) herbal medicinal products [48].

With many TCM herbal drug monographs are implemented in the Ph Eur, this will be a significantly contribution to the acceptance of TCM worldwide [50]. All aspects relevant to the quality parameters have to be achieved in an adequate manner, requiring a broad range of analytical methods to be applied for new herbal drug monographs in the Ph Eur [47].

Opportunity for economic globalization

First, due to the equivalent access for World Trade Organization (WTO) members, China's admission to the WTO gave it more opportunities to participate in international exchanges and cooperation, to promote the wider spread of Chinese medicinal culture, and to recommend TCM products with minimal side effects and high efficiency in treating both symptoms and causes of disease, which will establish a good foundation for popularizing TCM in the international community [25]. Second, Chinese medicine is becoming more popular for treating and preventing many diseases, especially incurable diseases and chronic diseases, in many countries due to the poor efficacy and obvious side effects of Western medicine. Third, due to a decline in tariffs [51], many enterprises are more able and more willing to introduce foreign advanced technologies and equipment into China, which will speed up the production technology and accelerate the internationalization of traditional Chinese medicine.

Chinese government policy support

In recent years, China has introduced a series of new policies and regulations to support the development of Chinese medicine, while increasing the support for international cooperation in Chinese medicine, indicating that the development of Chinese medicine has risen to a strategic governmental level. China attaches great importance to the inheritance and innovation of Chinese medicine, which will greatly promote the entry of Chinese medicine into the international market.

In addition, the implementation of the national strategy "One Belt and One Road" will create a new historical opportunity for Chinese medicine to move into the international community [52]. The development strategy of "One Belt and One Road", utilizes the ancient "Silk Road" historical symbols, actively develops economic cooperation partnerships along with the countries with geographical proximity and cultural similarities to create great opportunities for the development of Chinese medicine industry [52]. With the "One Belt and One Road" strategy, we can promote the communication of TCM cultures. Through constantly TCM cultural exchange, we can bridge the gap between Eastern and Western medical systems to enhance the TCM internationalization.

At the same time, the advantages of TCM and the international market demand provide great possibilities for TCM under the "One Belt and One Road" strategy. TCM has the feature of both humanity and medical sciences, therefore, its great resource in the economy, cultural and health care, should be regarded as one of the best mediums of cultural exchanges and international cooperations between China and the countries along the "One Belt and One Road". Moreover, "One Belt and One Road" strategy also provides the platform for inheritance and innovation of TCM, which will promote the further development of Chinese traditional medicine [53]. During this period, we can make full use of related resources and strengthen the international exchange and cooperation related to TCM. Cooperation and exchange include enhancing the policies and regulations for traditional medicine, improving herbal medicine quality standards and control indicators, and establishing administration regulations. There will be more exchanges between the Chinese government and international organizations, and the cooperation with foreign universities, research institutions, and hospitals as well, to co-establish academic and clinical research centres or groups to let more academic authority institutions accept and recognize TCM.

Continuous recognition of the advantages of TCM

The unique role of TCM has been widely recognized by the international community in the process of severe acute respiratory syndrome (SARS) prevention and control and has been highly praised by the World Health Organization. Chinese medicine can effectively reduce the mortality rate of SARS patients and the sequelae in the process of treating the SARS virus, and the treatment costs are significantly reduced. The specific function and significance of Chinese herbal medicine in treating SARS have been recognized by WHO experts and have also helped reduce prejudice against the supposed inaccurate efficacy of TCM in the international community [54, 55].

A researcher at the China Academy of Chinese Medical Science, Tu Youyou, was awarded the 2015 Nobel Prize in Physiology or Medicine for the development of artemisinin. Tu Youyou made an exploratory investigation of TCM and found that the components extracted from the plant *Artemisia annua* are effective in the treatment of malaria. By referring to ancient books and many studies, Tu Youyou found the best extraction method for artemisinin. Artemisinin is the invention not only of Tu Youyou but also of China and is an achievement of TCM heritage and innovation, which deserve popularization. This important invention created a sensation in the world [14].

Threat analysis of the internationalization of TCM

Threats posed by differences between Chinese and Western cultures

Due to differences between Chinese and Western cultures, China's TCM theory cannot be accepted by the international community [56]. TCM theories advocate "discontinuing medication when the patient is cured", oppose the long-term medication. Long-term medication or even increase of dose to several times of standard dose may inevitably lead to side effect [57]. This also exposes the differences between Chinese and Western cultures. Chinese medicine emphasizes the principle of syndrome differentiation. However, from Western medicine perspective the concept of TCM is hardly understood and accepted, therefore TCM is not well positioned and accepted [5].

Dual threats in Chinese and foreign markets

The officially entering of TCM to Europe Union (EU) market is at a slow rate, and there are only four products produced by Chinese enterprises registered in the EU; no real TCM is sold in the US; and the TCM industry is facing enormous challenges. China's botanical drugs have only a small share, less than 5%, of the international botanical market, 2% in the United Kingdom and the US, and 0.2% in Germany [58]. As natural medicine has been recognized by the international community, TCM and natural medicine have become the target of many large multinational companies. The international herbal medicine market is highly competitive. At present, Japan, South Korea and other countries are competitive with China in the international herbal medicine market and pose a great threat to China's exports.

In addition, a large number of foreign TCM companies based in Japan, South Korea and India have impacted the TCM market in China. China is the world's largest TCM market, and its demand for natural medicine is also very large. In recent years, due to the continuous opening of

China's pharmaceutical market, many large-scale foreign pharmaceutical enterprises have entered the Chinese market, and approximately 40 types of natural medicine manufactured in more than 10 countries and regions are successfully registered and listed in China [59].

Limitation of technical trade barriers
The practice standards of China's TCM industry remain in the progress of standardization. After entering the WTO, China had to align its standards with international standards. However, many countries and regions in the world, especially the Western developed countries, restrict foreign products entering their territory through various administrative measures and requirements, high-tech trade barriers and the "green trade barriers" threshold, including measures for medication safety and protection to strengthen the supervision of imported drugs; develop or improve relevant technical requirements, such as quality standards for heavy metal residues, pesticide residues, aflatoxin and others; standardize the technology of plant extracts and environmental standards; and so on [42].

Threats to intellectual property related to TCM
Chinese medicine has a 5000-year history in China, and in a traditional comprehensive theoretical system, the related intellectual property should belong to China. However, the implementation of patent protection and technical protection of the novel TCM drugs in China began late, and there is a lack of study of protection of TCM intellectual property rights; therefore, most Chinese medicine enterprises lack experience in patent applications in foreign countries and are not ready to protect their intellectual property. Most TCM can easily be imitated or limited by patents in foreign countries; thus, many valuable Chinese medicine product technologies and knowledge are under threat of advanced applications for patents by foreign enterprises. The developed countries, which have rich experience in drug patents, can not only obtain for TCM intellectual property rights but also compete for other resources related to Chinese medicine by using intellectual property advantages.

Summary and perspective
With the SWOT analysis of the internal and external environments, we can observe the advantages, disadvantages, opportunities and threats of TCM during the internationalization process (Table 2). Overall, the advantages outweigh the disadvantages, and the opportunities outweigh the threats.

To deal with these disadvantages and threats, we can provide some recommendations. First, we can strengthen the international communication on Chinese culture.

Table 2 SWOT analysis in traditional Chinese medicine internationalization

Subjects	Criteria description
Strength	TCM in theory and in treating diseases International demand for TCM Natural medicine resources The scale and power of TCM enterprises
Weakness	Cultural diversity Quality control of TCM Difficulty in identification of active principle from TCM composition Limited research input into TCM and challenge for technological innovation
Opportunity	Continuous improvement of attention to TCM by the international community Opportunity for economic globalization Chinese government policy support Continuous recognition of the advantages of TCM
Threat	Differences between Chinese and Western cultures Dual risks in Chinese and foreign markets Limitation of technical trade barriers Challenges in intellectual property related to TCM

We should make full use of related resources at home and strengthen the international exchange and cooperation related to TCM, thereby promoting the development of TCM culture. We should strengthen the exchange between the Chinese government and the leadership of international organizations; strengthen the cooperation with foreign institutions of higher educations and hospitals and co-establish clinical research centers or groups to make more academic authority institutions accept and recognize TCM.

Second, we can increase the input into TCM research. To align the foreign regulations concerning natural medicines, TCM can start with each individual medicinal materials. Enterprises can take some multi-herbal formula of TCM with specific curative effects, and take the effective part as an "effective body", then control the composition and contents of the "effective body", and gradually reach the purposes of "safe, effective, controllable, and stable". The "effective body" in individual medicinal material can also be analyzed and summarized with the "assistant and guide" theory of TCM. We should explore and investigate the traditional formulas and carry out secondary development with modern innovative technologies to develop and produce new products.

Third, we can enhance the standardization and modernization of TCM quality. We should issue TCM product quality standards that are applicable to both China and the world as soon as possible and establish strict management of planting and production, to ensure that the consistency of TCM quality can be controlled. We should regulate each step of the TCM industrial process, apply high and new technologies, use advanced equipment and adopt strict standards to transform the TCM production and reach the goals of modernizing the technologies for the extraction, formulation, and quality control of TCM based on related conventional theories.

Finally, we must carry out intellectual property protection training among the practitioners of the TCM industry and enhance the awareness of the whole industry regarding the protection of intellectual property. We must learn the domestic and international regulations on the protection of intellectual property. We may also achieve effective protection through the core technologies, trademarks, essence and inventions in TCM intellectual property.

In the process of the internationalization of TCM, we must emphasize the advantages to avoid the disadvantages, seize the opportunity to overcome the threats, carry out specific internationalization processes, avoid detours and promote a rapid internationalization process.

Abbreviations

TCM: traditional Chinese medicine; DM: diabetes mellitus; R&D: research and development; US: the United States; GMP: good manufacturing practice; GCP: good clinical practice; GLP: good laboratory practice; Ph Eur: European Pharmacopoeia; EDQM: European Directorate for the Quality of Medicines; WTO: World Trade Organization; SARS: severe acute respiratory syndrome; EU: Europe Union.

Authors' contributions

HT, WH, JM and LL conceived and designed the review. HT, JM and LL wrote the manuscript. All authors read and approved the final manuscript.

Author details

[1] China Pharmaceutical University, Longmian Road 639, Nanjing 211198, China. [2] Jiangsu Suzhong Pharmaceutical Group Co., Ltd., No. 1, Suzhong Road, Jiangyan District, Taizhou 225500, Jiangsu, China.

Acknowledgements

Not applicable.

Competing interests

The authors declare that they have no competing interests.

Consent for publication

All of authors consent to publication of this work in *Chinese Medicine*.

Funding

Not applicable.

References

1. Hoessel R, Leclerc S, Endicott JA, Nobel ME, Lawrie A, Tunnah P, et al. Indirubin, the active constituent of a chinese antileukaemia medicine, inhibits cyclin-dependent kinases. Nat Cell Biol. 1999;1(1):60.
2. Yin J, Zhang H, Ye J. Traditional chinese medicine in treatment of metabolic syndrome. Endocr Metab Immune Disord Drug Targets. 2008;8(2):99.
3. Cui GL, Xia Q, Zhang YB, et al. Berberine differentially modulates the activities of ERK, p38 MARK, and JNK to suppress Th17 and Th1 T cell differentiation in type 1 diabetic mice. J Biol Chem. 2009;284(41):28420–9.
4. Wang WJ. Prevention and treatment of metabolic syndrome with integrated traditional chinese and Western medicine. J Chin Integr Med. 2004;2(5):390–5.
5. Jiang WY. Therapeutic wisdom in traditional Chinese medicine: a perspective from modern science. Discov Med. 2005;5(29):455.
6. Vuksan V, Sievenpiper JL. Herbal remedies in the management of diabetes: lessons learned from the study of ginseng. Nutr Metab Cardiovasc Dis. 2005;15:149–60.
7. Xie JT, McHendale S, Yuan CS. Ginseng and diabetes. Am J Chin Med. 2005;33:397–404.
8. Yin J, Xing H, Ye J. Efficacy of berberine in patients with type 2 diabetes. Metabolism. 2008;57:712–7.
9. Kong W, Wei J, Abidi P, et al. Berberine is a novel cholesterol-lowering drug working through a unique mechanism distinct from statins. Nat Med. 2004;10:1344–51.
10. Khanna P, Jain SC, Panagariya A, Dixit VP. Hypoglycemic activity of polypeptide-p from a plant source. J Nat Prod. 1981;44:648–55.
11. Hu C, Wei H, Kong H, Bouwman J, Gonzalez-Covarrubias V, Van der Heijden R, et al. Linking biological activity with herbal constituents by systems biology-based approaches: effects of panax ginseng in type 2 diabetic goto-kakizaki rats. Mol Biosyst. 2011;7(11):3094.
12. Ehrman TM, Barlow DJ, Hylands PJ. Virtual screening of Chinese herbs with random forest. J Chem Inf Model. 2007;47(2):264.
13. Pan SY, Chen SB, Dong HG, et al. New perspectives on Chinese herbal medicine (Zhong-Yao) research and development. Evid Based Complement Altern Med. 2011;2011(1):1–11.
14. Klayman DL. Qinghaosu (artemisinin): an antimalarial drug from china. Science. 1985;228(4703):1049–55.
15. Li WL, Zheng HC, Bukuru J, et al. Natural medicines used in the traditional Chinese medical system for therapy of diabetes mellitus. J Ethnopharmacol. 2004;92(1):1–21.
16. Li J, Huang XY, Zou XZ, et al. Clinical curative effect of traditional Chinese medicine, Western medicine fuzheng attack comprehensive treatment of malignant tumor. Chin J Med Guide. 2014; 16(03):529–30, 532.
17. Zhang L, Wang L, Zhang G. Traditional Chinese medicine combined with insulin in the treatment of gestational diabetes clinical comparative study. J Med Theory Pract. 2014;27(24):3250–1.
18. Tobinick EL. The value of drug repositioning in the current pharmaceutical market. Drug News Perspect. 2009;22(2):119.
19. Schmid EF, Smith DA. R&D technology investments: misguided and expensive or a better way to discover medicines? Drug Discov Today. 2006;11(17–18):775.
20. Pan SY, Chen SB, Dong HG, et al. New perspectives on Chinese herbal medicine (Zhong-Yao) research and development. Evid Based Complement Altern Med (eCAM). 2011;2011(1):403709.
21. Xu JT, Wang LQ, Xu B. Research development of *Coptis chinensis*. Acta Acad Med Sin. 2004;26(6):704–7.
22. Xi Zeng. Chinese medicine is facing a good opportunity to the world. World Sci Technol Modernization Tradit Chin Med. 2004;6:71.
23. Balunas MJ, Kinghorn AD. Drug discovery from medicinal plants. Life Sci. 2005;78(5):431–41.
24. Efferth T, Li PC, Konkimalla VS, Kaina B. From traditional chinese medicine to rational cancer therapy. Trends Mol Med. 2007;13(8):353–61.
25. Cui X, Wang Y, Kokudo N, Fang D, Tang W. Traditional chinese medicine and related active compounds against hepatitis b virus infection. Biosci Trends. 2010;4(2):39–47.
26. Li X, Wang H. Chinese herbal medicine in the treatment of chronic kidney disease. Adv Chronic Kidney Dis. 2005;12(3):276–81.

27. Fu B. Analysis on the current situation of Chinese traditional medicine export. Int Technol Trade. 2007;6:69–70.

28. Chen SL, Hua Y, Luo HM, et al. Conservation and sustainable use of medicinal plants: problems, progress, and prospects. Chin Med. 2016;11(1):37.

29. Van der Greef J, Van Wietmarschen H, Schroën J, Wang M, Hankemeier T, Xu G. Systems biology-based diagnostic principles as pillars of the bridge between chinese and Western medicine. Planta Med. 2010;76(17):2036.

30. Schroën Y, Van Wietmarschen H, Wang M, et al. East is East; and West is West; and never the twain shall meet? Science. 2015;346(6216):1291–3.

31. Li WL, Zheng HC, Bukuru J, De Kimpe N. Natural medicines used in the traditional Chinese medical system for therapy of diabetes mellitus. J Ethnopharmacol. 2004;92:1–21.

32. Gao L, Wu X. Comparison of traditional chinese medicine with Western medicine cancer therapy. Cancer Biol Med. 2008;5(3):231–4.

33. Zhang L, Wu C, Zhang Y, Liu F, Zhao M, Bouvet M, et al. Efficacy comparison of traditional chinese medicine lq versus gemcitabine in a mouse model of pancreatic cancer. J Cell Biochem. 2013;114(9):2131–7.

34. Liang YZ, Xie P, Chan K. Quality control of herbal medicines. J Chromatogr B Anal Technol Biomed Life Sci. 2004;812(1–2):53–70.

35. Bent S, Ko R. Commonly used herbal medicines in the united states: a review. Am J Med. 2004;116(7):478.

36. Martins E. The growing use of herbal medicines: issues relating to adverse reactions and challenges in monitoring safety. Front Pharmacol. 2014;4(4):177.

37. Singhuber J, Ming Z, Prinz S, Kopp B. Aconitum in traditional chinese medicine—a valuable drug or an unpredictable risk? J Ethnopharmacol. 2009;126(1):18.

38. Wagner H, Bauer R, Melchart D. New analytical monographs on TCM herbal drugs for quality proof. Forsch Komplementarmed. 2016;23(Suppl 2):16.

39. Wang M, Lamers RJ, Korthout HA, et al. Metabolomics in the context of systems biology: bridging traditional Chinese medicine and molecular pharmacology. Phytother Res. 2005;19(3):173–82.

40. Zhang JW, Chen LB, Jing-Kai GU, Wei-Hong GE, Yang M. Novel theory and methods for chemomic multi-component release/dissolution kinetics of traditional chinese medicine. Chin J Nat Med. 2008;6(1):48–52.

41. Wang Y, Fan X, Qu H, Gao X, Cheng Y. Strategies and techniques for multi-component drug design from medicinal herbs and traditional chinese medicine. Curr Top Med Chem. 2012;12(12):1356.

42. Gong F, Liang YZ, Xie PS, et al. Information theory applied to chromatographic fingerprint of herbal medicine for quality control. J Chromatogr A. 2003;1002(1–2):25–40.

43. Normile D. The new face of traditional chinese medicine. Science. 2003;299(5604):188–90.

44. Jian J, Wu Z. Effects of traditional chinese medicine on nonspecific immunity and disease resistance of large yellow croaker, *Pseudosciaena crocea*, (Richardson). Aquaculture. 2003;218(1–4):1–9.

45. Zhao RH, Hao ZP, Zhang Y, Lian FM, Sun WW, Liu Y, et al. Controlling the recurrence of pelvic endometriosis after a conservative operation: comparison between chinese herbal medicine and Western medicine. Chin J Integr Med. 2013;19(11):820–5.

46. Ministry of Science and Technology. Outline of the International S & T Cooperation Program for Chinese Medicine (2006–2020). Asia Pacific Traditional. Medicine. 2006;8(7):1–9.

47. Franz G. Globalisation of TCM herbal drugs: quality monographs for the European Pharmacopoeia. Planta Med. 2011;77(12):1239.

48. Bauer R. The current status and prospects in the elaboration of monographs for the European Pharmacopoeia. Planta Med. 2014;80(16):WS3.

49. Franz G. Pharmacopoeia monographs for Chinese herbal drugs for quality assurance. Planta Med. 2015;81(16):RAW_02.

50. Wang M, Franz G. The role of the European Pharmacopoeia (Ph EU) in quality control of traditional Chinese herbal medicine in European member states. World J Tradit Chin Med. 2015;1(1):5–15.

51. Jixia Xiong. Opportunities, challenges and countermeasures of China's pharmaceutical industry after China's accession to WTO. J Nanjing Univ Tradit Chin Med. 2001;2(4):1–4.

52. Huo A, Wang Q. Study on transcultural communication of culture of traditional chinese medicine in countries along one belt one road. Serv Oriented Cloud Comput. 2015;9306(3–4):95–109.

53. Tian L, Wei JH, Lan C. Inheritance and innovation of Chinese traditional medicine in the background of "One Belt and One Road". Pop Sci Technol. 2016; 18(04):150–52, 157.

54. Chen Z, Nakamura T. Statistical evidence for the usefulness of chinese medicine in the treatment of sars. Phytother Res. 2004;18(7):592–4.

55. Leung Ping-Chung. The efficacy of chinese medicine for SARS: a review of chinese publications after the crisis. Am J Chin Med. 2007;35(4):575.

56. Dong XH, Dai RW. Traditional chinese medicine in views of system science and system complexity. Acta Simulata Syst Sin. 2002;14(11):1457–8.

57. Ma DY, Zhang FY, Fu XL. Study on the influencing factors and preventive methods of toxic and side effects of Chinese herbal medicine. Clin J Chin Med. 2016;8(12):136–8.

58. Mingde YU. The challenge to China's pharmaceutical enterprises after WTO entry. China Pharm. 2001;12(2):68–70.

59. Wang YJ, Zhang SH. Export of Chinese medicine: difficult to develop. China Cust. 2013;07:60–1.

4

Wentong decoction cures allergic bronchial asthma by regulating the apoptosis imbalance of EOS

Yue Yan[1†], Hai-Peng Bao[2†], Chun-Lei Li[1†], Qi Shi[1], Yan-Hua Kong[1], Ting Yao[1] and You-Lin Li[1*] (iD)

Abstract

Background: Eosinophils (EOS) is one of the most important cells involved in the pathogenesis of chronic airway inflammation in asthma, and its apoptosis is part of the mechanisms of asthma. Therefore, this study aimed to observe the effect of Chinese medicine Wentong decoction (WTD) in EOS apoptosis in asthmatic rats. This work also explored the mechanism of WTD regulation in EOS apoptosis and provided a new target for clinical treatment of asthma.

Methods: Asthmatic rats induced by ovalbumin were treated with WTD. Lung function of rats in each group was detected, and lung tissue pathology, EOS counts in blood and bronchoalveolar lavage fluid were observed. The degree of the EOS apoptosis in rats was detected. The expression content of interleukin (IL)-5, IL-10, chemokine (C–C motif) ligand 5 (CCL5), granulocyte–macrophage colony-stimulating factor (GM-CSF), transforming growth factor beta 1 (TGF-β1), interferon (IFN)-γ, and other cytokines in rat serum and the genes of Eotaxin mRNA, Fas mRNA, FasL mRNA, Fas/FasL and Bcl-2 mRNA in the lung tissues were determined.

Results: WTD can reduced airway resistance in rat models and improved airway compliance. The pathological changes of lung tissue in WTD group were significantly alleviated, at the same time, WTD could reduce the EOS count in the blood and BALF smears of the asthmatic model rats. Compared with the model group, the apoptosis degree of EOS significantly increased in rats in the WTD group. The expression of IL-5, CCL5, and GM-CSF in the serum and the expression of Eotaxin mRNA, Bcl-2 mRNA in the lung tissues in rats in the WTD group rats decreased. Moreover, the expression of IL-10, TGF-β1, and IFN-γ in the serum and the expression of Fas mRNA, FasL mRNA in the lung tissues in rats in the WTD group rats increased compared with that in rats in the model group.

Conclusions: Wentong decoction may accelerate EOS apoptosis, reduce asthma inflammation, and alleviate the disease through regulating and controlling the factors related to the anti-apoptosis and pro-apoptosis.

Keywords: Apoptosis, Eosinophil, Bronchial asthma, Wentong decoction

*Correspondence: lyl19610721@163.com
†Yue Yan, Hai-Peng Bao and Chun-Lei Li are co-first authors
[1] The 2nd Department of Pulmonary Disease in TCM, The Key Unit of SATCM Pneumonopathy Chronic Cough and Dyspnea, Beijing Key Laboratory of Prevention and Treatment of Allergic Diseases With TCM (No. BZ0321), Center of Respiratory Medicine, China-Japan Friendship Hospital, National Clinical Research Center for Respiratory Diseases, Beijing 100029, China
Full list of author information is available at the end of the article

Background

Bronchial asthma (BA) is a chronic inflammatory disease of the airway associated with multiple cells (such as eosinophils, mast cells, T-lymphocytes, neutrophils, and airway epithelial cells) and the cellular elements [1]. This inflammation causes the susceptible person to exhibit high-airway reactivity to each kind of motivating factor causing airway constriction, wherein eosinophil (EOS) infiltration of airway leads to airway inflammation and airway pathology change is an important sign of clinical changes of asthma disease [2, 3]. Asthma is currently incurable, but it can be controlled by appropriate medications, self-management education, and avoidance of exposure to environmental allergens and irritants [4]. Rapid development of global industrialization, environmental pollution, and the change of climate and ecological environments cause rapid increase in global respiratory diseases. Asthma prevalence rate is significantly different in different countries and regions, and the asthma prevalence rate in children is 3.3–29% [5, 6]. The prevalence rate of adult asthma is 1.2–25.5% [7].

Many inflammatory cell infiltrations exist in the bronchial lung tissues of asthmatic patients, and EOS with abnormally long life is the main inflammatory component of allergic reaction in asthmatic patients [8]. BA animal model [9] showed that EOS infiltration is specifically correlated to the increase of airway reactivity and continues to accumulate and activate in the lungs. EOS infiltration also plays an important role in the formation of airway inflammation and the asthma onset [10]. EOS apoptosis plays a key role in the elimination of BA airway inflammation [11], which is associated with the increase of apoptosis, the improvement of BA symptom, and the decrease of inflammation.

Apoptosis, also known as programmed cell death (PCD), is an energy-consuming process, wherein cells obtain a certain signal or undergo some stimulations and an active apoptotic-related gene interacting to produce cells dies out. Simon et al. [12] suggested that EOS may be regulated by both apoptotic and anti-apoptotic signals, and the imbalance of EOS' anti-apoptosis and pro-apoptosis mechanism may be the root cause of the delay of EOS apoptosis. Studies have shown that the expression of cytokines, growth factors, and cell-surface molecules and their ligands is directly related to EOS apoptosis. In addition, various factors can achieve the effect of resisting apoptosis and promoting apoptosis by different mechanisms, thereby constituting a complex regulatory network, which plays an important role in the occurrence, development, and outcome of asthma. Interleukin (IL)-5, granulocyte–macrophage colony-stimulating factor (GM-CSF), Eotaxin, Bcl-2 and chemokine (C–C motif) ligand 5 (CCL5) are the main factors that maintain the EOS survival and inhibit their apoptosis [13–15]. IL-10, transforming growth factor beta 1 (TGF-β1), interferon (IFN)-γ, and Fas antigens, Fas ligand are involved in the regulation of the EOS apoptosis. These cytokines can also promote EOS apoptosis [16–18].

This experiment reveals the biological effects of WTD on EOS apoptosis in asthmatic rat models and determines the molecular mechanism of WTD in EOS apoptosis by detecting IL-5, IL-10, GM-CSF, CCL5, TGF-β, IFN-γ, Eotaxin mRNA, Bcl-2 mRNA, Fas mRNA, FasL mRNA and other related factors.

Methods

The minimum standards of reporting checklist (Additional file 1) contains details of the experimental design, and statistics, and resources used in this study.

Herbal medicine and preparation of Wentong decoction

Twelve herbs, namely, *Astragalus membranaceus, cassia twig, Rhizoma zingiberis, bighead atractylodes rhizome, Fructus Corni, Rhizoma anemarrhenae, Aster tataricus Linn, Aceranthus sagittatus S. et Z., Inula britannica chinensis, Magnolia officinalis, Schisandra chinensis, liquorice,* for Wentong decoction were purchased from Tong Ren Tang (Tong Ren Pharmaceutical Co., Ltd., Beijing, China). Testing shows that the herbal medicines reached the Pharmacopoeia standard (version 2010). The extraction of active constituents from Wentong decoction was performed using water boiling method, and all herbs were made into medicinal extract according to the standard of the School of Chinese Materia Medica, Beijing University of Chinese Medicine.

Animal handling

Healthy male 4-week-old SD rats were purchased from Beijing Huafukang Bio-Tech Co., Ltd., Beijing, China (License No.: SCXK (Beijing) 2009-0007) and provided adaptive feeding, ambient temperature of 24 ± 2 °C, air humidity of 45–65%, separate cages for natural and artificial light, free diet, and drinking water. The experiment was started 1 week later. All experimental procedures were carried out in accordance with internationally recognized guidelines for the use and care of American Laboratory Animals (NIH Publication No. 85–23, revised in 1985).

Rats were randomly divided into four groups (10 per group) as follows: the normal control group (N), asthmatic rat model group (M), dexamethasone-positive control group (D), and Wentong decoction treatment group (W).

Establishment of asthmatic rat model

All rats except the normal control group were provided 0.2 mL 10% ovalbumin (OVA)/Al(OH)$_3$-mixed liquid (OVA, a16951, Alfa Aesar, Ward Hill, MS, USA; Al(OH)$_3$, a4682, Sigma Aldrich, St Louis, MO, USA) at the 1st and 8th days with five-point subcutaneous injection (bipedal, double groin, and peritoneal). At the same time, 0.0023‰ pertussis toxoid (p7208, Sigma-Aldrich) intraperitoneal injection was provided. After the initial sensitization, daily application of 1% OVA saline-atomization inhalation simulated for 1 h was performed using an ultrasonic atomizer (402ai; Yuyue Medical Equipment Co., Ltd., Jiangsu, China), and allergic asthmatic rat model was replicated for 9th–15th days. In the 16th–29th days, the dexamethasone control group and Wentong decoction treatment group were provided 0.5 mg/kg of dexamethasone (Sigma-Aldrich) and 1.34 g/kg of Wentong decoction, respectively, with daily lavage once each day. The normal control group and model group rats were provided equal saline (0.3 mL) for lavage. After 24 h of lavage, the lung tissue, BALF, abdominal aorta blood, and caudal venous blood were collected in rats.

Lung function test

After intraperitoneal injection of 4% pentobarbital sodium anesthesia in rats (2 mL/kg), rats were positioned in supine position in the enclosure, and 2 mm plastic tube was inserted into the trachea. The plastic tube was connected to a AniRes2005 small animal lung function analyzer (Beijing Bellambo High-tech Co., Ltd., Beijing, China). After 5 min, the inspiratory resistance, expiratory resistance, and dynamic compliance of the airway were observed.

Lung histopathology and detection of the EOS apoptosis

For lung histopathology and detection, the right lung middle lobe was used, and 4% of paraformaldehyde solution was added fixed for 24 h and paraffin-embedded at 4 μm thick continuous slices for routine hematoxylin and eosin (H&E) staining. In situ end labeling was performed using terminal deoxynucleotidyl transferase dUTP nick end labeling (TUNEL) alkaline phosphatase to detect the apoptotic cells, following the specific operation in strict accordance with the TUNEL reagent box manual (11684817910, Roche, United States). By combining the same H&E staining slices, one observer randomly selected five high-power fields in each slice to determine the index of EOS apoptosis and calculate its average as the representative value of the slice. The observation and analysis of the slices were performed under a light microscope (Olympus Corp., Tokyo, Japan).

EOS count in blood and BALF smears and flow cytometry technique for the detection of EOS apoptosis in blood

We took 20 μL of the rat tail vein blood, and 0.38 mL of the EOS count liquid was added at static pressure for 30 min. The EOS was counted on the cell count plate, and the procedure was repeated thrice to obtain the mean value.

The BALF was centrifuged (3500 r/min, 15 min), the centrifuged pellets were shaken with 8 mL PBS, and the supernatant was discarded by centrifugation and repeated three times. Take 0.1 mL liquid for smear, H&E staining, 200 cells were counted under a 400-fold light microscope, eosinophils were counted, repeated 3 times, and the average value was taken.

Up to 3 mL abdominal aorta blood was aseptically extracted from rats, and sodium citrate (130 mmol/L, ph 7.4) and 5% fetal bovine serum/Hanks liquid dilution were added for anti-coagulation. In a 15-mL centrifuge tube, we added 1 mL of Percoll liquid with a density of 1.100 and 1.085 g/mL successively. Finally, the diluted blood was added slowly to the cell suspension and horizontally centrifuged at $960 \times g$ for 15 min (20 °C). After centrifuging, we recycled the eosinophilic cell layer of Percoll liquid interfaces with different densities. D-Hanks liquid was used for centrifugal washing at 1500 rpm for 10 min twice. Then, using D-Hanks liquid of 1 mL heavy suspension, we calculated the absolute numbers of EOS under a microscope. We adjusted the cell count to approximately 2×10^6/mL and took 1 mL for flow detection.

Enzyme-linked immunosorbent assay (ELISA)

We took 2 mL of the rat's blood at room temperature, centrifuged at 3000 r/min for 15 min at static pressure for 2 h, and then stored at -80 °C after collecting the supernatant liquid. We performed the procedure in strict accordance with the ELISA Kit manual. We used the double antibody sandwich-ELISA assay test, to determine the IL-5, IL-10, GM-CSF, CCL5, TGF-β, and IFN-γ (Abcam, Cambridge, UK) in the serum.

RNA extraction and real-time polymerase chain reaction (PCR)

We evaluated the effect of Wentong decoction on the expression of Eotaxin mRNA and Fas mRNA in the lung tissues of asthmatic rats by using real-time fluorescent quantitative PCR. We determined the primer sequences using glyceraldehyde 3-phosphate dehydrogenase (GAPDH) and performed primer design (Table 1). We used Trizol total RNA extraction kit (DP405-02, Tiangen Biochemical Technology, Beijing Co., Ltd., Beijing, China) to extract total RNA from the 25 mg lung tissue

Tabel 1 Sense and antisense primer sequences of Eotaxin, Bcl-2, Fas, FasL and GAPDH

Equipment name	Primer sequence (5′–3′)	Product size (bp)
GAPDH upstream primer	CCTTCCGTGTTCCTACCCC	131
GAPDH downstream primer	GCCCAGGATGCCCTTTAGTG	
Eotaxin upstream primer	GCTACAAAAGAATCACCAACAACAG	95
Eotaxin downstream primer	CTTTTTCTTGGGGTCAGCACAG	
Bcl-2 upstream primer	GGGCTACGAGTGGGATACTGGAG	101
Bcl-2 downstream primer	CGGGCGTTCGGTTGCTCT	
Fas upstream primer	ATCAATAATCATGGCTGTGT	116
Fas downstream primer	TATTTGAGTGTATCCCTGCT	
FasL upstream primer	GGTGCTGGTGGCTCTGGTT	142
FasL downstream primer	TGTGCTGGGGTTGGCTATTT	

according to the manufacturer's instructions for inverse transcription of RNA samples to obtain the corresponding cDNA. After pretreatment of the upper machine mixture, we operated the real-time PCR device at 95 °C, 30 s, and 40 PCR loops (collected the fluorescence at 95 °C for 5 s and 60 °C for 40 s). The target and internal control genes of each sample underwent real-time PCR, and the data were analyzed using $2^{-\triangle\triangle CT}$ method.

Data analysis

All data were analyzed using SPSS software (version 17.0, SPSS, Inc., Chicago, IL, USA). The result of each group is shown in mean ± standard deviation. $P < 0.05$ indicates statistically significant difference. Single factor variance

analysis and Newman–Keuls test were used for group analysis. If the data do not conform to normal distribution, the nonparametric Kruskal–Wallis test was used for comparison.

Results
Lung function

Lung function examination plays an important role in evaluating the asthma severity, prognosis, and curative effect of drugs. To evaluate the effect of Wentong decoction in improving lung function in asthmatic rats, we tested the inspiratory resistance, expiratory resistance, and dynamic compliance of the airway in all groups of rats (Fig. 1). The results showed that compared with the normal group, the inspiratory resistance and expiratory resistance of rats in the model group increased significantly. Airway compliance significantly reduced, and the difference was statistically significant ($p < 0.05$). After drug intervention, dexamethasone (DXM) and WTD significantly reduced inspiratory resistance and expiratory resistance in rat models and improved airway compliance ($p < 0.05$). This finding suggested that WTD exhibited positive effect on the improvement of lung function of rats with OVA-sensitized asthma.

Pathology

The pathological changes of lung tissue in rats were evaluated using H&E staining in the paraffin section. In the model group, we can observe the irregular dark red hyperemia in the lung tissue, bronchial and vascular smooth muscle hyperplasia, airway and blood vessels with a large number of red-stained eosinophilic granulocyte and inflammatory cell infiltration taking purple-blue cluster-like lymphocytes as principal cells, lumen stenosis, tube wall thickening, arrangement disorder of

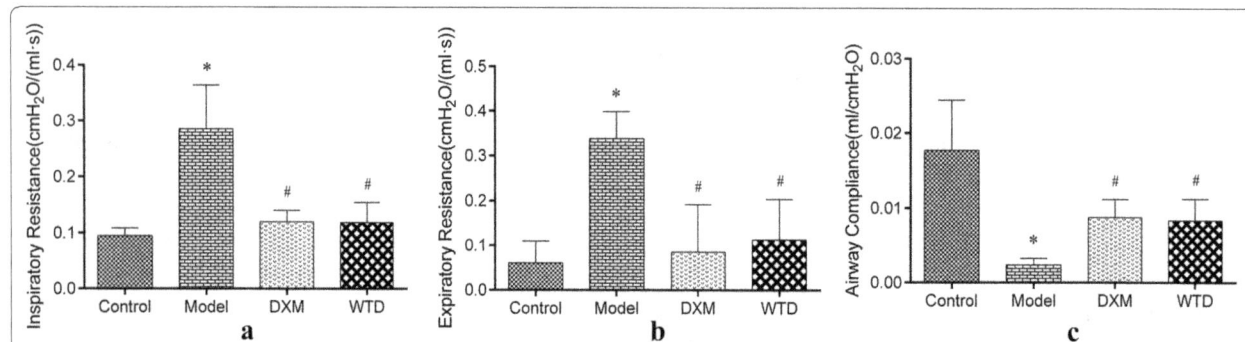

Fig. 1 Changes of lung function in rats in each group. **a** Changes in inspiratory resistance of the airway in rats. Inspiratory resistance of asthmatic rat model was significantly higher than that of the normal control group, and inspiratory resistance decreased after DXM and WTD treatments. **b** Changes in airway expiratory resistance in rats. The expiratory resistance of the asthmatic rat model was significantly higher than that in the normal control group, and the expiratory resistance decreased after DXM and WTD treatments. **c** Changes in the dynamic compliance of the airway in rats. Airway compliance in asthmatic rat model was significantly lower than that in the normal control group, and the expiratory resistance increased after DXM and WTD treatments (*$p < 0.05$, compared with the normal group; #$p < 0.05$, compared with the model group; $n = 8$)

bronchial mucosa epithelial cell, flakiness falling off, obvious goblet cell hyperplasia, and other typical pathological manifestations of BA. After the intervention of DXM and WTD, the pathological changes of the two groups significantly reduced, and the decrease in pathological changes in the DXM group was significant (Fig. 2). The results showed that WTD and DXM showed similar antiasthma effects in pathological changes of allergic asthma rats.

EOS count in blood and BALF

The inflammatory level of asthma was evaluated by calculating the EOS count of rat-tail-vein blood (Fig. 3a). Observation of BALF smears after HE staining (Fig. 4), counting the number of EOS per 200 cells (Fig. 3b). WTD and DXM can significantly reduce the level of EOS in the blood and BALF of OVA-sensitized-asthmatic rats. The results suggested that WTD may be able to reduce the

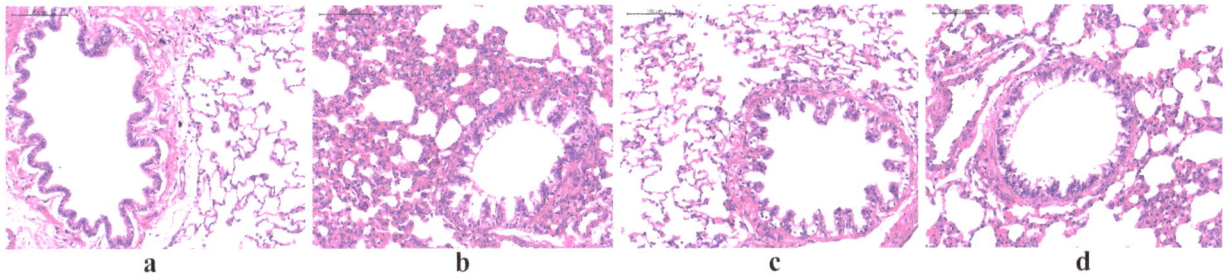

Fig. 2 Pathological changes of lung tissue in rats observed by a light microscope: **a** normal control group; **b** model group; **c** DXM group; **d** WTD group

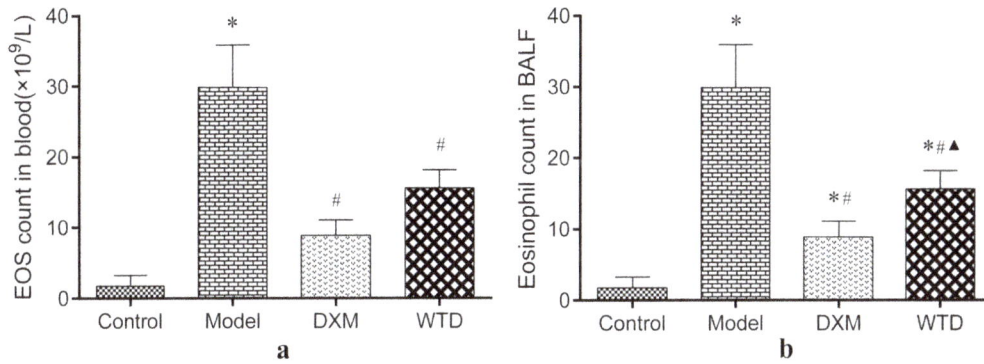

Fig. 3 Analysis results of EOS count showing that WTD can reduce the inflammatory level of asthma. **a** EOS count in blood (1×10^9/L; *$p < 0.05$, compared with the normal control group; #$p < 0.05$, compared with the model group; $n = 8$); **b** EOS count in BALF smears (*$p < 0.05$, compared with the normal control group; #$p < 0.05$, compared with the model group; ▲$p < 0.05$, compared with the DXM group; $n = 8$)

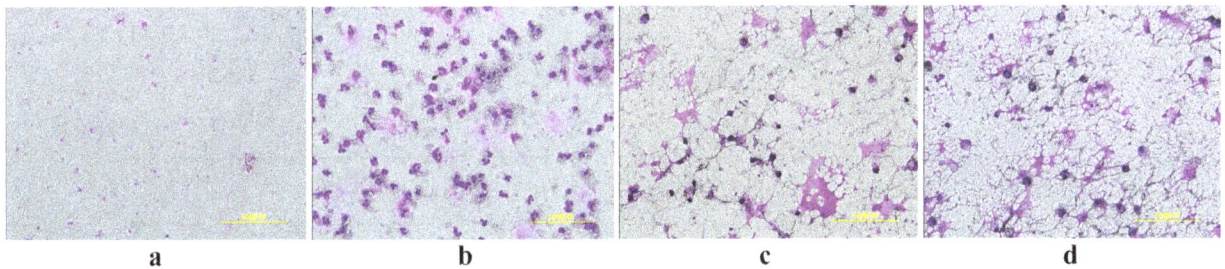

Fig. 4 Observation of EOS in BALF under the microscope. Eosinophils are round and 13–15 μm in diameter. The cytoplasm is filled with coarse, neat, even, and tightly arranged brick red or bright red eosinophilic particles. The nucleus is a characteristic lobular nucleus, usually 2–3 leaves, spectacle-shaped, dark purple. Eosinophils are easily broken and particles can be dispersed around the cells. Under the microscope, the expression of eosinophils from high to low was as follows: **b** asthma model group, **d** WTD group, **c** DXM group and **a** normal control group

inflammatory state of asthmatic rats to achieve the effect of antiasthma.

Detection of EOS apoptosis

To evaluate the EOS apoptosis in asthmatic rats and the effect of WTD on the degree of EOS apoptosis, we adopted flow cytometry and TUNEL method, respectively, to determine the EOS apoptosis in the arterial blood and lung tissues of rats (Figs. 5, 6). The results showed that the degree of EOS apoptosis in arterial blood and lung tissues of rats was obviously consistent. Compared with the normal control group, the percentage of EOS apoptosis in asthmatic rat model decreased significantly, and the difference was statistically significant ($p < 0.05$). Compared with the model group, the

WTD group could significantly increase the percentage of serum EOS in rats, and the difference was statistically significant ($p < 0.05$).

Expression of cytokines in the serum

Several kinds of cytokines will exhibit a certain effect on EOS apoptosis. To further clarify whether the WTD can adjust the apoptosis state of EOS to achieve the purpose of alleviating asthma, we use ELISA method to detect IL-5, IL-10, CSF, CCL5, TGF-β, and IFN-γ in rat serum (Fig. 7). The results show that WTD and DXM can significantly reduce the expression of IL-5, GM-CSF, and CCL5 and significantly enhance the expression of IL-10, TGF-β, and IFN-γ in asthmatic rats.

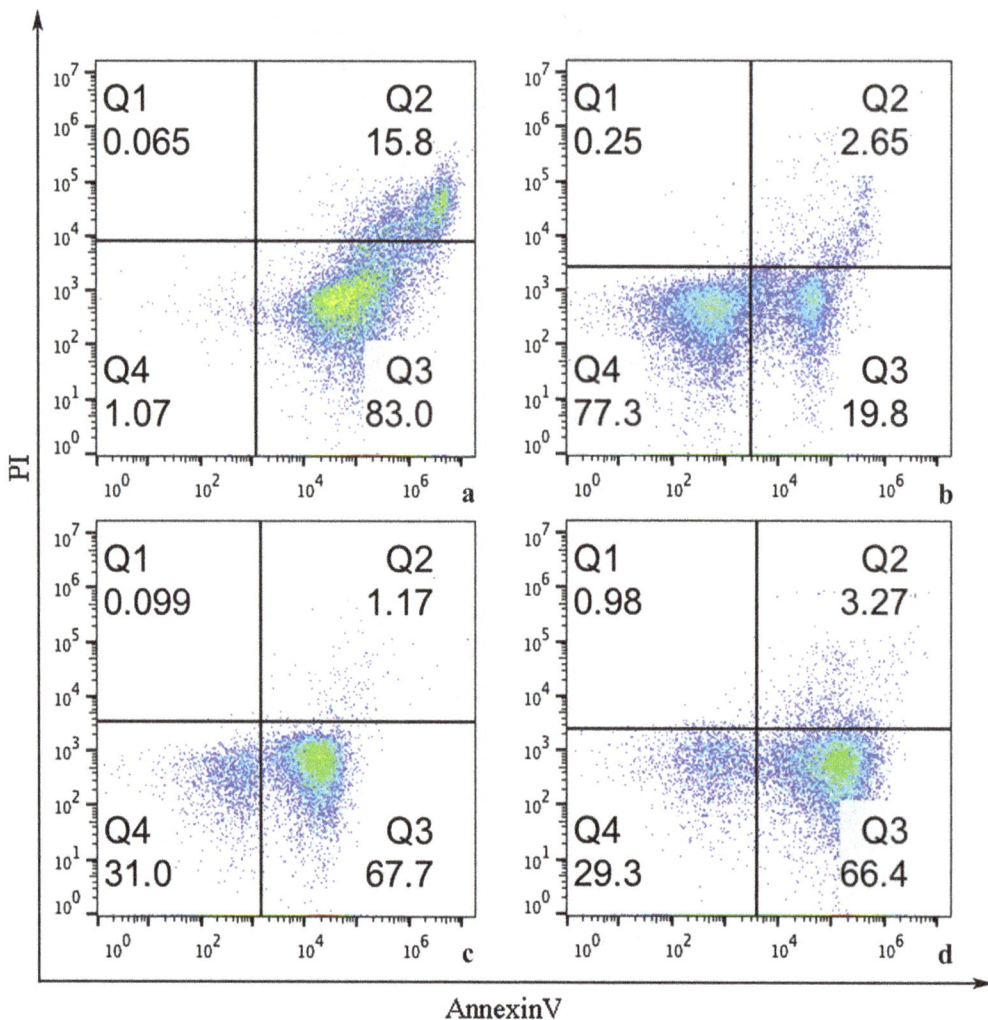

Fig. 5 EOS apoptosis in arterial blood of rats: Q3. Quadrant representing the EOS apoptosis; **a** normal control group; **b** model group; **c** DXM group; **d** WTD group

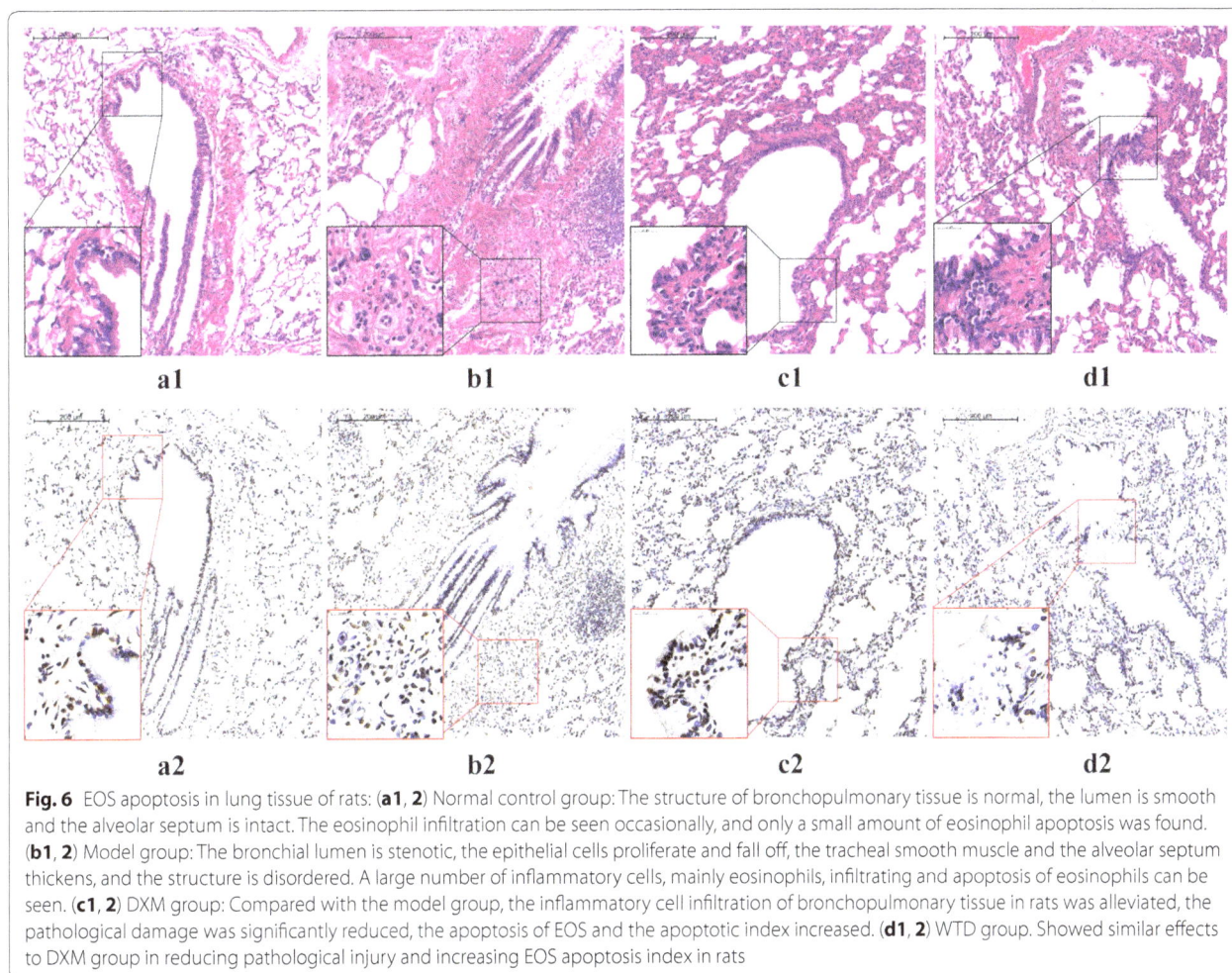

Fig. 6 EOS apoptosis in lung tissue of rats: (**a1**, **2**) Normal control group: The structure of bronchopulmonary tissue is normal, the lumen is smooth and the alveolar septum is intact. The eosinophil infiltration can be seen occasionally, and only a small amount of eosinophil apoptosis was found. (**b1**, **2**) Model group: The bronchial lumen is stenotic, the epithelial cells proliferate and fall off, the tracheal smooth muscle and the alveolar septum thickens, and the structure is disordered. A large number of inflammatory cells, mainly eosinophils, infiltrating and apoptosis of eosinophils can be seen. (**c1**, **2**) DXM group: Compared with the model group, the inflammatory cell infiltration of bronchopulmonary tissue in rats was alleviated, the pathological damage was significantly reduced, the apoptosis of EOS and the apoptotic index increased. (**d1**, **2**) WTD group. Showed similar effects to DXM group in reducing pathological injury and increasing EOS apoptosis index in rats

Expression of Eotaxin, Bcl-2, Fas and FasL mRNA in the lung tissues

Real-time PCR assay was used to detect the gene expression of Eotaxin, Bcl-2, Fas and FasL in lung tissues of rats. Quantitative results show that the expression of Eotaxin and Bcl-2 mRNA in lung tissue of the asthmatic model group significantly increased, whereas the expression of Fas and FasL mRNA decreased (compared with normal control group). Both DXM and WTD can significantly reduce the expression of Eotaxin and Bcl-2 mRNA in lung tissues of model rats and significantly increase Fas and FasL mRNA content in the lung tissues of rats (Fig. 8).

Discussion

In this experiment, we successfully established asthmatic rat model by OVA sensitization, weakened pulmonary-function state in the model group, deteriorated histopathological changes, and aggregated and infiltrated the EOS. These undertakings can prove the success of our asthmatic rat model. After the intervention of WTD

and DXM, the condition of rats improved obviously, indicating that WTD can achieve the asthma-like effect of DXM. In addition, we also found that WTD showed some anti-asthmatic effects in a dose-dependent manner. The WTD middle-dose group had more pronounced anti-asthma effects than the low-dose group, but the high-dose group and middle-dose groups had similar efficacy, Medium dose group is human equivalent group.

EOS infiltration is one of the important inflammatory mechanisms of asthma, and the activation and long-term survival of EOS are concentrated in the bronchial bronchi of allergic asthma [19], which induces a series of symptoms. However, the delay of EOS apoptosis maintained and aggravated the inflammatory state, which increased the difficulty of treatment. After bone marrow maturation, the EOS circulates briefly (~3 days) causing the PCD (apoptosis) in the peripheral blood [8]. Meanwhile, the apoptosis and necrosis are different, apoptosis indicating positive biological significance necessary for maintaining organism stability. The results of this experiment show that WTD can promote the EOS apoptosis in

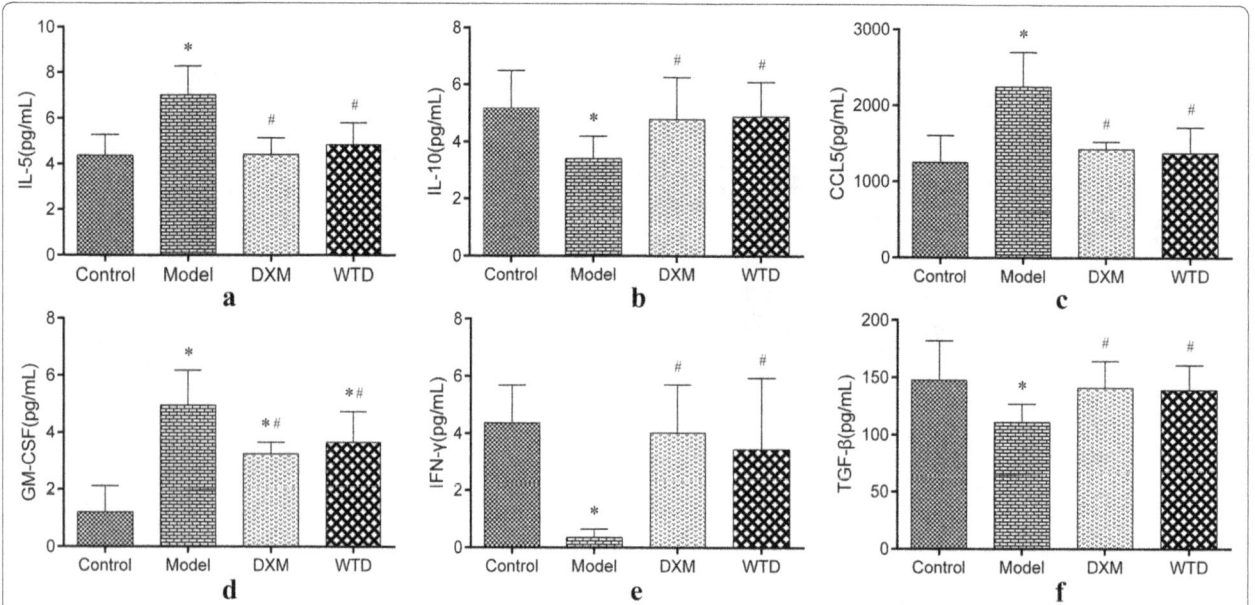

Fig. 7 Changes of cytokines in rat serum: **a**, **c**, and **d** Expression of IL-5, CCL5, and GM-CSF. The expression of IL-5, CCL5, and GM-CSF in asthmatic rat model was significantly higher than that in the normal control group, and the expression of IL-5, CCL5 and GM-CSF after DXM and WTD treatments significantly reduced. **b**, **e**, and **f** Expression of IL-10, IFN-γ, and TGF-β. The expression of IL-10, IFN-γ, and TGF-β in asthmatic rat model was significantly lower than that in the normal control group, and the expression of IL-10 and IFN-γ, and TGF-β significantly increased after DXM and WTD treatments. (*$p < 0.05$, compared with the normal group; #$p < 0.05$, compared with the model group; $n = 8$)

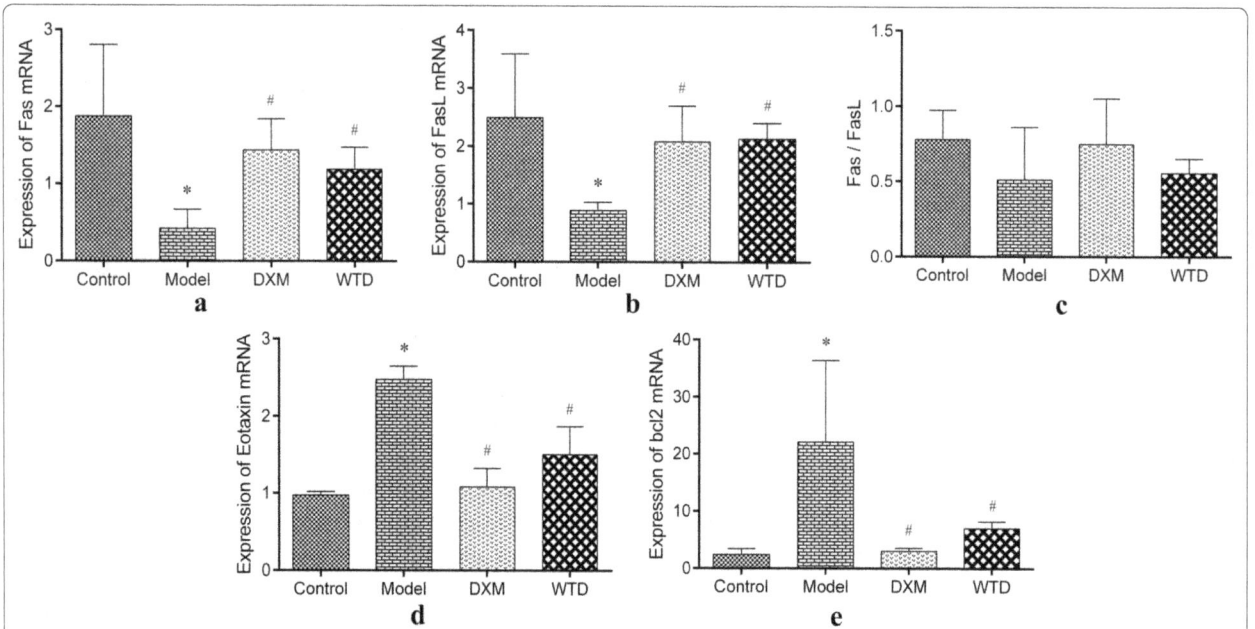

Fig. 8 Gene expression of Eotaxin, Bcl-2, Fas and FasL in lung tissues. **a**, **b** Compared with the normal control group, the expression of Fas and FasL mRNA in lung tissues of the asthmatic model group significantly lower, the Fas and FasL mRNA increased after DXM and WTD treatment; **c** the expression of Fas and FasL was consistent, and the ratio of Fas/FasL showed no significant difference among groups. **d**, **e** Both the expression of Eotaxin and Bcl-2 mRNA in lung tissues of the asthmatic model group was significantly higher than that of the normal group. The Eotaxin and Bcl-2 mRNA decreased after DXM and WTD treatment (*$p < 0.05$, compared with the normal group; #$p < 0.05$, compared with the model group; $n = 4$)

the lung tissue and blood and alleviate the inflammatory state of asthma.

IL-5 is a glycoprotein composed of 115 amino acids and mainly produced by T-helper cells and plays a biological effect through the binding of target cell surface of the specific receptor. IL-5 exhibits the role of promoting the proliferation, activation, and release of inflammatory mediators of EOS. IL-5 is also the most important eosinophil promoter. Suzuki [20] studies have confirmed that IL-5 inhibits EOS apoptosis. The high-affinity receptors on the EOS membrane combine with IL-5 to transmit the anti-apoptotic information into the cells, inhibit the apoptosis, and maintain the cell survival [13, 21].

CCL5 displays chemotaxis to EOS, which can show activation of EOS in vitro and increase EOS to express intercellular adhesion molecules. The study found that the CCL5 level in bronchoalveolar lavage fluid is significantly high in asthmatic patients [22], and the polymorphism of CCL5 gene is a risk factor for asthma by using meta-analysis of Huang et al. [23].

Eotaxin is one of the members of the CCL family. In normal respiratory tract, Eotaxin is mainly produced by epithelial cells. However, the exudation macrophages and EOS after antigen sensitization to some extent are the main sources of Eotaxin. This condition increases the Eotaxin formation [24]. Dexamethasone inhibits the production of Eotaxin mRNA in EOS, and IL-5 can induce Eotaxin expression in EOS [25]. Eotaxin increased synthesis after antigen stimulation, promoting the selective recruitment of EOS in local tissues. Once a large amount of EOS accumulated at the antigen-stimulating site, IL-5, together with other factors, causes the EOS to prolong survival and release a range of protein particles, leading to asthma attacks. Bcl-2 gene is a proto-oncogene that inhibits apoptosis. It not only plays an important role in the molecular regulation of apoptosis, but also has a close relationship with the occurrence and development of asthma. The high expression of Bcl-2 gene inhibits the apoptosis of eosinophils, causing a large number of eosinophils to infiltrate into the peripheral blood, lung tissue, and BALF. Eosinophils release inflammatory mediators and lead to asthma attacks.

GM-CSF is a cytokine closely related to asthma pathogenesis [26]. GM-CSF is mainly produced from T cells and macrophages. In asthma pathogenesis, GM-CSF can induce the growth of T cell precursors, cause EOS chemotaxis and activation, and promote EOS collection in the airway, causing airway-epithelial injury, inflammatory cell infiltration, and high-airway reactivity [27, 28].

In this study, we found that the content of serum IL-5, CCL5, GM-CSF, Eotaxin mRNA and Bcl-2 mRNA in asthmatic rat model was significantly higher than that in normal control group and negatively correlated with EOS apoptosis. WTD and DXM can effectively reduce the expression of the three cytokines in the serum of model rats. The effect of DXM on reducing CCL5 content was better than that of TCM Wentong decoction. However, no significant difference was observed between the two groups in IL-5, GM-CSF, and Eotaxin mRNA ($p > 0.05$).

IL-10 is an immunosuppressive agent with a multidirectional biological activity secreted by Th2 cells. IL-10 exhibits a direct inhibition effect on airway inflammatory cell activation, releases inflammatory factor in asthmatic patients [29, 30], can inhibit the IgE production, promotes IgG4 synthesis, and plays an important role in pathophysiology of allergic asthma [31]. Study found that IL-10 can inhibit the ability of Th2 cells to produce IL-5, and its inhibitory effect is concentration-dependent [32].

TGF-β induces EOS apoptosis and inhibits the IL-5, GM-CSF, and other cytokine-induced EOS to prolong the life cycle [33]. In addition to inhibiting cytokine synthesis and EOS survival, TGF-β also prevented EOS from releasing peroxidase and decreased the expression of EOS cell lines (Eol-1) CD_{23}^+, indicating that TGF-β shows an inhibiting effect on growing EOS, differentiation, function, and all aspects of survival [34]. IFN-γ mainly originates from Th1 cells. In vivo experiments showed that IFN-γ can inhibit the infiltration of eosinophilic cells caused by allergens in the lungs [35], and inhibit the synthesis of Th2 cytokine IL-5, and its mechanism may be that IFN-γ inhibits the EOS collection by blocking the IL-5 synthesis by inhibiting GATA3 expression [36].

Fas gene is encoded as one of the members of the TNF receptor family, and its activation can induce apoptosis. Study found that interferon combined with tumor necrosis factor promoted the Fas expression on the surface of EOS and enhanced the FasL-mediated EOS apoptosis in vitro [37]. The expression of Fas receptor and FasL is relatively high in the cells of the immune system, which mediates apoptosis/proliferation plays an important role in asthma T cells with dysregulation of apoptosis/proliferation, Th1/Th2 imbalance, airway inflammation, airway hyperresponsiveness (AHR) and airway remodeling.

In this study, we found that the content of IL-10, TGF-β1, IFN-γ in the serum, Fas and FasL mRNA in the lung tissues of asthmatic rat model was significantly lower than that of the normal control group, which was positively correlated with the EOS apoptosis. Both WTD and DXM can effectively improve the expression of IL-10, TGF-β1, IFN-γ in the serum, and Fas mRNA in the lung tissues of model rats. This condition inhibits the EOS infiltration and promotes the EOS apoptosis to reduce the inflammatory response of asthma and achieve the goal of treating the disease.

In the complex internal environment, the local EOS apoptosis is not determined by a single factor but is controlled by the complex network system consisting of many cytokines, cell surface molecules, ligands, and chemokines. Maintaining homeostasis between pro-apoptotic factors and anti-apoptotic factors is the key to determine the EOS apoptosis.

Conclusions
Wentong decoction may promote the EOS apoptosis and reduce airway inflammation by increasing the expression of pro-apoptotic factors of IL-10, TGF-β1, IFN-γ, Fas mRNA and FasL mRNA and decreasing the anti-apoptotic factors of IL-5, GM-CSF, CCL5, Eotaxin mRNA and Bcl-2 mRNA. Thus, asthma prevention is achieved.

Abbreviations
TCM: traditional Chinese medicine; EOS: eosinophil; WTD: Wentong decoction; IL: interleukin; CCL5: chemokine (C–C motif) ligand 5; TGF-β1: transforming growth factor beta 1; GM-CSF: granulocyte–macrophage colony-stimulating factor; IFN-γ: interferon-γ; BA: bronchial asthma; PCD: programmed cell death; DXM: dexamethasone.

Authors' contributions
YY and YLL conceived and designed the research; CLL and TY performed the experiments; YHK and QS analyzed the data; HPB and YY wrote the first draft of the manuscript and other authors participated in revision. All authors read and approved the final manuscript.

Author details
[1] The 2nd Department of Pulmonary Disease in TCM, The Key Unit of SATCM Pneumonopathy Chronic Cough and Dyspnea, Beijing Key Laboratory of Prevention and Treatment of Allergic Diseases With TCM (No. BZ0321), Center of Respiratory Medicine, China-Japan Friendship Hospital, National Clinical Research Center for Respiratory Diseases, Beijing 100029, China. [2] Beijing University of Chinese Medicine, Beijing 100029, China.

Acknowledgements
Not applicable.

Competing interests
The authors declare that they have no competing interest.

Consent for publication
The manuscript is approved by all authors for publication.

Funding
This study was supported by the National Natural Science Foundation of China (No. 81173245); NSFC Youth Foundation (No. 81302943); Class A Promotion Project of Young Scientific Talents in 2015 (No. 2015-QNYC-A-07); Beijing Ten Disease of Ten Drugs (No. Z151100003815025).

References
1. Ray A, Kolls JK. Neutrophilic inflammation in asthma and association with disease severity. Trends Immunol. 2017. https://doi.org/10.1016/j.it.2017.07.003.
2. Kay AB. The role of eosinophils in the pathogenesis of asthma. Trends Mol Med. 2005;11(4):148.
3. Kulkarani NS, Hollins F, Sutcliffe A, et al. Eosinophil protein in airway macrophages: a novel biomarker of eosinophilic inflammation in patients with asthma. J Allergy Clin Immun. 2010;126(1):61.
4. Kliegman RM, Behrman RE, Jenson HB, Stanton BF. Nelson textbook of pediatrics. 18th ed. Philadelphia: Saunders Elsevier; 2007.
5. Akinbami LJ, Moorman JE, Garbe PL, et al. Status of childhood asthma in the Untied States. 1980–2007. Pediatrics. 2009;123(Suppl 3):S131–45.
6. Bai J, Zhao J, Shen KL, Xiang L, Chen AH, Huang S, Huang Y, Shu C, Wang JS, Rong-Wei YE. Prevalence of childhood asthma in Beijing, Chongqing, and Guangzhou. Chin J Allergy Clin Immunol. 2010;4:010.
7. Al Ghobain MO, Al-Hajjai MS, Al Moamary MS. Asthma prevalence among 16–18 year old adolescents in Saudi Arabia using the ISAAC questionnaire. BMC Public Health. 2012;12:239.
8. Oh J, Malter JS. Pin1-FADD interactions regulate Fas-mediated apoptosis in activated eosinophils. J Immunol. 2013;190(10):4937–45.
9. Blain JF, Sirois P. Involvement of LTD(4) in allergic pulmonary inflammation in mice: modulation by cysLT(1)antagonist MK-571. Prostaglandins Leukot Essent Fatty Acids. 2000;62(6):361–8.
10. Zietkowski Z, Tomasiak-Lozowska MM, Skiepko R, et al. Eotaxin-1 in exhaled breath condensate of stable and unstable asthma patients. Respir Res. 2010;11:110.
11. Kankaanranta H, Lindsay MA, Giembycz MA, Zhang X, Moilanen E, Barnes PJ. Delayed eosinophil apoptosis in asthma. J Allergy Clin Immunol. 2000;106(1 Pt 1):77–83.
12. Simon HU, Blaser K. Inhibition of programmed eosinophil death: a key pathogenic event for eosinophilia? Immunol Today. 1995;16(2):53–5.
13. Tai PC, Sun L, Spry CJ. Effects of IL-5, granulocyte/macrophage colony-stimulating factor (GM-CSF) and IL-3 on the survival of human blood eosinophils in vitro. Clin Exp Immunol. 1991;85(2):312–6.
14. Ganzalo JA, Jia GQ, Aguirre V, Friend D, Coyle AJ, Jenkins NA, Lin GS, Katz H, Lichtman A, Copeland N, et al. Mouse Eotaxin expression parallels eosinophil accumulation during lung allergic inflammation but it is not restricted to a Th2-type response. Immunity. 1996;4(1):1–14.
15. Lintomen L, Franchi G, Nowill A, Condino-Neto A, de Nucci G, Zanesco A, Antunes E. Human eosinophil adhesion and degranulation stimulated with Eotaxin and RANTES in vitro: lack of interaction with nitric oxide. BMC Pulm Med. 2008;8:13.
16. Beauvais F, Michel L, Dubertret L. The nitric oxide donors, azide and hydroxylamine, inhibit the programmed cell death of cytokine-deprived human eosinophils. FEBS Lett. 1995;361(2–3):229–32.
17. Aggarwal S, Gupta S. Increased apoptosis of T cell subsets in aging humans: altered expression of Fas (CD95), Fas ligand, Bcl-2, and Bax. J Immunol. 1998;160(4):1627–37.
18. Liu C, Wang Z, Feng Y, Lei S. A kinetic study on the relationship between of IL-5, IL-10 and eosinophil apoptosis in asthmatic airway inflammation. J West China Univ Med Sci. 2001;32(1):55–8.
19. Maret M, Ruffie C, Letuve S, Phelep A, Thibaudeau O, Marchal J, Pretolani M, Druilhe A. A role for bid in eosinophil apoptosis and in allergic airway reaction. J Immunol. 2009;182(9):5740–7.
20. Suzuki S, Okubo M, Kaise S, Ohara M, Kasukawa R. Gold sodium thiomalate selectivity inhibits interleukin-5-mediated eosinophil survival. J Allergy Clin Immunol. 1995;96(2):251–6.
21. Yousefi S, Hoessli DC, Blaser K, Mills GB, Simon HU. Requirement of Lyn and Syk tyrosine kinases for the prevention of apoptosis by cytokines in human eosinophils. J Exp Med. 1996;183(4):1407–14.

22. Alam R, York J, Boyars M, Stafford S, Grant JA, Lee J, Forsythe P, Sim T, Ida N. Increased MCP-1, RANTES, and MIP-1α in bronchoalveolar lavage fluid of allergic asthmatic patients. Am J Respir Crit Care Med. 1996;153(4 Pt 1):1398–404.

23. Huang H, Nie W, Zang Y, Chen J, Xiu Q. Association between CC motif chemokine ligand 5 (CCL5) polymorphisms and asthma risk: an updated meta-analysis. J Investig Allergol Clin Immunol. 2015;25(1):26–33.

24. Kampen GT, Stafford S, Adachi T, Jinquan T, Quan S, Grant JA, Skov PS, Poulsen LK, Alam R. Eotaxin induces degranulation and chemotaxis of eosinophils through the activation of ERK2 and p38 mitogen-activated protein kinases. Blood. 2000;95(6):1911–7.

25. Han SJ, Kim JH, Noh YJ, Chang HS, Kim CS, Kim KS, Ki SY, Park CS, Chung IY. Interleukin (IL)-5 downregulates tumor necrosis factor (TNF)-induced Eotaxin messenger RNA (mRNA) expression in eosinophils. Induction of Eotaxin mRNA by TNF and IL-5 in eosinophils. Am J Respir Cell Mol Biol. 1999;21(3):303–10.

26. Esnault S, Malter JS. Granulocyte macrophage-colony-stimulating factor mRNA is stabilized in airway eosinophils and peripheral blood eosinophils activated by TNF-alpha plus fibronectin. J Immunol. 2001;166(7):4658–63.

27. Weller PF, Lim K, Wan HC, Dvorak AM, Wong DT, Cruikshank WW, Kornfeld H, Center DM. Role of the eosinophil in allergic reactions. Eur Respir J Suppl. 1996;22:109s–15s.

28. Corrigan CJ, Hamid Q, North J, Barkans J, Moqbel R, Durham S, Gemou-Engesaeth V, Kay AB. Peripheral blood CD4 but not CD8 t-lymphocytes in patients with exacerbation of asthma transcribe and translate messenger RNA encoding cytokines which prolong eosinophil survival in the context of a Th2-type pattern: effect of glucocorticoid therapy. Am J Respir Cell Mol Biol. 1995;12(5):567–78.

29. Moniuszko M, Grubczak K, Kowal K, Eljaszewicz A, Rusak M, Jeznach M, Jablonska E, Dabrowska M, Bodzenta-Lukaszyk A. Development of asthmatic response upon bronchial allergen challenge is associated with dynamic changes of interleukin-10-producing and interleukin-10-responding CD4 + T cells. Inflammation. 2014;37(6):1945–56.

30. Palomares O, Martin-Fontecha M, Lauener R, Traidl-Hoffmann C, Cavkaytar O, Akdis M, Akdis CA. Regulatory T cells and immune regulation of allergic diseases: roles of IL-10 and TGF-β. Genes Immun. 2014;15(8):511–20.

31. Takeuchi M, Sato Y, Ohno K, Tanaka S, Takata K, Gion Y, Orita Y, Ito T, Tachibana T, Yoshino T. T helper 2 and regulatory T-cell cytokine production by mast cells: a key factor in the pathogenesis of IgG4-related disease. Mod Pathol. 2014;27(8):1126–36.

32. Codolo G, Mazzi P, Amedei A, Del Prete G, Berton G, D'Elios MM, de Bernard M. The neutrophil-activating protein of Helicobacter pylori down-modulates Th2 inflammation in ovalbumin-induced allergic asthma. Cell Microbiol. 2008;10(11):2355–63.

33. Komai M, Tanaka H, Nagao K, Ishizaki M, Kajiwara D, Miura T, Ohashi H, Haba T, Kawakami K, Sawa E, et al. A novel CC-chemokine receptor 3 antagonist, Ki19003, inhibits airway eosinophilia and subepithelial/peribronchial fibrosis induced by repeated antigen challenge in mice. J Pharmacol Sci. 2010;112(2):203–13.

34. Alam R, Forsythe P, Stafford S, Fukuda Y. Transforming growth factor beta abrogates the effects of hematopoietins on eosinophils and induces their apoptosis. J Exp Med. 1994;179(3):1041–5.

35. Iwamoto I, Nakajima H, Endo H, Yoshida S. Interferon gamma regulates antigen-induced eosinophil recruitment into the mouse airways by inhibiting the infiltration of CD4+ T cells. J Exp Med. 1993;177(2):573–6.

36. Li Q, Zhang YD, Sun CW, Chen YL, Du YH, Zhao GJ, Zhang DL. Treatment of allergic rhinitis rats by intranasal interferon gamma. Chin J Otorhinolaryngol Head Neck Surg. 2008;43(2):134–8.

37. Luttmann W, Dauer E, Schmidt S, Marx O, Hossfeld M, Matthys H, Virchow JC Jr. Effects of interferon-gamma and tumour necrosis factor-alpha on CD95/Fas ligand-mediated apoptosis in human blood eosinophils. Scand J Immunol. 2000;51(1):54–9.

5

The therapeutic effect of scalp acupuncture on natal autism and regressive autism

Chuen Heung Yau*, Cheuk Long Ip and Yuk Yin Chau

Abstract

Background: Autism spectrum disorders (ASD) is a common disease and the incidence has been rising constantly. Acupuncture is one of the most widely used complementary and alternative medicine therapies. Despite studies had been done on the effectiveness of acupuncture on ASD children, how factors such as chronological age and the onset pattern influence the effectiveness of the therapy remains unclear. The aim of this retrospective study is to know how symptomatology of ASD alters upon the introduction of scalp acupuncture and how do age and onset type affect the effectiveness of the therapy.

Methods: ASD children aged 2–11 years old were invited to join the study. In the course of the investigation, they received a total of 30 sessions of scalp acupuncture therapy. They were then evaluated to compare the performance on various aspects before and after the treatment. The influence on the therapeutic effect by factors including chorological age and onset pattern were further taken into consideration and analyzed. In addition, investigation on the relationship between allergies and onset pattern of ASD was performed by statistically analyzing the received epidemiologic data from the participants.

Results: 68 children with ASD participated in the study. It is found that the significant effective rate of scalp acupuncture on ASD is 97%. Scalp acupuncture can improve verbal communication problems the most while noise sensitivity improves the least. The therapeutic effectiveness decreases with increasing age and children with natal autism benefit more from acupuncture than those with regressive autism. In the latter part of the study, we observe a positive correlation between the family history of allergy and onset pattern.

Conclusion: Scalp acupuncture is an effective treatment for alleviating the symptomatology of ASD. The therapeutic effectiveness is expected to be higher for those patients with natal or early onset of the disorder, and at a younger age when they receive the therapy. The study result helps to formulate an ideal regimen for ASD patients and allow therapists and parents to make appropriate expectation towards the therapeutic outcome of acupuncture. Early intervention of scalp acupuncture therapy recommended. The relationship between the family history of allergic disorder and the onset type of ASD hints that the etiologies of natal and regressive ASD are discrete. It shows a great significance in differentiating the onset pattern in carrying out clinical assessments or researches on ASD patients.

Keywords: Natal autism, Regressive autism, Scalp acupuncture

*Correspondence: annyau@hkbu.edu.hk
School of Chinese Medicine, Hong Kong Baptist University, Kowloon Tong, Hong Kong

Background

According to World Health Organization, it was estimated that 1 in 160 children is suffering from autism spectrum disorders (ASD) worldwide and the prevalence has been rising over the past 50 years [1]. The diagnosis of ASD emphasizes few essential features, includes reciprocal social interaction, communication, and restricted and repetitive behaviors [2, 3]. In terms of onset pattern, two types of autism can be observed clinically. Children showing abnormal social development and speech delay around 1 year-old are identified as early-onset or natal autism [4]; while some children might develop normally in the first few years but lose the previously acquired skills upon the onset of autism, are known as regressive or acquired autism [5].

Since there is no definitive cure for ASD, numerous treatment methods claim to be beneficial to autistic children. Complementary and alternative medicine (CAM) treatments have been commonly used in treating ASD. Study reported that 74% of the children diagnosed with autism use one or more than one type of CAM treatments as they perceive CAM interventions to be safe and natural [6]. Among all the CAM available, scalp acupuncture has been widely used for treating ASD. In common practice of acupuncture, needles are inserted into specific points (acupoints) on the body of the patients. For scalp acupuncture, acupoints along different scalp lines or zones are selected.

Controlled trials on the effect of scalp acupuncture and electro-acupuncture on ASD patients have showed significant improvement in language comprehension and self-care ability [7, 8]. Despite the advantages of acupuncture therapy on ASD children was demonstrated in previous studies, no investigations has currently been made on how age and onset type of ASD influence the therapeutic effect of acupuncture treatment.

Study design

A pragmatic study was conducted in a typical community based outpatient setting, from May 2010 to June 2013 at Hong Kong Baptist University Mr. & Mrs. Chan Hon Yin Chinese Medicine Specialty Clinic and Good Clinical Practice Centre. Institutional review and approval was secured by the Committee on the Use of Human and Animal Subjects in Teaching and Research, Hong Kong Baptist University (Approval number: HASC/Student/17-18/0115). The Minimum Standards of Reporting Checklist contains details of the experimental design, and statistics, and resources used in this study (Additional file 1).

Subjects and methods

Participants

ASD patients who consulted for acupuncture treatment at Hong Kong Baptist University Mr. & Mrs. Chan Hon Yin Chinese Medicine Specialty Clinic and Good Clinical Practice Centre were invited to join the study. Eligibility criteria included children of both gender, aged 2–11 years old, with a current medical diagnosis of ASD by a recognized specialist such as pediatrician, psychiatrist or psychologist. No cut-off exclusion criteria concerning the severity of the ASD symptoms were set.

Therapist and treatment

Both assessment and acupuncture treatments were carried out by principal investigator (Yau Chuen Heung), who is an experienced traditional Chinese medicine practitioner specialized in acupuncture for ASD children for 18 years.

A standardized scalp acupuncture therapy was applied to all participants. Fourteen acupoints were selected based on traditional Chinese medicine theory or functional areas of the brain; including BaiHui (GV20), SiShenChong (EX-NH3), mid line of forehead, lateral line 2 of forehead, posterior lateral line of vertex, primary auditory cortex, and auditory speech area.

Participants were held and positioned properly by their parents. Their scalps were disinfected with 75% alcohol cotton ball, followed by subcutaneous insertions of 0.20×25 mm needles obliquely onto the acupoints, into the depth of 10 mm between aponeurosis layer and loose areolar connective tissue layer. Needles were twirled every 15 min for three times with "neutral supplementation and draining method" before all the needles were removed after an hour. Scalp acupuncture treatments were performed twice a week and the whole course consisted of 30 sessions of treatment.

Measurement of outcome

Participants were assessed by a clinician-rated inventory on ASD-related symptoms. In light of Blatt-Kupperman index, we designed a set of rating scale for quantifying symptoms of ASD [9]. By means of a semi-structured interview with the participants and their parents, therapist would be able to score a total mark of 20, based on 5 subscale domain items rated on a 5 point scale (Table 1) that reflects the frequency and intensity of the ASD-related symptoms in aspects of social problem, verbal communication problem, behavioral problems, food selectivity and noise sensitivity.

The measurement of the score was administered at the 1st and 30th session of acupuncture treatment.

Table 1 Marking criteria for score

Score	Marking criteria
0	No symptoms
1	Minimal symptoms, seldom shown
2	Mild symptoms, often shown
3	Moderate symptoms, usually shown
4	Severe symptoms, always shown

Table 2 Overall therapeutic effect evaluated by effective rate

Effective rate	Significance
> 20%	Highly effective
5–20%	Effective
< 5%	Ineffective

Participants' past medical history and demographic information was also recorded. Materials concerning the onset of ASD, familial and personal history of allergic diseases were also collected and manipulated. Participants who lose the previously acquired language skills were categorized into regression group, otherwise will be included into the natal group.

Therapeutic effect of acupuncture on ASD patient is evaluated by the effective rate by the following equation:

$$\text{Effective rate} = \frac{(\text{Total score 1st acupuncture} - \text{Total score 30th acupuncture})}{\text{Total score 1st acupuncture}} \times 100\%$$

The overall therapeutic effectiveness is then concluded by categorizing patients into groups of highly effective, effective and ineffective by comparing their effective rate (Table 2).

An average improvement of one level across all domains would show the score decrease by 20% or above, which we consider to be a remarkable improvement and states the high effectiveness of the treatment. An improvement of 5% of less represents it has no improvement or only been beneficial in sole domain by a level; therefore considered to be an ineffective treatment.

Statistical analysis

Data analyses were conducted on all treatment responders. An alpha level of 0.05 was used for all statistical tests. The mean score and standard deviation at the 1st and 30th treatment section were analyzed using paired t test. The effect of acupuncture on natal and regressive ASD patients of different ages was evaluated by means of

independent t-test and analyses of variance (ANOVAs). Pearson Chi square tests were used to show the correlation among the type of onset of ASD, personal history of allergic disorder and family history of allergy. All the calculations were performed on software IBM SPSS Statistics (Windows, version 21).

Results

Participant characteristics

Among 68 patients with autism spectrum disorders, there were 11 female and 57 male. Ages ranged from 2 to 10 years old. The oldest child was 10 years and 7 months old while the youngest one was 2 years and 1 month old. 47 (69%) natal autism cases and 21 (31%) regressive autism cases were included.

Comparison of clinical manifestation before the 1st and after the 30th acupuncture treatment on both natal and regressive autism

In the first section, we tried to investigate the effect of acupuncture on ASD patients, and the results are shown in Table 3 and Fig. 1. Before acupuncture, item of verbal communication problems scored the highest mark with the mean score of 3.06, followed by social problems and behavioral problems scoring 2.50 and 2.34, respectively. While food selectivity and noise sensitivity scored the least marks of 1.85 and 1.71, respectively.

The scores of five symptoms decreased after the thir- tieth acupuncture, and the improvement is significant ($p < 0.05$). Among all domains, improvement made on social problems (-35.9%) and verbal communication problems (-34.6%) have been most prominent. Other items such as behavioral problems (-26.4%), food selectivity (-19.8%) and noise sensitivity (-12.9%) showed relatively less effective towards acupuncture treatment.

Comparison of the change in clinical manifestation after acupuncture between natal and regressive autism of different age

Verbal communication problems

Table 4 shows the data about the communication performance in natal and regressive ASD children of different age. It was found that p-value comparing the score of pretreatment and post-treatment in all ages of natal group was smaller than 0.05; whereas for regressive autism, age groups other than five or above showed a p-value greater than 0.05. Results indicates a general significant

Table 3 Comparison of clinical manifestation before the 1st and after the 30th acupuncture treatment in natal and regressive autism of different age

Items	Pre-treatment		Post-treatment		Percentage change (-%)	P-value
	Mean	SD	Mean	SD		
All	11.46	2.37	8.29	2.03	27.60	0.000
Verbal communication problems	3.06	1.01	2.00	0.90	34.62	0.000
Social problems	2.50	0.78	1.60	0.69	35.88	0.000
Social problems	2.34	1.07	1.72	0.77	26.42	0.000
Social problems	1.85	0.70	1.49	0.63	19.84	0.000
Noise sensitivity	1.71	0.88	1.49	0.76	12.93	0.003

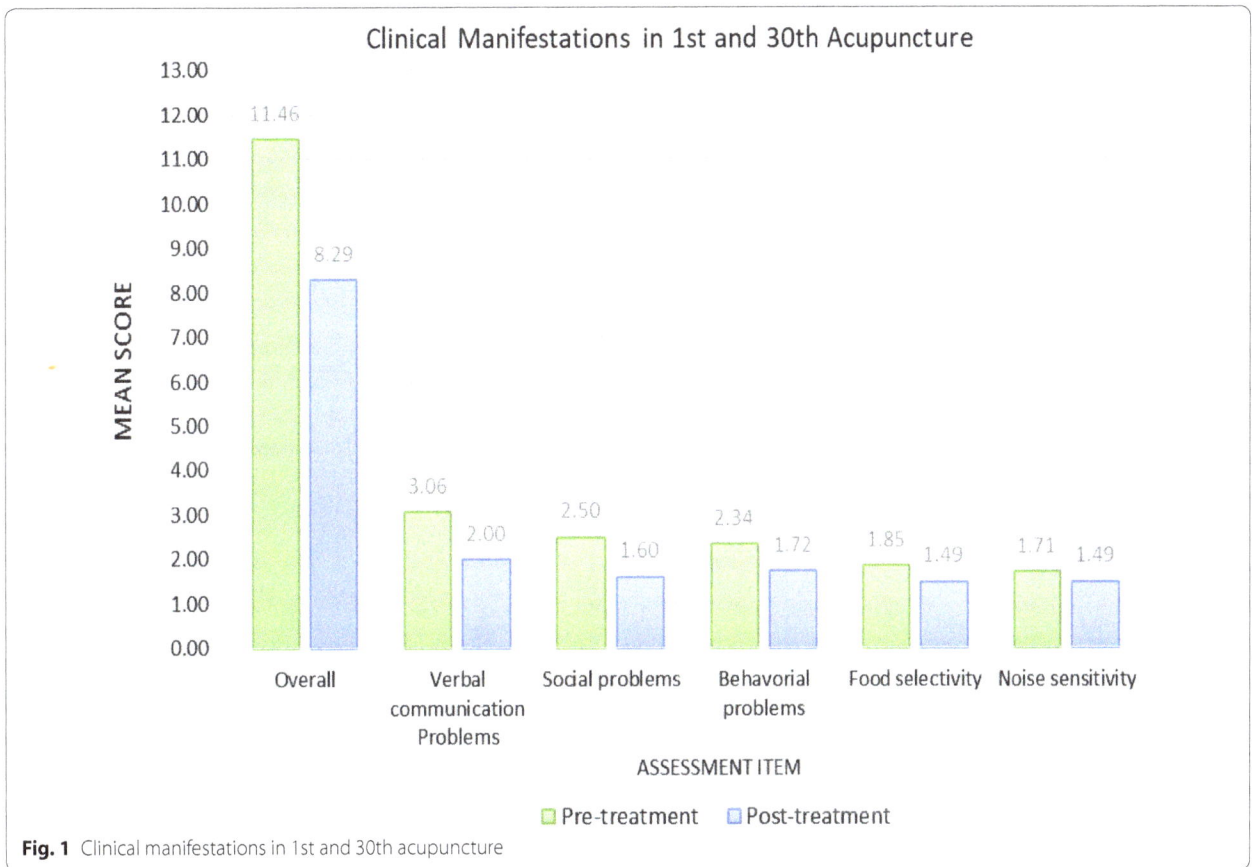

Fig. 1 Clinical manifestations in 1st and 30th acupuncture

improvement in verbal communication problems for both onset types across all age groups after acupuncture therapy.

More specifically, natal onset ASD children with age of 2 to 3 improved the most and their mean scores were reduced by 1.2–1.0, while the score of 4 years old children decreased by 0.94. The children above 5 years old improved the least and their score decrease 0.5 only. In regressive group, both scores of children of 2 years old and 3 years old reduced by 1.25 and 1.38, respectively while that of children of 4 years old decreased by 0.8. The score of children with age above five reduced a mark of 1.25. Concerning the problems in verbal communication in both natal and regression ASD, we observed a better improvement in children of younger age to receive acupuncture treatment.

Social problems
Table 5 shows the improvement in social problems in natal and regressive ASD children of different age. In natal onset group, p-value of all age groups are less than 0.05. In group of regressive autism, only the p-value of age above five is greater than 0.05, while the remaining groups obtained the value smaller than 0.05. Patients performed significantly better in social interaction after acupuncture treatment.

The score of natal ASD children with age of 2 and 3 decreased by 1.38 and 1.15, respectively while the score of 4 year-old children fell by 0.77. With the least decrease,

the score of "above 5 year-old" group reduced by 0.50. The pattern of improvement across different age groups in regressive autism group is similar to that of natal group. The improvement in score of children with age of 2 and 3 are 1.00 and 0.87, respectively. The score of children with age of 4 fell by 0.80. The score of children with age of 5 or above reduced the least of 0.50 marks.

Behavioral problems
Table 6 shows how behavior problems changed in natal and regressive ASD patients of different age. In group of natal autism, p-value for the 5 year-old group is larger

Table 4 Comparison of verbal communication problems before the 1st and after the 30th acupuncture treatment in natal and regressive autism of different age

Age (year)	Natal						Regressive					
	Pre-treatment			Post-treatment			Pre-treatment			Post-treatment		
	n	Mean	SD	Mean	SD	p-value	n	Mean	SD	Mean	SD	p-value
All	47	2.87	0.99	1.87	0.80	0.000	21	3.48	0.93	2.29	1.06	0.000
2	8	3.25	1.16	2.25	0.89	0.001	4	4.00	0.00	2.75	0.50	0.015
3	14	2.93	0.83	1.57	0.76	0.000	8	3.63	0.74	2.25	1.04	0.008
4	17	2.82	1.01	1.88	0.78	0.000	5	3.00	1.00	2.20	0.84	0.016
5	8	2.50	1.07	2.00	0.76	0.033	4	3.25	1.50	2.00	1.83	0.141

Table 5 Comparison of social problems before the 1st and after the 30th acupuncture treatment in natal and regressive autism of different age

Age (year)	Natal						Regressive					
	Pre-treatment			Post-treatment			Pre-treatment			Post-treatment		
	n	Mean	SD	Mean	SD	p-value	n	Mean	SD	Mean	SD	p-value
All	47	2.47	0.83	1.53	0.72	0.000	21	2.57	0.68	1.76	0.62	0.000
2	8	2.63	0.52	1.25	0.46	0.001	4	3.00	0.00	2.00	0.00	0.015
3	14	2.36	1.01	1.21	0.43	0.000	8	2.75	0.46	1.88	0.64	0.000
4	17	2.59	0.80	1.82	0.88	0.003	5	1.80	0.45	1.00	0.00	0.016
5	8	2.25	0.89	1.75	0.71	0.033	4	2.75	0.96	2.25	0.50	0.182

Table 6 Comparison of behavioral problems before the 1st and after the 30th acupuncture treatment in natal and regressive autism of different age

Age (year)	Natal						Regressive					
	Pre-treatment			Post-treatment			Pre-treatment			Post-treatment		
	n	Mean	SD	Mean	SD	p-value	n	Mean	SD	Mean	SD	p-value
All	47	2.38	1.09	1.72	0.77	0.000	21	2.24	1.04	1.71	0.78	0.004
2	8	2.88	1.13	1.88	0.64	0.007	4	2.00	0.82	1.25	0.50	0.058
3	14	1.86	0.95	1.50	0.65	0.014	8	2.50	1.20	2.13	0.99	0.197
4	17	2.59	1.00	1.82	0.88	0.001	5	1.80	1.10	1.60	0.55	0.621
5	8	2.38	1.30	1.75	0.89	0.180	4	2.50	1.00	1.50	0.58	0.092

than 0.05 while the rest of the age groups are lesser than 0.05. On the contrary, no groups obtain a p-value below 0.05 in regressive autism. However, in the calculation, the p-value in paired t-test in regressive ASD regardless of the age group is below 0.05. Therefore, we suggest that improvement in behavioral problems is significant in both natal and regressive autistic children in general, despite it is reasonable to expect that natal ASD individual are more likely to make more remarkable progress in behavior aspect when compared with regressive individuals.

As shown in Table 6, in natal autism group, the score of children with age of 2 fell by 1.00 while that of children with age of 3 reduced by 0.36. The scores of children who are 4 years old and above 5 years old decreased by 0.77 and 0.63, respectively.

Food selectivity

In Table 7, it shows the data about food selection problems in the patients. p-values of 2 groups in natal autism were smaller than 0.05 and they were the groups of "2 year-old to 2 year-old and 11 months" and group of "3 year-old to 3 year-old and 11 months". The p-value of group "4 year-old to 4 year-old and 11 months" and group of "above 5 year-old" was greater than 0.05. Besides, all p-value of groups in regressive autism cannot

show a value smaller than 0.05. Despite the difference within each age groups might not be statistically significant, when we consider the overall p-value across all age groups of natal and regressive group, p-value is below 0.05, indicating an overall significance effect of acupuncture in different onset types.

It shows that the improvement of food selectivity fell with increasing age in natal group. The improvement has been most remarkable in age group of 2 years old with a score decrement of 0.75. The drop in score of children with age of 3 and 4 are both 0.35; followed by that of children with age of above 5 scoring a 0.25-point decrease.

Noise sensitivity

In Table 8, it shows the score indicating noise sensitivity issues. In the item of noise sensitivity, only p-values of 4 year-old children with natal autism and 3 year-old children with regressive autism were smaller than 0.05 and the p-values of remaining children were larger than 0.05.

For natal group, the score of 4 years old children dropped the most with a descent of 0.41, followed by age of 2 which decreased 0.38. Children with age of 3 score 0.22 less. Sound sensitivity in children above 5 years old shows no changes upon the treatment. In regressive autism group, the score of 2 years old children decreased by 0.75 while 4 years old decreased by 0.4. The score of

Table 7 Comparison of food selectivity before the 1st and after the 30th acupuncture treatment in natal and regressive autism of different age

Age (year)	Natal						Regressive					
	Pre-treatment			Post-treatment			Pre-treatment			Post-treatment		
	n	Mean	SD	Mean	SD	p-value	n	Mean	SD	Mean	SD	p-value
All	47	1.85	0.69	1.45	0.62	0.000	21	1.86	0.73	1.57	0.68	0.030
2	8	1.75	0.71	1.00	0.00	0.020	4	1.50	0.58	1.00	0.00	0.182
3	14	1.64	0.63	1.29	0.47	0.009	8	1.88	0.83	1.88	0.83	0.080
4	17	2.06	0.75	1.71	0.69	0.055	5	2.40	0.55	1.80	0.45	0.208
5	8	1.88	0.64	1.63	0.74	0.170	4	1.50	0.58	1.25	0.50	0.391

Table 8 Comparison of food selectivity before the 1st and after the 30th acupuncture treatment in natal and regressive autism of different age

Age (year)	Natal						Regressive					
	Pre-treatment			Post-treatment			Pre-treatment			Post-treatment		
	n	Mean	SD	Mean	SD	p-value	n	Mean	SD	Mean	SD	p-value
All	47	1.74	0.90	1.53	0.78	0.024	21	1.62	0.86	1.38	0.74	0.056
2	8	2.13	0.89	1.75	1.04	0.351	4	1.75	0.96	1.00	0.00	0.215
3	14	1.43	0.65	1.21	0.58	0.083	8	1.63	0.92	1.63	0.92	0.011
4	17	2.06	1.14	1.65	0.86	0.029	5	1.60	0.89	1.20	0.45	0.178
5	8	1.63	0.52	1.63	0.52	NA	4	1.50	1.00	1.50	1.00	0.215

children with age of 3 and above 5 remains constant after all the treatment sessions.

Overall score and effect

From Table 9, the overall therapeutic effect of acupuncture on natal and regressive autism along with the age of the patients is observed. P-values of all the groups in both natal autism and regressive autism were smaller than 0.05. Therapeutic effect of acupuncture is significant on both natal and regressive ASD patients of all the age groups. From Fig. 2a, the overall effectiveness of scalp acupuncture on natal ASD patients dropped with the increment of the age. In Fig. 2b shows the overall effectiveness on regressive group is highest at the age of 2, tumbled to the lowest at 3 years old and then retained a slight and steady increase when the patients are older.

From Table 10, among 68 children with ASD, 51 of them had highly significant improvement while 15 of them had significant improvement. Only 2 of them did not have significant improvement. The highly significant rate was 75% and the significant rate was 22%. The total significant rate was 97%.

Relationship between allergy and ASD

17 (25%) participants had shown various degree of allergic disorders such as allergic rhinitis, asthma and eczema, while the remaining (75%) showed not history or relevant disorders. Concerning the family history of allergy-related disease, 29.4% (n=20) participants' father or mother had a history of respiratory or dermatologic allergic disorder, while the rest of 70.6% (n=48) participants' parents did not.

Figure 3a, b represents the percentage of patients having allergic disorder and Graph Fig. 3c, d shows the percentage of patients having a family history of allergic disorder. By means of Pearson's Chi square tests, the interrelations among family history, personal allergies, and onset type (natal or regressive) were evaluated. Results show a significant correlation between family and

personal history of allergy diseases (p=0.000), and also between family history of allergies and the onset type of ASD (p=0.000). However, no significant correlation between personal history of allergies and the type of ASD can be statistically drawn (p=0.293).

Discussion

In the first section, we looked into the baseline symptomatology of the participants before acupuncture treatment. Considering the background score across the measuring domains, we observed that verbal communication problems and social problems showed the greatest improvement while food selectivity and noise sensitivity showed the least progress.

Age is a predictor for treatment outcome. Studies have shown that patients of 5 years old or younger benefit from a more promising treatment outcome from applied behavior analysis treatment [10–12]. To date, there was no research on how the age of the children affect the therapeutic outcome of acupuncture to ASD. Yet it is well perceived clinically that younger patients are more responsive to scalp acupuncture. Our investigation reassures that sooner the treatment starts; better the therapeutic effect can be achieved. Thus, early intervention of acupuncture is encouraged for ASD patients, especially those with commanding speech and social problems. It is important to state that although therapeutic effect reduces with age, older patients still benefit from acupuncture.

Scalp acupuncture is effective with statistical significance on treating both natal and regressive autism. Our clinical experience tells natal ASD patient generally benefit more from acupuncture than regressions ASD. We manipulated a series of independent t-test to investigate how natal and regressive ASD patients manifest and response to treatment differently. Despite natal ASD patients show a better response to acupuncture on average, the calculation displays no significant discrepancies (p > 0.05) between the two onset

Table 9 Comparison of Overall manifestation before the 1st and after the 30th acupuncture treatment in natal and regressive autism of different age

| Age (year) | Natal | | | | | | Regressive | | | | | |
| | Pre-treatment | | | Post-treatment | | | Pre-treatment | | | Post-treatment | | |
	n	Mean	SD	Mean	SD	p-value	n	Mean	SD	Mean	SD	p-value
All	47	11.32	2.49	8.11	2.09	0.000	21	11.76	2.10	8.71	1.87	0.000
2	8	12.25	1.91	8.13	1.25	0.000	4	12.25	1.26	8.00	0.00	0.007
3	14	10.21	2.36	6.79	1.25	0.000	8	12.38	2.20	9.75	2.49	0.002
4	17	12.12	2.62	8.88	2.29	0.000	5	10.60	2.70	7.80	1.30	0.025
5	8	10.63	2.33	8.75	2.60	0.001	4	11.50	1.73	8.50	1.29	0.001

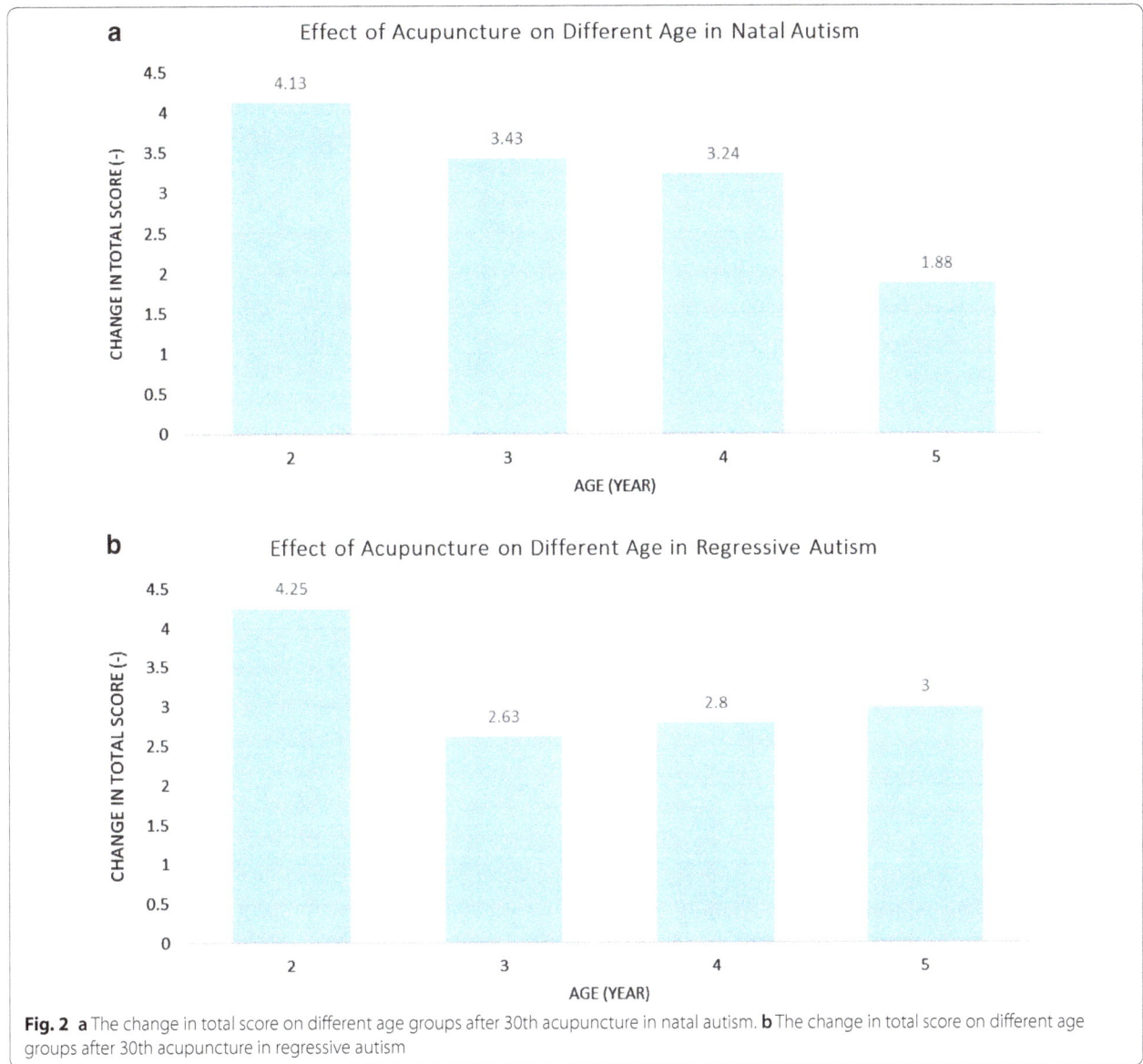

a Effect of Acupuncture on Different Age in Natal Autism

b Effect of Acupuncture on Different Age in Regressive Autism

Fig. 2 **a** The change in total score on different age groups after 30th acupuncture in natal autism. **b** The change in total score on different age groups after 30th acupuncture in regressive autism

Table 10 Overall effect of scalp acupuncture on ASD

	n	Percentage (%)
Total	68	100
Highly significant	51	75
Significant	15	22
Not significant	2	3

types in pre-treatment score or change in score across all items except verbal communication problems. Analysis reveals that that natal group performs significantly better in language use than regressive group (p = 0.021). We therefore reasonably propose that

despite successful acquisition of language skills prior to the regression does not provide any protective values; it assists a more rapid re-mastering of precedent learnt abilities or brings about better progress upon effective treatments or recovery.

In the second part of the study, we looked into the relationship between allergy and ASD. Strong correlation between familial and maternal atopic history and ASD had been well-recognized [13–16]. Furthermore, Molloy [17] revealed familial autoimmune disease such as thyroid disease is a significant risk factor to the regressive onset of ASD. Our investigation hints that familial atopies apart from thyroid disease, such as asthma, rhinitis and eczema, also exhibit similar

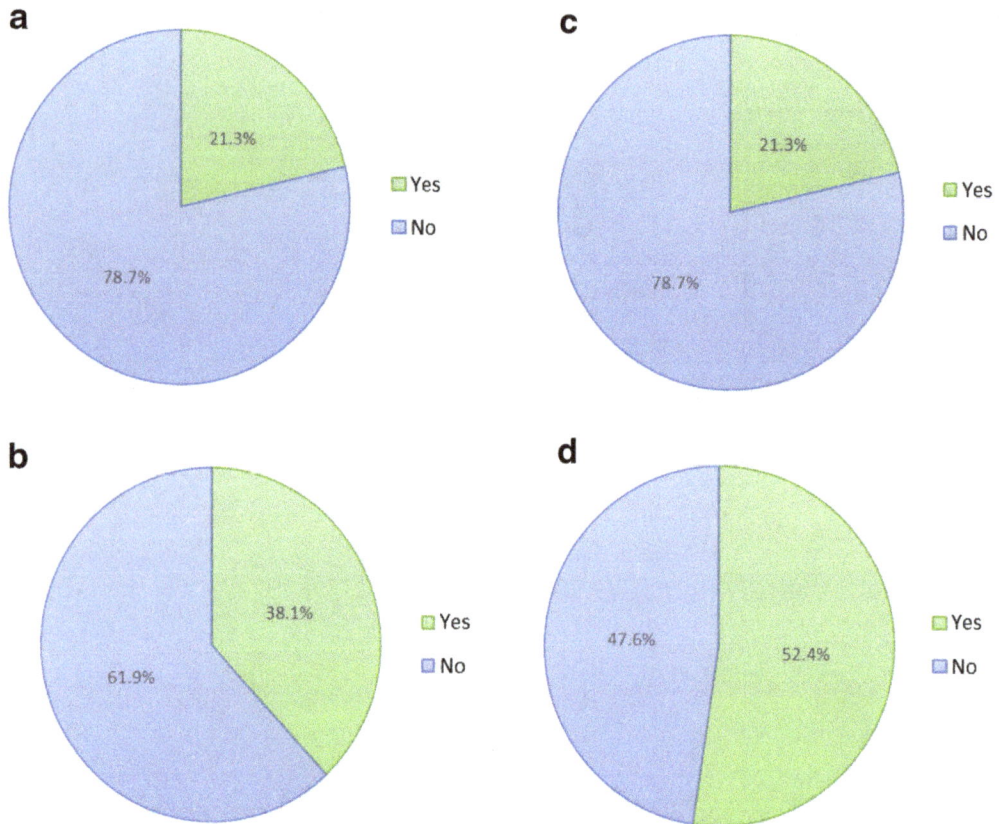

Fig. 3 **a** History of allergic disorder in natal ASD. **b** History of allergic disorder in regressive ASD. **c** Family history of allergic disorder in natal ASD. **d** Family history of allergic disorder in regressive ASD

relationships. Thus individual with a family history of allergies are more likely to develop into regressive rather than natal ASD.

The reason of late onset of autism remains unclear and we still cannot completely rule out the possibilities that environment factors including vaccination such as measles, mumps and rubella (MMR) shots, might contribute to the occurrence of regressive ASD. On the other hand, we clinically observe abnormal immune response status on ASD individuals. It is demonstrated as a vigorous response to mosquito bites or frequent cold and fever experienced by patients. It is therefore postulated that attenuated immune system might be involved in the onset or the presentation of ASD.

The biological mechanism beneath the working of acupuncture on ASD patients remains unclear. We believed that acupuncture on scalp can stimulate and activate the release of neuron transmitter and therefore assist in "rewiring" the defective neuron pathways. Experiments on mouse models suggested that

the stimulation at specific scalp areas can increase the expression of a postsynaptic density protein 95 (PSD-95) and activate nitric oxide synthase (NOS), result in improving learning memory ability and intelligence respectively [18, 19]. Different areas and lines can be drawn on the scalp as a projection of functional areas of cerebrum according to reflexology. For example, midline and the lateral line 2 of forehead are in response to the prefrontal cortex of frontal lobes; posterior lateral line of vertex in response to posterior parietal lobe; auditory speech area is in response to the Brodmann area 22, etc. Acupuncture at these areas was performed in order to stimulate the activity of the corresponding cerebral function.

There are few limitations in the present study. Firstly, 68 patients joined the study and a larger size of sample is more preferable. Secondly, it is desirable to obtain laboratory data such as functional magnetic resonance imaging (fMRI) for spotting any alteration in brain function throughout the course of acupuncture treatment.

Conclusion

ASD manifestations of some aspects such as verbal communication, social, and behavioral problems obtained a highly significant improvement upon the introduction of acupuncture; whereas domains of food selectivity and auditory sensitivity benefit less in the process. Age and the onset type are predictors for the therapeutic effect of acupuncture. We shall expect better therapeutic effect on natal onset ASD children with a younger age of two. Therefore, early intervention is always encouraged for ASD children.

Due the discrepancies between the effect of acupuncture on natal and regressive onset ASD, we postulated deviation in the etiology or the mechanisms between the two onset types. Our result showing the correlation between family history of atopy and onset type coheres with our hypothesis stating the difference in nature of natal and regressive ASD. Yet much more effort is required to reveal the underlying mechanisms for autism.

Despite the rapid development of modern science, the incidence rate of ASD shows no sign of decline and remains to be an incurable disorder. Only if we could reveal factors or incidences that would cause or induce the onset of the ASD, i.e., regressive ASD, preventive measure or effective treatments could be applied. Whilst the mechanism of ASD remains unsettled, we should remain skeptical about the use of medical manipulations such as vaccination on infants and young kids.

Abbreviation
ASD: autism spectrum disorder; CAM: complementary and alternative medicine; fMRI: functional magnetic resonance imaging; MMR: measles—mumps—rubella; NOS: nitric oxide synthase; PSD-95: postsynaptic density protein 95.

Authors' contributions
CHY participated in data collection and designed the study. YYC participated in data analysis and drafted the manuscript. CLI participated in data analysis and drafted the manuscript. All authors read and approved the final manuscript.

Acknowledgements
We would like to express our sincere gratitude to all people who have been associated with this project and all the children and their parents for being co-operative throughout the study. Also thanks go to School of Chinese Medicine, Hong Kong Baptist University for providing supports to the project.

Competing interests
The authors declare that they have no competing interests.

Consent for publication
Not applicable.

Funding
Not applicable.

References
1. World Health Organization (WHO. Autism spectrum disorders: Fact sheet. Accessed 21 May 2017. 2017.
2. World Health Organization. The ICD-10 classification of mental and behavioural disorders: clinical descriptions and diagnostic guidelines. Geneva: World Health Organization; 1992.
3. American Psychiatric Association. Diagnostic and statistical manual of mental disorders (DSM-5®). Washington DC: American Psychiatric Pub; 2013.
4. Ozonoff S, Heung K, Byrd R, Hansen R, Hertz-Picciotto I. The onset of autism: patterns of symptom emergence in the first years of life. Autism Res. 2008;1(6):320–8.
5. Hoshino Y, Kaneko M, Yashima Y, Kumashiro H, Volkmar FR, Cohen DJ. Clinical features of autistic children with setback course in their infancy. Psychiatry Clin Neurosci. 1987;41(2):237–45.
6. Hanson E, Kalish LA, Bunce E, Curtis C, McDaniel S, Ware J, Petry J. Use of complementary and alternative medicine among children diagnosed with autism spectrum disorder. J Autism Dev Disord. 2007;37(4):628–36.
7. Allam H, Eldine NG, Helmy G. Scalp acupuncture effect on language development in children with autism: a pilot study. J Altern Complement Med. 2008;14(2):109–14.
8. Wong VC, Chen WX, Liu WL. Randomized controlled trial of electro-acupuncture for autism spectrum disorder. Altern Med Rev. 2010;15(2):136–46.
9. Alder E. The Blatt-Kupperman menopausal index: a critique. Maturitas. 1998;29(1):19–24.
10. Fenske EC, Zalenski S, Krantz PJ, McClannahan LE. Age at intervention and treatment outcome for autistic children in a comprehensive intervention program. Anal Interv Dev Disabil. 1985;5(1–2):49–58.
11. Rogers SJ. Brief report: early intervention in autism. J Autism Dev Disord. 1996;26(2):243–6.
12. Harris SL, Handleman JS. Age and IQ at intake as predictors of placement for young children with autism: a four-to six-year follow-up. J Autism Dev Disord. 2000;30(2):137–42.
13. Comi AM, Zimmerman AW, Frye VH, Law PA, Peeden JN. Familial clustering of autoimmune disorders and evaluation of medical risk factors in autism. J Child Neurol. 1999;14(6):388–94.
14. Sweeten TL, Bowyer SL, Posey DJ, Halberstadt GM, McDougle CJ. Increased prevalence of familial autoimmunity in probands with pervasive developmental disorders. Pediatrics. 2003;112(5):e420.
15. Croen LA, Grether JK, Yoshida CK, Odouli R, Van de Water J. Maternal autoimmune diseases, asthma and allergies, and childhood autism spectrum disorders: a case-control study. Arch Pediatr Adolesc Med. 2005;159(2):151–7.
16. Atladóttir HÓ, Pedersen MG, Thorsen P, Mortensen PB, Deleuran B, Eaton WW, Parner ET. Association of family history of autoimmune diseases and autism spectrum disorders. Pediatrics. 2009;124(2):687–94.
17. Molloy CA, Morrow AL, Meinzen-Derr J, Dawson G, Bernier R, Dunn M, Hyman SL, McMahon WM, Goudie-Nice J, Hepburn S, Minshew N.

Familial autoimmune thyroid disease as a risk factor for regression in children with autism spectrum disorder: a CPEA study. J Autism Dev Disord. 2006;36(3):317.

18. Zhang XJ, Wu Q. Effects of electroacupuncture at different acupoints on learning and memory ability and PSD-95 protein expression on hippocampus CA1 in rats with autism. Zhongguo zhen jiu = Chin Acupunct Moxib. 2013;33(7):627–31.

19. Cui L, Sun GJ, Zhou H, Du YJ. Influence of pre-stimulation with acupuncture and moxibustion on learning and memory ability and the activity of sod, nos in hippocampal area of alzheimer disease model rats. J Hubei Univ Chin Med. 2009;3:003.

6

Jiangtang decoction ameliorate diabetic nephropathy through the regulation of PI3K/Akt-mediated NF-κB pathways in KK-Ay mice

Jin-Ni Hong[1†], Wei-Wei Li[1†], Lin-Lin Wang[1], Hao Guo[2], Yong Jiang[3], Yun-Jia Gao[3], Peng-Fei Tu[3] and Xue-Mei Wang[1*]

Abstract

Background: Jiangtang decoction (JTD) is a China patented drug which contains *Euphorbia humifusa* Willd, *Salvia miltiorrhiza* Bunge, *Astragalus mongholicus* Bunge, *Anemarrhena asphodeloides* Bunge, and *Coptis chinensis* Franch. For decades, it has also been used clinically to treat diabetic nephropathy (DN) effectively; however, the associated mechanisms remain unknown. Thus, the present study aimed to examine the protective efficacy of JTD in DN and elucidate the underlying molecular mechanisms.

Methods: A diabetic model using KK-Ay mice received a daily administration of JTD for 12 weeks. Body weight, blood glucose, triglycerides (TGs), total cholesterol (TC), urea nitrogen (UN), creatinine (Cr), and microalbumin/urine creatinine (MA/UCREA) was measured every 4 weeks. Furthermore, on the day of the sacrifice, blood, urine, and kidneys were collected to assess renal function according to general parameters. Pathological staining was performed to evaluate the protective renal effect of JTD. In addition, the levels of inflammatory cytokines (tumor necrosis factor-α [TNF-α], interleukin [IL]-6 and intercellular adhesion molecule [ICAM]-1), insulin receptor substrate [IRS]-1, advanced glycation end products [AGEs], and receptor of glycation end products [RAGE] were assessed. Finally, the phosphoinositide 3-kinase (PI3K)/protein kinase B (Akt) signaling pathway and involvement of nuclear factor-κB (NF-κB) was further analyzed.

Results: After 12 weeks of metformin and JTD administration, the mice exhibited a significant amelioration in glucose and lipid metabolism dysfunction, reduced morphological changes in the renal tissue, decreased urinary albumin excretion, and normalized creatinine clearance. JTD treatment also reduced the accumulation of AGEs and RAGE, up-regulated IRS-1, and increased the phosphorylation of both PI3K (p85) and Akt, indicating that the activation of the PI3K/Akt signaling pathway was involved. Additionally, JTD administration reduced the elevated levels of renal inflammatory mediators and decreased the phosphorylation of NF-κB p65.

Conclusions: These results demonstrate that JTD might reduce inflammation in DN through the PI3K/Akt and NF-κB signaling pathways.

Keywords: Diabetic nephropathy, Jiangtang decoction, Inflammation, Traditional Chinese Medicine

*Correspondence: wangxuemeibjmu@163.com
†Jin-Ni Hong and Wei-Wei Li contributed equally to this work and share the first authorship
[1] Integrated Laboratory of Traditional Chinese Medicine and Western Medicine, Peking University First Hospital, Beijing, People's Republic of China
Full list of author information is available at the end of the article

Background

Diabetes mellitus (DM) is an endocrine-based metabolic disease characterized by hyperglycemia due to insufficient insulin or/and insulin resistance (IR) [1]. Glucose glycates proteins and generates advanced glycation end products (AGEs), which can induce cellular effects via interactions with specific cellular receptors. Receptor of glycation end products (RAGE) is an important signal transduction receptor that activates an array of signaling transduction cascades in response to AGE-binding [2]. Moreover, elevated levels of RAGE were found to activate pro-inflammatory nuclear factor-κB (NF-κB) and other inflammatory responses, so as to induce diabetic complications [3]. DN is one of these complications, for which early progression is notoriously difficult to detect and quantify prior to the occurrence of substantial histological damage, manifesting as microalbumin (MA) and declining glomerular filtration rate. Diabetic nephropathy (DN) is considered to be an inflammatory disease, and increased inflammatory factors contribute significantly to the development of DN [3, 4]. Moreover, NF-κB is a critical signaling pathway which mediates several inflammatory processes [5]. As an upstream mediator of NF-κB, the phosphoinositide 3-kinase (PI3K)/protein kinase B (Akt) signaling pathway has been confirmed to play a vital role in proliferation, cell cycle progression, and cell viability in DN [6]. In addition, rats with streptozotocin (STZ)-induced DN exhibit a significant decrease in the PI3K and Akt [7]. Moreover, podocyte apoptosis can be inhibited by stabilizing the PI3K/Akt signaling pathway [8]. These findings indicate that the PI3K/Akt signaling pathway might play a role in DN, and alternative approaches which activate the PI3K/Akt signaling pathway and inhibit NF-κB-dependent inflammation might be a potential method of protecting against renal injury.

In China, the incidence of DN ranges from 25 to 40% [9]. In addition, DN is both the strongest predictor of mortality in diabetic patients worldwide and the leading cause of end-stage renal disease, with limited effective therapies available. Therefore, further study of the mechanisms of DN, as well as prevention and treatment strategies are required. Based on the associated clinical manifestations, DM has been defined as "Xiao-Ke," a sign of a Yin-Yang imbalance, characterized by yin vacuity with fire flaming upward, as well as qi vacuity [10]. Physically, "Xiao-Ke" patients experience dryness, thirst, and weight loss due to exhaustion. Based on the etiology and pathogenesis of DM, scholars in Traditional Chinese Medicine (TCM) have reported the main cause of DM to be heat toxins [10]. Specifically, the internal blazing of heat and stagnation of qi damage the yin, making it deficient [10]. In addition to "excessive fire consuming qi," damage to yin and qi via internal heat has also been

proposed as the primary mechanism of DM [10]. Thus, the effects of heat toxins on qi, yin, and blood stasis are thought to be key pathogenic factors in DM [10]. Other studies of TCM also indicate that diabetes may be an inflammatory disease and the inhibition of inflammation might be useful to prevent its development [11]. Moreover, previous studies found that Chinese herbal medicine, such as berberine [11], astragaloside IV [11], salvianolic acid B [12], and timosaponin B-II [13], one of the main components of *Coptis chinensis Franch, Astragalus mongholicus Bunge, Salvia miltiorrhiza Bunge*, and *Anemarrhena asphodeloides Bunge*, respectively, might exert hypoglycemic effects that are partially mediated by anti-inflammatory mechanisms. JTD, a Chinese patented drug (Patent Number: 20141002188.3) containing *Euphorbia humifusa* Willd, *S. miltiorrhiza* Bunge, *A. mongholicus* Bunge, *A. asphodeloides* Bunge, and *C. chinensis* Franch was specifically formulated to clear heat, promote blood circulation, supplement the qi, and nourish the Yin, has been used clinically for decades to effectively treat DN; however, the mechanisms remain unclear. Therefore, the aim of the present study was to examine the hypothesis that JTD ameliorates DN by inhibiting inflammation through the PI3K/Akt and NF-κB signaling pathways.

Methods

The Minimum Standards of Reporting Checklist contains details of the experimental design, and statistics, and resources used in this study (Additional file 1).

Preparation and quality control of JTD

Euphorbia humifusa Willd, *S. miltiorrhiza* Bunge, *A. mongholicus* Bunge, *A. asphodeloides* Bunge, and *C. chinensis* Franch were purchased at the Chinese Medicine Pharmacy at Peking University First Hospital (No. 8, Xishiku Street, Xicheng District, Beijing, PRC). The medicinal components of JTD are listed in Table 1. Ethanol extracts were prepared in six volumes of 60% alcohol, then soaked for 30 min, and then refluxed twice for 1 h. The herbs were then filtered, condensed, and dried. Metformin HCl (1 g) was dissolved in 40 mL ddH$_2$O and mixed. The components of JTD were detected using high-performance liquid chromatography (HPLC; Agilent 1100, USA).

Appropriate amounts of JTD ethanol extract were dissolved and diluted with methanol to a concentration of 25 mg/mL. The sample solutions were then filtered through a 0.22-μm polytetrafluoroethylene membrane prior to performing HPLC analysis. Chromatographic separation was carried out in a Gemini-NX C18 column (250 mm × 4.6 mm, 5.0 μm, Phenomenex Inc.) at 30 °C with an acetonitrile (solvent A) and 15% acetonitrile-0.01% phosphoric acid aqueous solution (solvent B; 0.15 g SDS and 0.68 g monosodium phosphate were added to 500 mL

Table 1 Composition of JTD

Species	Chinese name	Plant part	Family	Mass (g)
Euphorbia humifusa Willd	Dijincao	Leaf	Euphorbiaceae	15
Salvia miltiorrhiza Bunge	Danshen	Root	Lamiaceae	20
Astragalus mongholicus Bunge	Huangqi	Root	Leguminosae	10
Anemarrhena asphodeloides Bunge	Zhimu	Root	Asparagaceae	10
Coptis chinensis Franch	Huanglian	Root	Ranunculaceae	5
Total amount				60

of solvent B) as the mobile phases. The chromatographic conditions were optimized to acquire good separation within 60 min at a flow rate of 1.0 mL/min. The gradient program was set as follows: 0–5 min, 0% A; 5–20 min, 0–25% A; 20–30 min, 25–35% A; 30–40 min, 35–50% A; 40–50 min, 50–60% A; and 50–60 min, 60–80% A. The wavelength used for detection was 250 nm.

Animal grouping and drug administration

All animal experiments were performed with the approval of the Institutional Animal Care and Use Committee of Peking University First Hospital (Approval Number: J201534). Male KK-Ay mice ($N = 50$) and C57BL/6J mice ($N = 10$) were purchased from Beijing HFK Bioscience Co., Ltd. [License No. SCXK (Jing) 2012-0001]. The mice were aged 8–9 weeks old and weighed 30 ± 2 g. Blood glucose was measured via the glucose oxidase method. All KK-Ay mice with PPG $\geq$11.1 mmol/L or FG $\geq$7.0 mmol/L and MA tested in the urine were used as DN samples, and all others were excluded. The mice recruited were randomly divided into six groups as follows: (1) control (untreated C57BL/6J mice); (2) model (untreated KK-Ay mice); (3) metformin (KK-Ay mice treated with 250 mg/kg metformin); (4) low JTD (KK-Ay mice treated with 2 g/kg ethanol extract of JTD); (5) medium JTD (KK-Ay mice treated with 4 g/kg ethanol extract of JTD); and (6) high JTD (KK-Ay mice treated with 8 g/kg JTD ethanol extract). All drugs were administered orally once per day for 12 weeks.

Metabolic parameters and renal function analysis

After 4, 8 and 12 weeks of treatment, the mice were placed in metabolic cages for 24-h urine collection, food, and water intake calculations. The blood was collected from the mouse caudal veins. Blood glucose, triglycerides (TGs), total cholesterol (TC), urea nitrogen (UN), creatinine (Cr), and microalbumin/urine creatinine (MA/UCREA) in the urine and/or serum were measured using a Hitachi 7180 biochemical analyzer (Hitachi Ltd., Tokyo, Japan). The kidneys were removed and frozen at -80 °C until processed for Western blotting and RNA extraction.

The remaining kidney was used for analysis by light and electronic microscopy.

Histopathological analysis

After 12 weeks of treatment, the kidneys were removed and fixed in 10% formaldehyde and embedded in paraffin. Sections (4-μm thick) were cut and stained with hematoxylin and eosin (H&E) and periodic schiff-methenamine (PASM) modified trichrome histological stains. The stained sections were examined at 400× magnification by an observer blinded to the treatment group of the tissue slices. In each section, 20 glomeruli were randomly selected, and the ratio of the mesangial matrix area to the total glomerular area (M/G) in the PASM-stained sections was determined using Image-Pro Plus quantitative software (Pax-it; Paxcam, Villa Park, IL, USA).

Immunohistochemistry analysis

The kidneys were immersed in 4% paraformaldehyde for 4 h and then transferred to 70% ethanol. Then the samples were cut into 4-μm-thick paraffin-embedded kidney sections and were incubated at 4 °C with AGEs (Abcam, UK) or RAGE (Abcam, UK) overnight. The sections were then incubated with a goat anti rabbit secondary antibody (Beijing Zhong Shan Golden Bridge Biotechnology Co., Ltd., China), for 1 h at room temperature. A negative control was included, in which the primary antibody was preincubated with a control peptide. Sections were examined using an Olympus DY07 microscope (Olympus, Tokyo, Japan) and digitized with a high-resolution camera (magnification 400×). Glomeruli or tubulointerstitial areas ($N = 20$, each) were randomly selected from each section and immunostaining was performed on the AGEs and RAGE. Immunostaining signals within each selected glomerular or tubulointerstitial area were highlighted and quantified using Image-Pro Plus quantitative software (Pax-it; Paxcam, Villa Park, IL, USA). Regions with positive staining were quantified and expressed as a percentage of the entire glomerulus.

Ultrastructural analysis

After 12 weeks of treatment, the renal cortexes of the mice were removed and fixed in 3% glutaraldehyde at 4 °C and embedded in an epoxy resin. Ultrathin sections were double-stained with 1.25% uranium acetate and 0.4% lead citrate, and examined under a JEM-100C X II electron microscope (JEOL Ltd., Tokyo, Japan).

ELISA analysis

After 12 weeks of treatment, the sera were collected. The concentrations of TNF-α (Nanjingjiancheng Inc., Nanjing, China), IL-6 (Nanjingjiancheng Inc., Nanjing, China), AGEs (Abbexa Ltd., UK), and RAGE (RnD biotechne, USA) in the serum were measured using commercial ELISA kits according to the manufacturer's protocol.

Western blot analysis

After 12 weeks of treatment, the kidneys from each of the mice were collected and prepared using a protein extraction kit (KetGEN Biotech Inc., Nanjing, China) according to the manufacturer's protocol. Equal quantities of protein were separated using sodium dodecyl sulfate (SDS)-polyacrylamide gel electrophoresis and transferred to a polyvinylidene fluoride membranes. The membranes were blocked with 5% bovine serum albumen (Amresco, Inc. USA) and incubated with the primary antibodies: AGEs (Abcam, UK), RAGE (Abcam, UK), PI3K p85 (cell signaling technology, USA), p-PI3K p85 (cell signaling technology, USA), Akt (pan) (cell signaling technology, USA), p-Akt (Ser473) (cell signaling technology, USA), IκBα (cell signaling technology, USA), NF-κB p65 (cell signaling technology, USA), p-NF-κB p65 (Santa Cruz Biotechnology, Glostrup, Denmark) and GAPDH (Beijing Zhong Shan Golden Bridge Biotechnology Co., Ltd., China), with a dilution of 1:1000, overnight at 4 °C. Following incubation with a horseradish peroxidase-labeled secondary antibody (Beijing Zhong Shan Golden Bridge Biotechnology Co., Ltd.,) at room temperature for 1 h, the membranes were developed with enhanced chemiluminescence (Thermo Scientific, USA) and visualized using a digital imaging system (BIO-RAD Laboratories, Inc., USA).

Real-time PCR analysis

The total RNA was extracted from the kidneys using Trizol Reagent (Invitrogen, USA). The cDNA was synthesized using a High-Capacity cDNA Reverse Transcription Kit (Applied Biosystems, CA, USA). Quantitative real-time PCR was performed using the Power SYBR Green PCR Master MIX (Applied Biosystems, CA, USA) with the primers presented in Table 2 using the Fast Real-Time PCR System 7500 (Applied Biosystems, CA, USA). The

Table 2 Nucleotide sequences of the primers used for real-time PCR

	Forward nucleotide sequence 5′–3′	Reverse nucleotide sequence 5′–3′
IRS-1	GGCAGCAATGAGGGCAACT	TGGAAGCTGATGCTGGCATA
IL-6	GTTGCCTTCTTGGGACTGAT	GCCATTGCACAACTCTTTTCT
TNF-α	GCCATTGCACAACTCTTTTCT	AGTTGGTCCCCCTTCTCC
ICAM-1	GCTTCACACTTCACAGTTACTT	AGAGGACCTTAACAGTCTACAAC
PI3K	CGGCGTGACATGTAGGCTCTCA	ACGGCCCGCACTGTAACCTAT
Akt	TGTGACCATGAACGAGTTTGA	GTCGTGGGTCTGGAATGAGTA
IKKβ	TGCTGCCCAAGGTAGAAGAGGTAG	AGGCACTGGAAGGCTGGGACATTA
NF-κB	CACCTCACCGGCCTCATCCACA	AGTCCCCGCGCTGCTCCTCTAT
GAPDH	GGTGGAGCCAAAAGGGTCAT	CGTGGTTCACACCCATCACA

relative level of mRNA expression was calculated using the $2^{-\Delta\Delta Ct}$ method. The expression of GAPDH mRNA was used as the endogenous reference control.

Statistical methods

All data were analyzed with SPSS 19.0 statistical software, and the data are reported as the mean ± standard deviation (SD). The statistical analysis between the different groups was performed using a one-way analysis of variance (ANOVA) with a Dunnets's multiple comparison post hoc test. $P < 0.05$ was considered to be statistically significant.

Results

Content of the JTD ethanol extract

After repeating the HPLC examination for JTD, the fingerprint revealed that the following seven of the components listed below are the main constituents of JTD. The HPLC profile of JTD ethanol extract (Fig. 1) exhibits peaks corresponding to calycosin-7-O-β-D-glucoside, which is the main component of *A. mongholicus* Bunge; salvianolic acid B, the main component of *S. miltiorrhiza* Bunge; quercetin, the main component of *E. humifusa* Willd; coptisine, palmatine, and berberine, three main components of *C. chinensis* Franch; Timosaponin BII, the main component of *A. asphodeloides* Bunge. And the quantification of JTD are listed in Table 3.

JTD reduces urinary albumin excretion, as well as ameliorates kidney function and metabolism

As shown in Fig. 2a, MA/UCREA was notably elevated in the DN model group over time compared to the control group, while the combined metformin and JTD treatment were able to alleviate the increase of MA/UCREA

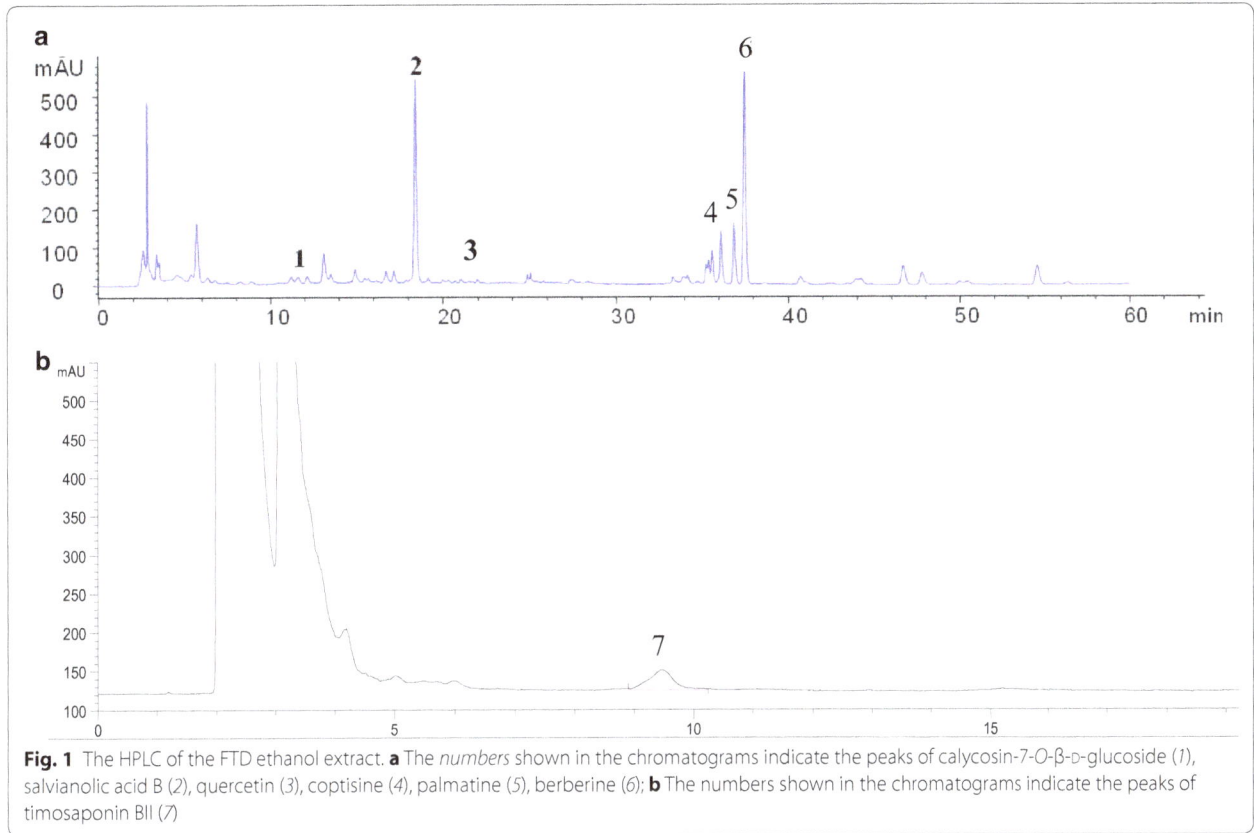

Fig. 1 The HPLC of the FTD ethanol extract. **a** The *numbers* shown in the chromatograms indicate the peaks of calycosin-7-O-β-ᴅ-glucoside (*1*), salvianolic acid B (*2*), quercetin (*3*), coptisine (*4*), palmatine (*5*), berberine (*6*); **b** The numbers shown in the chromatograms indicate the peaks of timosaponin BII (*7*)

Table 3 Quantification of JTD

Component	Ratio (mg/g JTD)
Calycosin-7-O-β-ᴅ-glucoside	0.15
Salvianolic acid B	1.89
Quercetin	0.05
Coptisine	14.12
Palmatine	0.61
Berberine	2.53
Timosaponin BII	0.68

in the urine. After 12 weeks of treatment with metformin and JTD, there was a significant decrease in MA/UCREA compared to the model group (Fig. 2b). Furthermore, treatment with JTD were found to down-regulate the concentration of UN and Cr in the urine (Fig. 2c, e) over time, thereby normalizing the concentration of UN in the urine in a dose-dependent manner (Fig. 2d) and decreasing the level of Cr excretion in the urine (Fig. 2f) after 12 weeks of treatment. The level of UN and Cr in the serum were tested after 12 weeks of treatment. Metformin and JTD treatment were found to significantly reduce UN and Cr in the serum (Fig. 2g, h). In addition, the mice were put into metabolic cages for 24 h, and the

level of food intake, water intake, and urine volume were calculated. The results showed that after 12 weeks of treatment with JTD and metformin, there was decreased food intake, water intake, and urine volume (Fig. 2i–k). It is interesting to note that treatment with a low dose of JTD can significantly normalize metabolism when compared with the model group.

JTD alleviates renal histopathology and ultrastructural pathology of the kidneys

Electron microscopy of the renal cortex ultrastructure revealed mesangial expansion, mesangial matrix deposition, podocyte fusion, and glomerular basement membrane thickening in the model group; however, these changes were significantly alleviated in the JTD and metformin-treated groups (Fig. 3a).

Both H&E and PASM staining revealed that compared to the control group, KK-Ay in the model group exhibited more severe pathological changes. From H&E staining, we found that the glomerular capillaries were dilated and filled with large amounts of red blood cells, and plasma proteins had extravasated from the renal capsules (Fig. 3b). From the PASM staining, notable glomerular hypertrophy, basement membrane thickening, increased mesangial matrix area, and glycogen, as

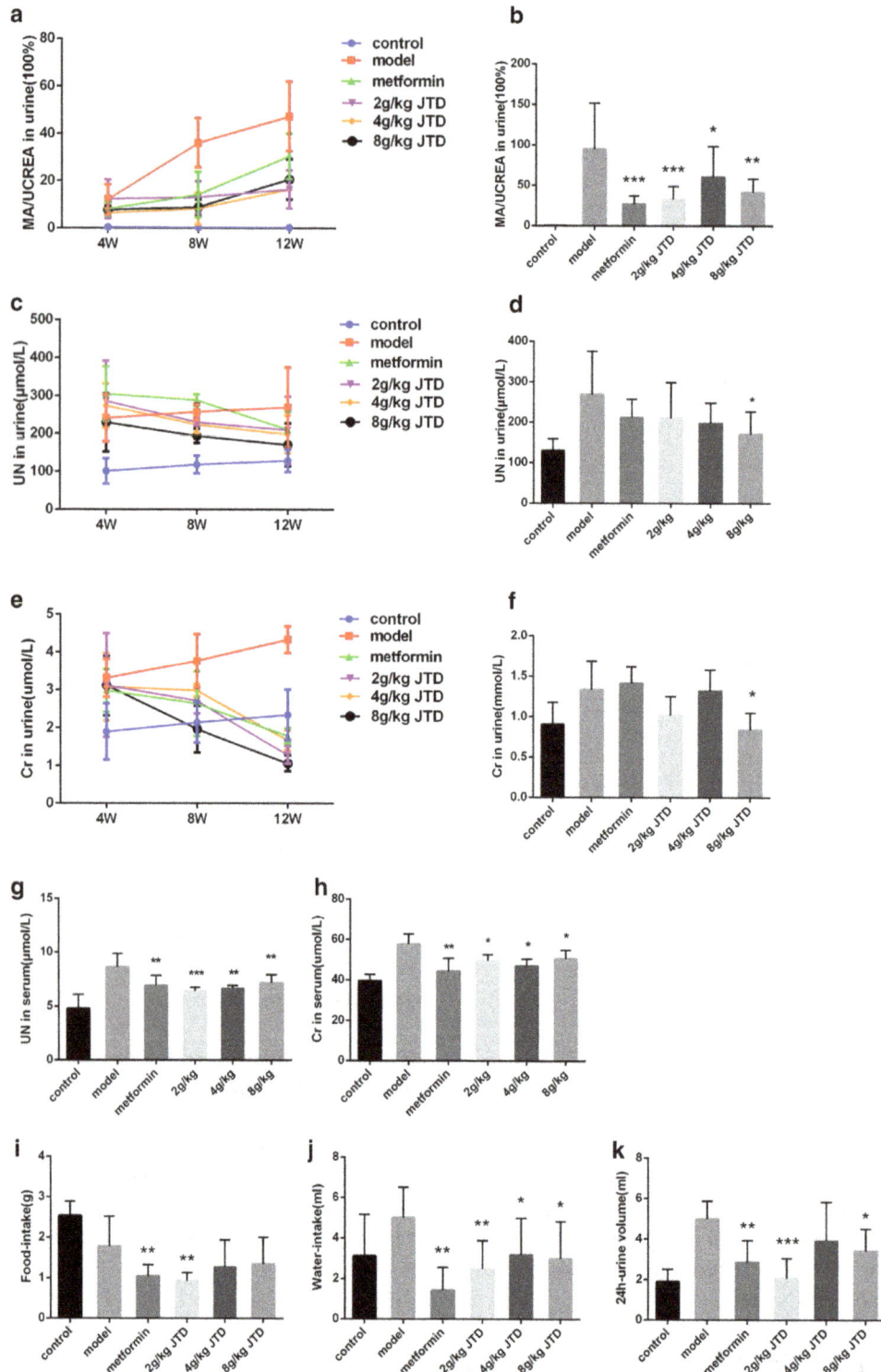

Fig. 2 JTD reduces urinary albumin excretion, as well as ameliorates the kidney function and metabolism of KK-Ay mice. **a** Changes of MA/UCREA in the urine during the treatment period. **b** JTD reduces the level of MA/UCREA in the urine. **c** Changes in the level of UN in the urine during the treatment period. **d** JTD reduces the level of UN in the urine. **e** Changes of Cr in the urine during the treatment period; **f** JTD reduces Cr in the urine. **g** JTD reduces the level of UN in the serum. **h** JTD reduces Cr in the serum. **i** JTD reduces food intake. **j** JTD reduces water intake. **k** JTD reduces the 24-h urine volume. Data are expressed as the mean ± S.D.; $N = 10$; *$P < 0.05$; **$P < 0.01$; and ***$P < 0.001$ compared to the model group

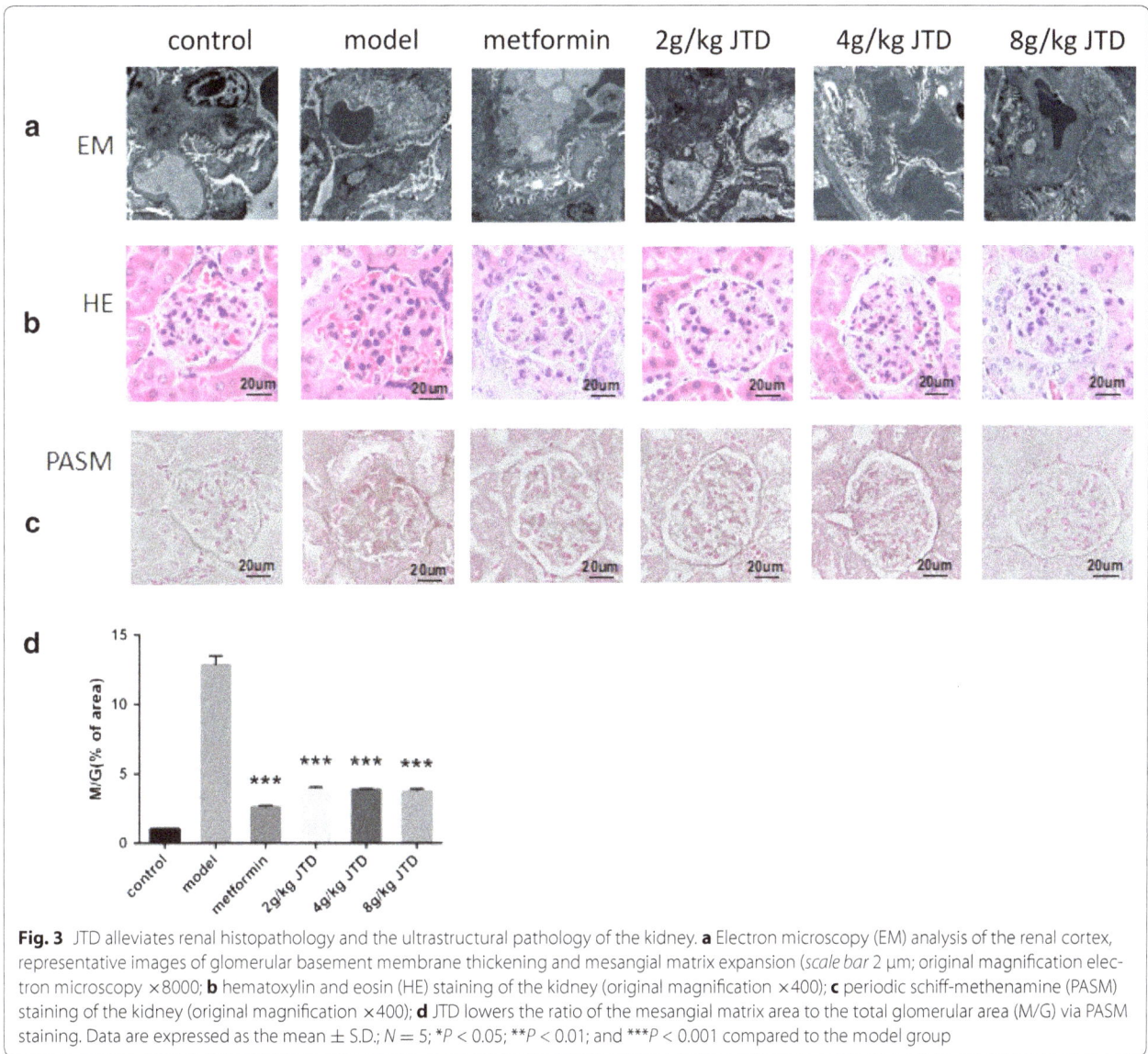

Fig. 3 JTD alleviates renal histopathology and the ultrastructural pathology of the kidney. **a** Electron microscopy (EM) analysis of the renal cortex, representative images of glomerular basement membrane thickening and mesangial matrix expansion (*scale bar* 2 μm; original magnification electron microscopy ×8000; **b** hematoxylin and eosin (HE) staining of the kidney (original magnification ×400); **c** periodic schiff-methenamine (PASM) staining of the kidney (original magnification ×400); **d** JTD lowers the ratio of the mesangial matrix area to the total glomerular area (M/G) via PASM staining. Data are expressed as the mean ± S.D.; $N = 5$; *$P < 0.05$; **$P < 0.01$; and ***$P < 0.001$ compared to the model group

well as vacuolation and deformation of the renal tubules were observed in the model group. Moreover, treatment with JTD or metformin significantly ameliorated these changes (Fig. 3c). Additionally, PASM staining showed that the M/G ratios were higher in the model group than the controls, whereas treatment with JTD and metformin significantly lowered the M/G ratio (Fig. 3d).

JTD reduce the increase in blood glucose, weight, and lipid metabolism

DM is a metabolic disease characterized by a high concentration of blood glucose. Thus, we examined the glucose levels of mice every 4 weeks and found that treatment with an oral administration of metformin and JTD decreased the increased levels of glucose (Fig. 4a,

b). As shown in Fig. 4a, a significant increase in postprandial glucose (PPG) in KK-Ay mice was decreased by metformin and JTD. Additionally, the effect of a low and medium dose of JTD was more potent than that of metformin. As shown in Fig. 4b, JTD can also reduce elevated levels of fasting glucose (FG), with a low and medium dose of JTD demonstrating a greater effect than a high dose of JTD. Moreover, JTD can reduce the area under the curve (AUC) of both the oral glucose tolerance test (OGTT) and insulin tolerance test (ITT) in KK-Ay mice (Fig. 4c, d). From Fig. 4c, it is observed that metformin and low doses of JTD can reduce OGTT (AUC), whereas a medium and a high dose of JTD have no positive effect. In Fig. 4d, both metformin and JTD are shown to significantly down-regulate ITT (AUC), compared to

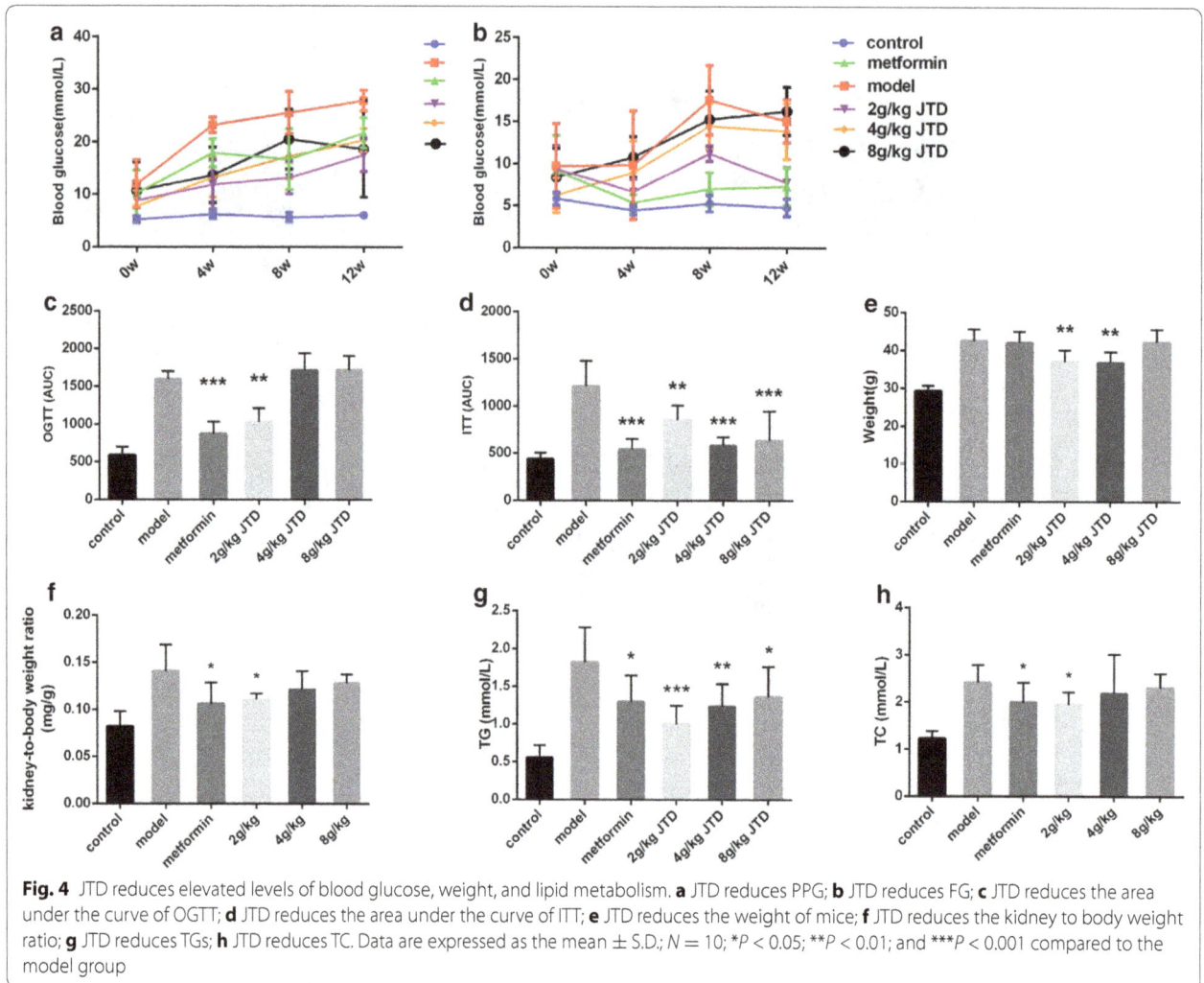

Fig. 4 JTD reduces elevated levels of blood glucose, weight, and lipid metabolism. **a** JTD reduces PPG; **b** JTD reduces FG; **c** JTD reduces the area under the curve of OGTT; **d** JTD reduces the area under the curve of ITT; **e** JTD reduces the weight of mice; **f** JTD reduces the kidney to body weight ratio; **g** JTD reduces TGs; **h** JTD reduces TC. Data are expressed as the mean ± S.D.; $N = 10$; *$P < 0.05$; **$P < 0.01$; and ***$P < 0.001$ compared to the model group

the model group. In addition, after 12 weeks of administration, body weight was found to be markedly increased in the model mice compared to the other groups (Fig. 4e). Furthermore, metformin and JTD were found to down-regulate the kidney to body ratio after 12 weeks of JTD administration (Fig. 4f). Additionally, we found that treatment with JTD significantly lowered the level of TGs and TC, which were elevated in the model group in a dose-dependent manner (Fig. 4g, h).

JTD reduces the accumulation of AGEs and RAGE

Non-enzymatic glycation of proteins by reducing saccharides is a post-translational modification leading to the formation of AGEs, which accumulate during aging and are involved in the pathogenesis of many diseases (e.g., DM) [14]. Studies on the pathological mechanisms of glycation-related diseases (e.g., DM) have shown that AGEs can induce cellular effects through interacting with specific cellular receptors [14]. In addition, RAGE

is an important signal transduction receptor which activates an array of signal transduction cascades in response to AGE-binding [2]. Furthermore, both AGEs and RAGE have been identified as key regulators of DN [2]. Thus, we next examined whether AGEs and RAGE accumulate in diabetic kidneys and whether JTD can alleviate this accretion. As presented in Fig. 5a, b, immunohistochemistry staining of AGE and RAGE in renal tissue were performed to assess the regional changes of AGEs and RAGE accumulation in diabetic kidneys. It was apparent that treatment with JTD and metformin could reduce the ratio of the area of AGE and RAGE accumulation to the total glomerular area (Fig. 5c, d). To elucidate the detailed mechanisms of this effect, we examined the impact of JTD on the expression of AGEs and RAGE in diabetic kidneys using an ELISA and Western blot. Figure 5e, f reveal that after 12 weeks of treatment, AGEs and RAGE in the serum were lower in the mice treated with JTD in a dose-dependent manner,

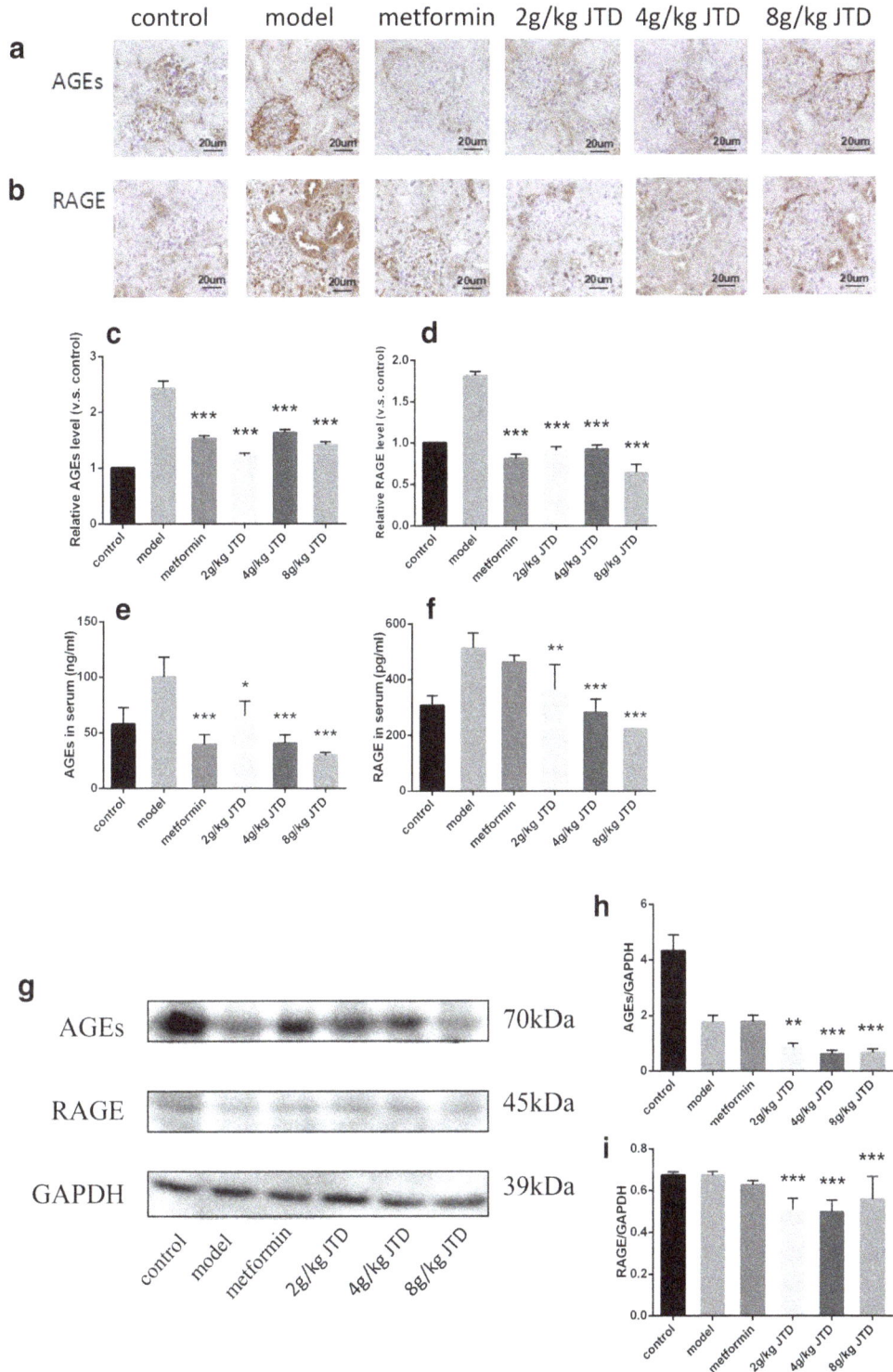

Fig. 5 JTD reduces the accumulation of AGEs and RAGE. **a** Immunohistochemistry of AGEs (original magnification ×400); **b** immunohistochemistry of RAGE (original magnification ×400); **c** JTD reduces the ratio of the area with AGEs accumulation to the total glomerular area; **d** JTD reduces the ratio of the area with RAGE accumulation to the total glomerular area; **g** Western blot analysis of AGEs and RAGE; **h** JTD can down-regulate the expression of AGEs; **i** JTD can down-regulate the expression of RAGE. Data are expressed as the mean ± S.D.; N = 10; *P < 0.05; **P < 0.01; and ***P < 0.001 compared to the model group

compared to the model group. Furthermore, when detecting the expression of AGEs and RAGE in the kidney by Western blot, we found that JTD alleviated the accumulation of both (Fig. 5h, i).

JTD down-regulates inflammatory factors

DN is confirmed to be an inflammatory disease, and pro-inflammatory cytokines are closely related to the pathology of DN. The increased production of free radicals and pro-inflammatory mediators (e.g., lipid mediators and cytokines) aggravates inflammation and damages host tissues. Thus, we detected the concentration of inflammatory factors to determine whether JTD treatment affects renal inflammation under diabetic conditions. The levels of IRS-1, TNF-α, IL-6, and ICAM-1 were detected with real-time PCR or an ELISA. As shown in Fig. 6e, IRS-1 expression was decreased in the model group, while the 12-week administration of metformin and JTD up-regulated IRS-1. Additionally, treatment with JTD down-regulated the expression of IL-6 in the serum (Fig. 6a), which was increased in the model group. Furthermore, treatment with JTD decreased the level of IL-6 mRNA in the kidney in a dose-dependent manner (Fig. 6d). TNF-α was highly expressed in the model group, while the

administration of metformin and JTD was found to normalize both the mRNA and protein expression of TNF-α in the serum and kidney (Fig. 6b, c). In addition, ICAM-1 mRNA was found to be down-regulated by treatment with metformin and JTD (Fig. 6f).

JTD activates the PI3K/Akt signaling pathway and inhibits NF-κB signaling pathways

PI3K/Akt is closely related to the progression of DN, which is considered to be an inflammatory disease [4]. Moreover, NF-κB serves as a vital mediator of the inflammatory response. IKKβ and IκBα are two important modulators upstream of the NF-κB signal transduction cascade. IKKβ acts as a protein subunit of IκBα, and IκBα retains NF-κB in an inactive state in the cytoplasm. Thus, we detected the effect of JTD on the PI3K/Akt and NF-κB signaling pathways. The level of p-PI3K (Tyr 458), PI3K p65, p-Akt (Ser 473), Akt (pan), p-NF-κB p65, NF-κB p65, IκBα, and IKKβ were detected via Western blotting or real-time PCR. Figure 7d, e show that in mice treated with metformin and JTD group for 12 weeks, the level of PI3K and Akt were up-regulated, and there was a statistically significant difference between the group that received the medium dose of JTD and the model

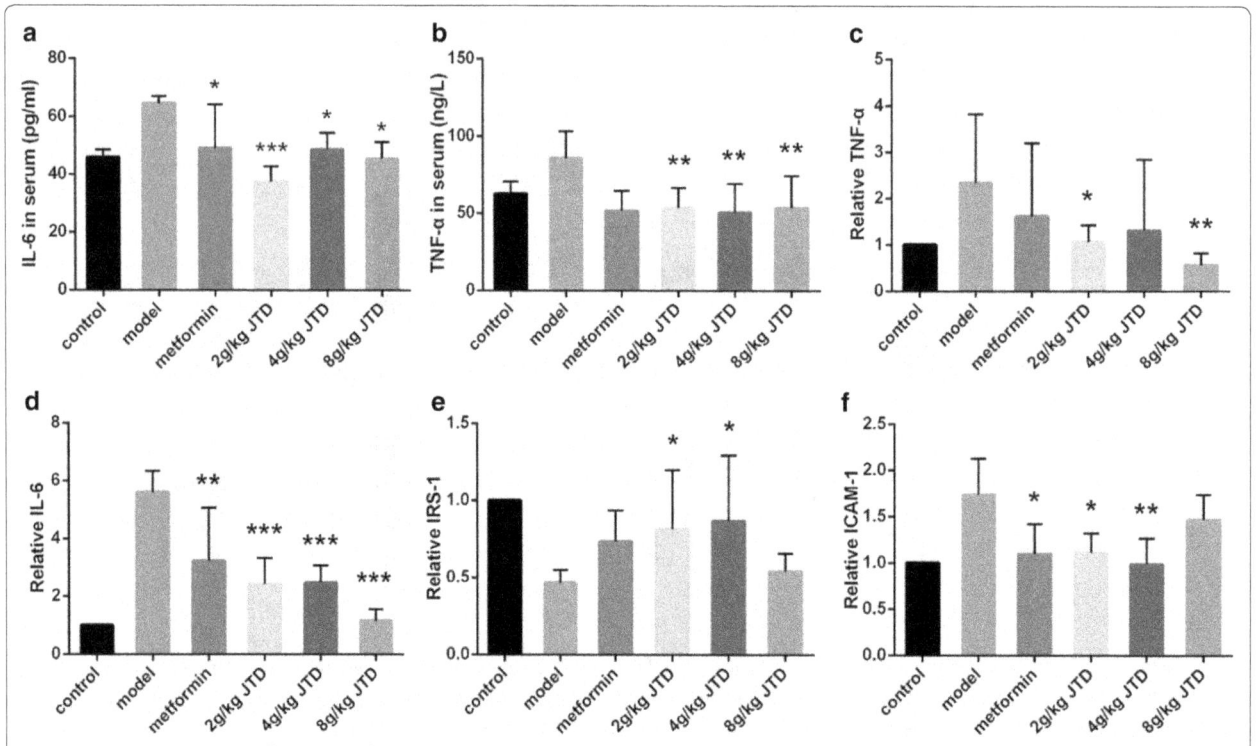

Fig. 6 JTD down-regulates inflammatory factors. **a** JTD reduces the level of IL-6 in the serum; **b** JTD reduces the level of TNF-α in the serum; **c** JTD reduces the expression of TNF-α mRNA in the kidney; **d** JTD reduces the expression of IL-6 mRNA in the kidney; **e** JTD reduces the expression of IRS-1 mRNA in the kidney; **f** JTD reduces the expression of ICAM-1 mRNA in the kidney. Data are expressed as the mean ± S.D.; N = 10; *P < 0.05; **P < 0.01; and ***P < 0.001 compared to the model group

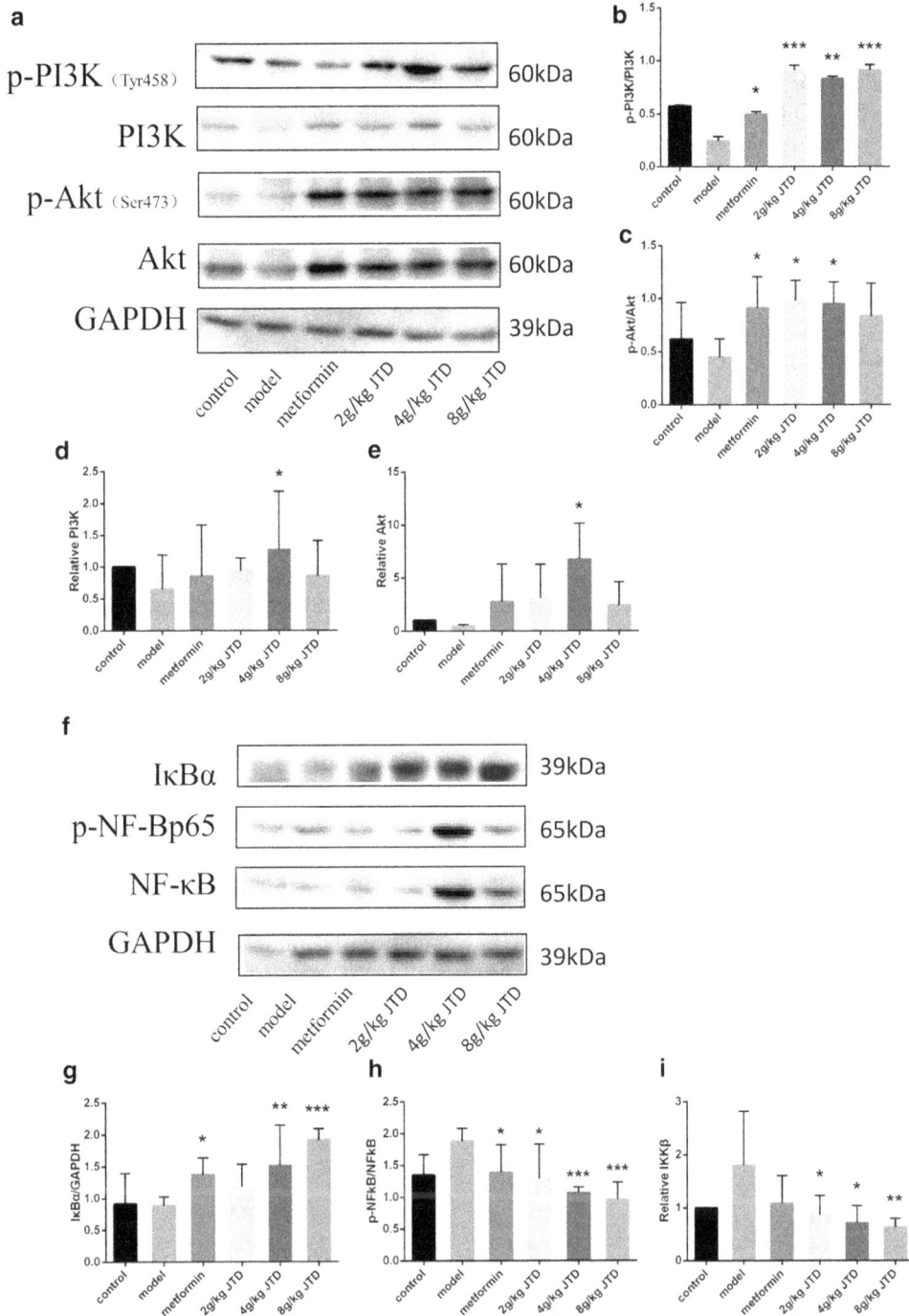

Fig. 7 JTD activates the PI3K/Akt signaling pathway and inhibits NF-κB signaling pathways. **a** Representative Western blots of phosphorylated PI3K (Tyr 458), PI3K p85, phosphorylated Akt (Ser 473), Akt (pan), and GAPDH proteins isolated from the mouse kidneys of different groups. Protein bands shown are representative of >3 independent experiments with similar results. **b** JTD up-regulates the phosphorylation of PI3K; **c** JTD up-regulates the amount of phosphorylated Akt (Ser473); **d** JTD up-regulates PI3K p85mRNA expression; **e** JTD up-regulates the mRNA expression of Akt (pan); **f** representative Western blots of IκBα as well as phosphorylated NF-κB p65, NF-κB p65, and GAPDH proteins isolated from the mouse kidneys of different groups. The protein bands are representative of >3 independent experiments with similar results. **g** JTD down-regulates the protein expression of IκBα in the kidney; **h** JTD downregulates the phosphorylation of NF-κB p65; **i** JTD down-regulates the mRNA expression of IKKβ. Data are expressed as the mean ± S.D.; $N = 10$; *$P < 0.05$; **$P < 0.01$; and ***$P < 0.001$ compared to the model group

group. Furthermore, p-PI3K/PI3K and p-Akt/Akt were also up-regulated in the group treated with metformin and JTD (Fig. 7a–c). Treatment with JTD can up-regulate the expression of PI3K and Akt. Figure 7g showed that in the mice treated with JTD for 12 weeks, the level of IκBα was up-regulated, while the level of IKKβ mRNA and p-NF-κB/NF-κB protein are down-regulated (Fig. 7h, i).

Discussion

DN is a leading cause of end-stage renal disease with limited effective therapies, and affects up to 40% of patients with type 1 or type 2 DM [15]. As DN is the strongest predictor of mortality in diabetic patients worldwide [15], it is critical to study the mechanism of DN in conjunction with strategies for prevention and treatment. Although knowledge regarding the molecular mechanisms of DN has progressed in recent years [16–18], efficient therapeutic approaches that prevent or reverse the progression of DN are lacking, highlighting the need to identify new treatment strategies.

In China, TCMs are known to produce remarkable results and some TCMs are recommended for the treatment of DN [19–21]. Unlike single compounds with only one active chemical ingredient, TCMs are typically complex combinations of chemicals that act in concert. Moreover, any one of the active components of a TCM alone cannot reflect the ultimate therapeutic effect of the entire medicine [22, 23]. Previous studies show that TCMs that exhibit heat- and toxin-clearing effects can down-regulate blood glucose, promote circulation, and relieve the clinical indicators of DN [20]. Several studies suggest that TCMs might exert hypoglycemic effects through anti-inflammatory mechanisms, including the modulation of inflammatory factors, AGEs,

renin-angiotensin systems, and lipid metabolism [11]. In addition, JTD contains various plant components that are widely used in TCM, many of which are effective in reducing both glucose and inflammation (Fig. 8). *Euphorbia humifusa* Willd is one of the elements of JTD thought to reduce FG and enhance insulin sensitivity in KK-Ay mice [24]. Additionally, it can inhibit NF-κB activity and down-regulate the production of inflammatory mediators, such as nitric oxide (NO) and TNF-α [25, 26]. *Salvia miltiorrhiza* Bunge has been reported to improve the quantity and amount of pancreatic islet cells, repair their structure and function, increase glucose transporter 4 (GLUT4) and glycogen synthase protein expression in the skeletal muscle, as well as suppress the secretion of NO, TNF-α, and IL-6 in RAW264.7 macrophages stimulated with LPS [12]. Additionally, it has been reported that *S. miltiorrhiza* Bunge inhibits platelet activation and arterial thrombosis via regulation of the PI3K and NF-κB signaling pathways [24]. Raw *A. mongholicus* Bunge, which tonifies qi, was commonly used clinically to reduce diabetic symptoms, such as fatigue; it was also found to increase serum levels of total adiponectin, as well as alleviate hyperglycemia, glucose intolerance, and IR in obese mice [27]. It was also reported to attenuate DN by reducing endoplasmic reticulum stress [28]. Similarly, *A. asphodeloides* Bunge was reported to reduce FG and improve impaired glucose tolerance in type 2 DM rats, and the flavonoids of *A. asphodeloides Bunge* are thought to reduce glucose and TGs [13]. Furthermore, TB-II, a main ingredient of *A. asphodeloides* Bunge, notably ameliorated IR and inflammation, and significantly improved cell viability decreased TNF-α and IL-6 levels, and the expression of p-NF-κBp65, p-IKKβ, p-IRS-1, p-PI3K, and p-Akt [13]. *Coptis chinensis Franch*

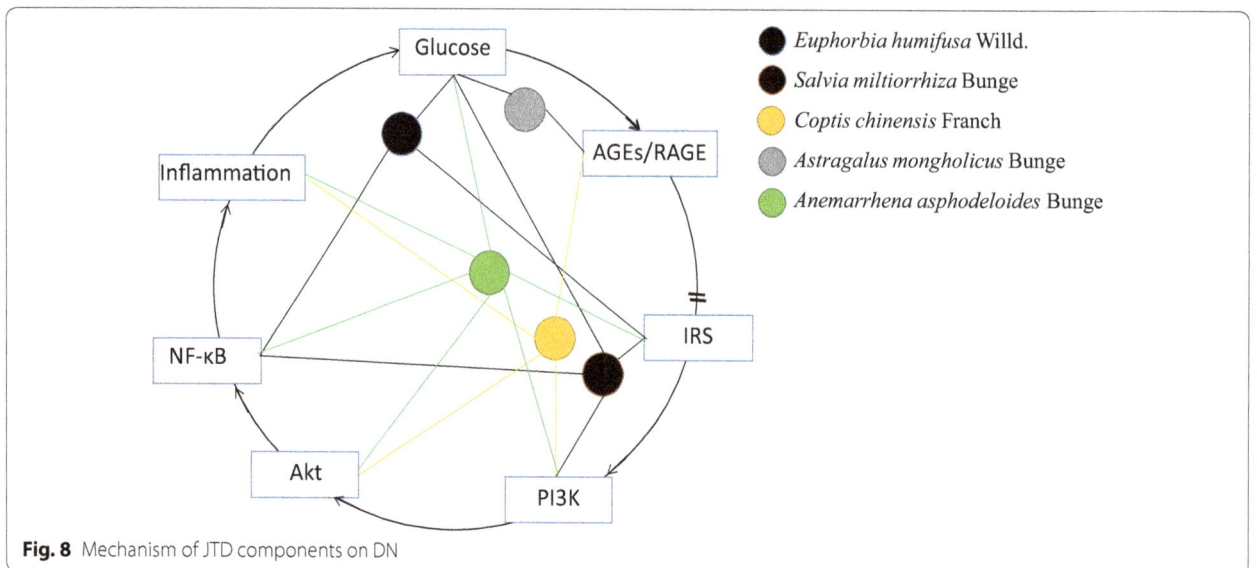

Fig. 8 Mechanism of JTD components on DN

was confirmed to significantly inhibit all the three periods of nonenzymatic protein glycation in vitro, including amadori products, dicarbonyl compounds, and AGEs formation [29]. It is also reported to attenuate myocardial ischemia–reperfusion by regulating the PI3K/Akt signaling pathway and the subsequent reduction of inflammatory factors, including IL-6, IL-18, and TNF-α [30]. In our previous random control trials and animal experiments, we confirmed that JTD is safe and effective at reducing glucose and MA/UCREA in both patients and KK-Ay mice (accepted). In this study, we found that JTD can reduce the morphological changes in renal tissue, ameliorate glucose and lipid metabolism dysfunction, as well as decrease MA, UN, and Cr. Moreover, JTD can also decrease the enhanced levels of blood glucose and the accumulation AGEs and RAGE, thereby normalizing IR. In our study, the increased phosphorylation of PI3K-Akt and IκBα expression decreased IKKβ, and reduced phosphorylation of NF-κB was observed in the kidneys of JTD-treated KK-Ay mice. In addition, we found that alterations in a number of indexes of renal inflammation (e.g., increased ICAM-1, TNF-α, and IL-6 expression) in KK-Ay mice were alleviated by JTD treatment. These results suggest that the activation of PI3K/Akt, inhibition of the NF-κB signaling pathway, and NF-κB-dependent inflammation may be a key mechanism by which JTD attenuates DN (Fig. 9).

DM is considered to be a group of metabolic diseases characterized by a high concentration of blood glucose, and glucose glycates proteins that give rise to AGEs, which induce cellular effects through interacting with specific cellular receptors. RAGE is an important signal transduction receptor known to activate an array of signal transduction cascades in response to the binding of AGEs [31]. Moreover, AGEs and RAGE play critical roles in the pathogenesis of DN [31]. AGEs result in cellular oxidative stress and IR, which have been implicated

as causative factors in diabetic complications [4]. The accumulation of AGEs and RAGE can induce harmful changes to some protein structures, thereby decreasing their enzymatic activity and interfering matrix protein connection, which can cause dysfunction in renal cells and induce histological changes, including inflammation, focal glomerulosclerosis, mesangial expansion, tubulointerstitial fibrosis, and epithelial- to- mesenchymal transdifferentiation [3]. It has been confirmed that elevated levels of AGEs and RAGE have been found to activate pro-inflammatory NF-κB, an initial step in type 2 DM evolution that contributes to both β-cell apoptosis and IR [32], and induces the release of inflammatory factors [33]. IRS-1 and PI3K are key insulin signaling molecules critically involved in glucose metabolism and IR [34, 35]. One of the key mechanisms observed in the tissues impacted by type 2 DM is that the phosphorylation of serine residues in the insulin receptor and IRS-1 molecule results in diminished enzymatic activity in the PI3K/Akt pathway [33]. When insulin binds to the insulin receptor (InsR), it stimulates InsR intrinsic kinase activity and subsequently activates PI3K and Akt in succession [33]. Therefore, due to an increase in insulin receptor activity, PI3K/Akt signaling is activated in the renal cortex of db/db mice during the early phase of DM [33]. Additionally, PI3K/Akt signaling was found to be lower in the glomeruli of 12-week-old db/db mice, which has been linked to the death of podocytes in db/db mice [36]. The down-regulation of PI3K/Akt signaling contributes to renal tubular apoptosis in the kidneys of STZ-induced diabetic mice and apoptosis in the proximal tubular cells of the kidney [37]. Mounting evidence has highlighted that DM activates NF-κB signaling, which regulates the expression of numerous genes that play key roles in the inflammatory response during kidney injury [5, 38, 39]. Moreover, the inhibition of NF-κB has been shown to result in the significant improvement of DN [40, 41]. Therefore, we postulated that the inactivation of NF-κB was involved in the JTD-mediated protection against DN. Under steady-state conditions, NF-κB is present in the cytoplasm and bound to its inhibitory protein, IκB; however, when IκB is phosphorylated by IKKβ, NF-κB is then released from the inhibitory unit, translocated into the nucleus, and undergoes phosphorylation. Finally, NF-κB promotes the transcription of pro-inflammatory cytokines, such as TNF-α, IL-6, and ICAM-1 [42]. A growing number of studies have revealed that the serum and urinary concentrations of TNF-α in patients with DN are substantially higher than that found in non-diabetic individuals, and TNF-α levels are implicated in the process of renal hypertrophy and hyperfunction during the initial stages of DN [43]. IL-6 is confirmed to be increased in patients with DN, and its levels are higher in patients with overt proteinuria

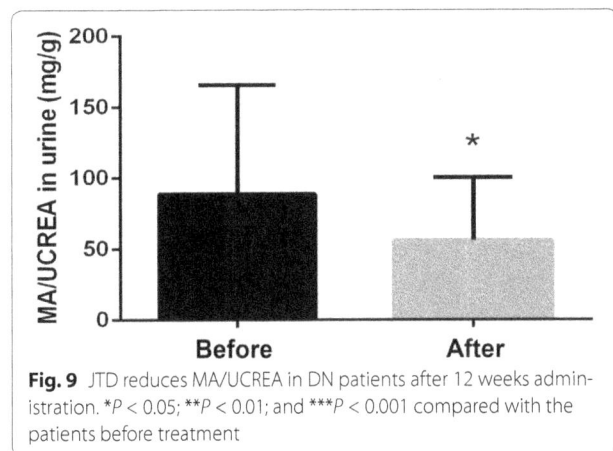

Fig. 9 JTD reduces MA/UCREA in DN patients after 12 weeks administration. *$P < 0.05$; **$P < 0.01$; and ***$P < 0.001$ compared with the patients before treatment

compared to those exhibiting microalbuminuria or normoalbuminuria [44]. Additionally, recent work also found that increased IL-6 is associated with glomerular basement membrane (GBM) thickening and mesangial expansion in the kidney biopsies of DM patients [45]. Produced by renal mesangial cells, IL-6 is thought to mediate endothelial permeability and mesangial proliferation [46]. Additionally, an ICAM-1 deficiency in transgenic mice results in a substantial decrease in macrophage accumulation in the glomeruli and a reduction in glomerular hypertrophy [42].

In our study, we found that the concentration of AGEs and RAGE in a KK-Ay mouse model were higher than that of the normal controls. In addition, the expression of IRS-1, PI3K/Akt, and NF-κB, as well as the histological changes observed in the KK-Ay model group, are consistent with previous reports [3, 24, 36]. The findings of the present study suggest that JTD can relieve DN by down-regulating increased levels of blood glucose, so as to reduce the accumulation of AGEs and RAGE, as well as alleviate inflammation via activation of the PI3K/Akt signaling pathways and inhibiting NF-κB signaling. Additionally, this study demonstrates that PI3K/Akt-mediated NF-κB signaling might be a mechanism for the treatment of DN, and use of multiple herbal compounds may be a useful therapeutic approach. While unlike single compounds with only one active chemical ingredient, Traditional Chinese Medicine, especially compounds are typically complicated combinations of chemicals that act in concert. The ultimate therapeutic effect of the compound is multi-targets and the effect might vary as the concentration change. Thus the effect of compound might not all be in a dose dependent manner. However, since the evidence demonstrating the effect of JTD on DN was obtained from studies using animal models, these findings should be confirmed with further research in diabetic patients.

Conclusion

JTD is a promising agent for the treatment of DN, and its therapeutic mechanism is likely related to the regulation of AGEs, RAGE, and PI3K/Akt-mediated NF-κB signaling pathways.

Abbreviations

JTD: jiangtang decoction; DM: diabetes mellitus; DN: diabetic nephropathy; TGs: triglycerides; TC: total cholesterol; FG: fasting glucose; PPG: postprandial glucose; OGTT: oral glucose tolerance test; ITT: insulin tolerance test; AUC: area under the curve; MA: microalbumin; MA/UCREA: microalbumin/urine creatinine; UN: urea nitrogen; Cr: creatinine; IL-6: interleukin-6; TNF-α: tumor necrosis

factor-alpha; ICAM-1: intercellular adhesion molecule-1; p-PI3K: phosphorylated phosphatidylinositol 3-kinase; PI3K: phosphatidylinositol 3-kinase; p-Akt: phosphorylated protein kinase B; Akt: protein kinase B; IKKβ: IκB kinase-beta antibody; IκBα: nuclear factor of kappa light polypeptide gene enhancer in B-cells inhibitor, alpha; p-NF-κB: phosphorylated nuclear factor kappa-B; NF-κB: nuclear factor kappa-B; AGEs: advanced glycation end products; RAGE: receptor of glycation end products; H&E: hematoxylin-eosin staining; PASM: periodic schiff-methenamine; EM: electronic microscopy; GLUT4: glucose transporter 4; NO: nitric oxide; GBM: glomerular basement membrane.

Authors' contributions

Conceived and designed the experiments: WWL, XMW. Carried out the experiment: JNH, WWL, HG, LLW. Analyzed the data: JNH, LLW, WWL, XMW. Contributed reagents/materials/analysis tools: JNH, WWL, XMW. Wrote the paper: JNH, WWL. All authors read and approved the final manuscript.

Author details

[1] Integrated Laboratory of Traditional Chinese Medicine and Western Medicine, Peking University First Hospital, Beijing, People's Republic of China. [2] Institute of Basic Medical Sciences, Xiyuan Hospital, China Academy of Chinese Medical Sciences, Beijing, People's Republic of China. [3] School of Pharmaceutical Science, Peking University, Beijing, People's Republic of China.

Acknowledgements

We are grateful to the Integrated Laboratory of Traditional Chinese Medicine and Western Medicine, Peking University First Hospital, Beijing, P.R. China, the Laboratory Animal Facility and College of Pharmacy in Peking University Health Science Center, and professor TengXiang Zeng in School of Pharmaceutical Science, Peking University, Beijing, P.R. China for their assistance.

Competing interests

The authors declare that they have no competing interests.

Funding

This work was supported by the National Natural Science Foundation of China (Grant Numbers 81573763, 81530099), the Beijing Traditional Chinese Medicine Science and Technology Development Fund (Grant Number JJ2015-69), the Beijing Municipal Natural Science Foundation (Grant Numbers 7172221), and the National Key Technology R&D Program "New Drug Innovation" of China (Grant Number 2012ZX09301002-002-002).

References

1. Dronavalli S, Duka I, Bakris GL. The pathogenesis of diabetic nephropathy. Nat Clin Pract J Clin Endocr Metab. 2008;4:444–52. doi:10.1038/ncpendmet0894.
2. Ramasamy R, Yan SF, Herold K, Clynes R, Schmidt AM. Receptor for advanced glycation end products: fundamental roles in the inflammatory response: winding the way to the pathogenesis of endothelial dysfunction and atherosclerosis. Ann N Y Acad Sci. 2008;1126:7–13. doi:10.1196/annals.1433.056.
3. Han C, Lu Y, Wei Y, Wu B, Liu Y, He R. D-ribosylation induces cognitive impairment through RAGE-dependent astrocytic inflammation. Cell Death Dis. 2014;5:e1117. doi:10.1038/cddis.2014.89.

4. Tuttle KR. Linking metabolism and immunology: diabetic nephropathy is an inflammatory disease. J Am Soc Nephrol. 2005;16(6):1537–8. doi:10.1681/ASN.2005040393.

5. Navarro-González JF, Mora-Fernández C, De Fuentes MM, García-Pérez J. Inflammatory molecules and pathways in the pathogenesis of diabetic nephropathy. Nat Rev Nephrol. 2011;7:327–40. doi:10.1038/nrneph.2011.51.

6. Cantley LC. The phosphoinositide 3-kinase pathway. Science. 2002;296:1655–7. doi:10.1126/science.296.5573.1655.

7. Zhu J, Sun N, Aoudjit L, Li H, Kawachi H, Lemay S, Takano T. Nephrin mediates actin reorganization via phosphoinositide 3-kinase in podocytes. Kidney Int. 2008;73:556–66. doi:10.1038/sj.ki.5002691.

8. Yu S, Li Y. Dexamethasone inhibits podocyte apoptosis by stabilizing the PI3K/Akt signal pathway. Biomed Res Int. 2013. doi:10.1155/2013/326986 **(Article ID: 326986)**.

9. Zhu J, Wu Y, Wang Y. Multivariate analysis of Chinese medicine syndrome type and its correlated factors of diabetic nephropathy. Mod J Integr Tradit Chin West Med. 2012;21(1):18–20. doi:10.3969/j.issn.1008-8849.2012.01.008.

10. Hu J, Pang W, et al. Hypoglycemic effect of polysaccharides with different molecular weight of *Pseudostellaria heterophylla*. Complement Altern Med. 2013;13:267. doi:10.1186/1472-6882-13-267.

11. Xie W, Du L. Diabetes is an inflammatory disease: evidence from traditional Chinese medicines. Diabetes Obes Metab. 2011;13:289–301. doi:10.1111/j.1463-1326.2010.01336.x.

12. Huang MQ, Zhou CJ, Zhang YP, et al. Salvianolic acid B ameliorates hyperglycemia and dyslipidemia in db/db mice through the AMPK pathway. Cell Physiol Biochem. 2016;40(5):933–43. doi:10.1159/000453151.

13. Yuan YL, Lin BQ, Zhang CF, et al. Timosaponin B-II ameliorates palmitate-induced insulin resistance and inflammation via IRS-1/PI3K/Akt and IKK/NF-κB pathways. Am J Chin Med. 2016;44(4):755–69. doi:10.1142/S0192415X16500415.

14. Pugliese G, Pricci F, Romeo G, Pugliese F, Mene P, Giannini S, et al. Upregulation of mesangial growth factor and extracellular matrix synthesis by advanced glycation end products via a receptor-mediated mechanism. Diabetes. 1997;46:1881–7. doi:10.2337/diab.46.11.1881.

15. Martinez-Castelao A, Navarro-Gonzalez JF, Gorriz JL, de Alvaro F. The concept and the epidemiology of diabetic nephropathy have changed in recent years. J Clin Med. 2015;4(6):1207–16. doi:10.3390/jcm4061207.

16. Reidy K, Kang HM, Hostetter T, Susztak K. Molecular mechanisms of diabetic kidney disease. J Clin Investig. 2014;124(6):2333–40. doi:10.1172/JCI72271.

17. Zoja C, Zanchi C, Benigni A. Key pathways in renal disease progression of experimental diabetes. Nephrol Dial Transplant. 2015;30(Suppl 4):54–9. doi:10.1093/ndt/gfv036.

18. Forbes JM, Cooper ME. Mechanisms of diabetic complications. Physiol Rev. 2013;93(1):137–88. doi:10.1152/physrev.00045.2011.

19. The Microvascular Complications Group of Diabetes Association of the Chinese Medical Association. The expert consensus of diabetic kidney disease prevention and control. Chin J Diabetes Mellit. 2014;6(11):792–801. doi:10.3760/cma.j.issn.1674-5809.2014.11.004.

20. Sun GD, Li CY, Cui WP, Guo QY, Dong CQ, Zou HB. Review of herbal traditional chinese medicine for the treatment of diabetic nephropathy. J Diabetes Res. 2016. doi:10.1155/2016/5749857 **(Article ID: 5749857)**.

21. Liu X, Liu L, Chen P, Zhou L, Zhang Y, Wu Y, et al. Clinical trials of traditional Chinese medicine in the treatment of diabetic nephropathy—a systematic review based on a subgroup analysis. J Ethnopharmacol. 2014;151(2):810–9. doi:10.1016/j.jep.2013.11.028.

22. Gao H, Sun W, Zhao J, et al. Tanshinones and diethyl blechnics with anti-inflammatory and anti-cancer activities from *Salvia miltiorrhiza* Bunge (Danshen). Sci Rep. 2016;6:33720. doi:10.1038/srep33720.

23. Hu L, Luan LJ, Cheng YY. Study on establishing the correlativity between fingerprint peaks and the effective fraction of traditional Chinese medicine prescription and its relevant herbs. Chin Pharm J. 2004;12(39):895–8. doi:10.3321/j.issn:1001-2494.2004.12.005.

24. Wang LL, Fu H, Li WW, Song FJ, Song YX, Yu Q, et al. Study of the effect of Euphorbia Herb on alleviating insulin resistance in type 2 diabetic model KK-Ay mice. China J Chin Materia Med. 2015;40(10):1994–9. doi:10.4268/cjcmm20151028

25. Shin SY, Kim CG, Jung YJ, et al. *Euphorbia humifusa* Willd exerts inhibition of breast cancer cell invasion and metastasis through inhibition of TNFα-induced MMP-9 expression. BMC Complement Altern Med. 2016;16(1):413. doi:10.1186/s12906-016-1404-6.

26. Luyen BT, Tai BH, Thao NP, et al. Anti-inflammatory components of *Euphorbia humifusa* Willd. Bioorg Med Chem Lett. 2014;24(8):1895–900. doi:10.1016/j.bmcl.2014.03.014.

27. Xu A, Wang H, Hoo RL, et al. Selective elevation of adiponectin production by the natural compounds derived from a medicinal herb alleviates insulin resistance and glucose intolerance in obese mice. Endocrinology. 2009;150(2):625–33. doi:10.1210/en.2008-0999.

28. Wang ZS, Xiong F, Xie XH, et al. Astragaloside IV attenuates proteinuria in streptozotocin-induced diabetic nephropathy via the inhibition of endoplasmic reticulum stress. BMC Nephrol. 2015;16:44. doi:10.1186/s12882-015-0031-7.

29. Yang Y, Li Y, Yin D, et al. *Coptis chinensis* polysaccharides inhibit advanced glycation end product formation. J Med Food. 2016;19(6):593–600. doi:10.1089/jmf.2015.3606.

30. Qin-Wei Z, Yong-Guang LI. Berberine attenuates myocardial ischemia reperfusion injury by suppressing the activation of PI3K/AKT signaling. Exp Ther Med. 2016;11(3):978–84. doi:10.3892/etm.2016.3018.

31. Wei Y, Han CS, Zhou J, Liu Y, Chen L, He RQ. D-ribose in glycation and protein aggregation. Biochim Biophys Acta. 2012;1820(4):488–94. doi:10.1016/j.bbagen.2012.01.005.

32. Mark AB, Poulsen MW, Andersen S, et al. Consumption of a diet low in advanced glycation end products for 4 weeks improves insulin sensitivity in overweight women. Diabetes Care. 2014;37:88–95.

33. Navarro-González JF, Mora-Fernández C. The role of inflammatory cytokines in diabetic nephropathy. J Am Soc Nephrol. 2008;19:433–42. doi:10.1681/ASN.2007091048.

34. Zhu Y, Pereira RO, O'Neill BT, et al. Cardiac PI3K-Akt impairs insulin-stimulated glucose uptake independent of mTORC1 and GLUT4 translocation. Mol Endocrinol. 2012;27(1):172–84. doi:10.1210/me.2012-1210.

35. Fukushima T, Arai T, Ariga-Nedachi M, et al. Insulin receptor substrates form high-molecular-mass complexes that modulate their availability to insulin/insulin-like growth factor-I receptor tyrosine kinases. Biochem Biophys Res Commun. 2011;404(3):767–73. doi:10.1016/j.bbrc.2010.12.045.

36. Feliers D, Duraisamy S, Faulkner JL, Duch J, Lee AV, Abboud HE, Choudhury GG, Kasinath BS. Activation of renal signaling pathways in db/db mice with type 2 diabetes. Kidney Int. 2001;60:495–504. doi:10.1046/j.1523-1755.2001.060002495.x.

37. Tejada T, Catanuto P, Ijaz A, Santos JV, Xia X, Sanchez P, Sanabria N, Lenz O, Elliot SJ, Fornoni A. Failure to phosphorylate AKT in podocytes from mice with early diabetic nephropathy promotes cell death. Kidney Int. 2008;73:1385–93. doi:10.1038/ki.2008.109.

38. Sanz AB, Sanchez-Niño MD, Ramos AM, Moreno JA, Santamaria B, Ruiz-Ortega M, Egido J, Ortiz A. NF-κB in renal inflammation. J Am Soc Nephrol. 2010;21:1254–62. doi:10.1681/ASN.2010020218.

39. Rane MJ, Song Y, Jin S, Barati MT, Wu R, Kausar H, Tan Y, Wang Y, Zhou G, Klein JB, et al. Interplay between Akt and p38 MAPK pathways in the regulation of renal tubular cell apoptosis associated with diabetic nephropathy. Am J Physiol Renal Physiol. 2010;298:49–61. doi:10.1152/ajprenal.00032.2009.

40. Ohga S, Shikata K, Yozai K, et al. Thiazolidinedione ameliorates renal injury in experimental diabetic rats through anti-inflammatory effects mediated by inhibition of NF-κB activation. Am J Physiol Renal Physiol. 2007;292(4):1141–50. doi:10.1152/ajprenal.00288.2005.

41. Lee FT, Cao Z, Long DM, et al. Interactions between angiotensin II and NF-κB-dependent pathways in modulating macrophage infiltration in experimental diabetic nephropathy. J Am Soc Nephrol. 2004;15:2139–51. doi:10.1097/01.ASN.0000135055.61833.A8.

42. Chow FY, Nikolic-Paterson DJ, Ozols E, Atkins RC, Tesch GH. Intercellular adhesion molecule-1 deficiency is protective against nephropathy in type 2 diabetic db/db mice. J Am Soc Nephrol. 2005;16:1711–22. doi:10.1681/ASN.2004070612.

43. Navarro JF, Mora-Fernández C. The role of TNF-α in diabetic nephropathy: pathogenic and therapeutic implications. Cytokine Growth Factor Rev. 2006;17(6):441–50. doi:10.1016/j.cytogfr.2006.09.011.

44. Aso Y, Yoshida N, Okumura K, et al. Coagulation and inflammation in overt diabetic nephropathy: association with hyperhomocysteinemia. Clin Chim Acta. 2004;348(1–2):139–45. doi:10.1016/j.cccn.2004.05.006.

45. Dalla M, Mussap M, Gallina P, et al. Acute-phase markers of inflammation and glomerular structure in patients with type 2 diabetes. J Am Soc Nephrol. 2005;16(Suppl 1):S78–82 **(PMID: 15938041)**.

46. Lim AK, Tesch GH. Inflammation in diabetic nephropathy. Mediat Inflamm. 2012;2012(5):146154. doi:10.1155/2012/146154.

Internationalization of Traditional/ Complementary Medicine products: market entry as medicine

Jiatong Li[1†], Jianfan Zhu[1†], Hao Hu[1], Joanna E. Harnett[2], Chi Ieong Lei[3], Ka Yin Chau[4], Ging Chan[1*] and Carolina Oi Lam Ung[1,2,3*] (ORCID)

Abstract

Internationalization of Traditional/Complementary Medicine (T&CM) products is important for initiating and sustaining developments in this field. Particularly for traditional Chinese medicines (TCMs), the global market continues to expand due to an interest in the potential clinical benefits of traditional approaches that are largely considered lower risk and lower cost than many conventional treatments. While the benefits of internationalization hold clear advantages for the business of T&CM products, keeping abreast of regulatory processes in different countries and regions that regularly revise market entry requirements is challenging. At present, the regulations of T&CM products are country specific and largely based on a risk-based assessment with a focus on protecting the consumer. To date, systematic analysis of these regulatory differences between countries and regions is limited. Publically available information about the legal requirements for the market entry of T&CM products were obtained from the relevant regulatory authority's websites for selected countries and regions (Macau-China, Hong Kong-China, Singapore, Australia, Canada, the European countries and the US). The market entry requirements in terms of quality, safety and efficacy of T&CM products for each country were analyzed and compared. Major differences were identified in the classification of T&CM products, market entry pathways, requirements of compliance with Good Manufacturing Practices; and level of evidence to demonstrate safety and efficacy based on historical use, non-clinical and clinical studies. Variations in the evaluation standards adopted by regulatory authorities pose a number of barriers and opportunities for the internationalization of T&CM products and have great implications for internationalization of TCMs from the sponsors' and the regulators' perspectives.

Keywords: Traditional Chinese medicines, Chinese patent medicines, Proprietary Chinese medicines, Traditional and Complementary Medicine, Registration, Internationalization, Quality, Safety, Efficacy

Background

Chinese Medicine is considered a traditional medicine practice and a popular approach to health care adopted by many individuals throughout the world [1–4]. It refers to both traditional Chinese medical practices and traditional Chinese medicines (TCMs) [4]. In China, an ageing population, increased prevalence of chronic conditions, a rising GDP, and accommodating medical insurance programs are all considered drivers of the a growing TCMs market [5]. This has prompted the Chinese government to identify Chinese Medicine as a priority and they have issued supportive measures to support Chinese Medicine in a strategic attempt to provide universal health coverage. The State Council in the 13th Five-Year Plan (2016–2020) aim to ensure all citizens are covered with health care by 2020 and that Chinese Medicine will be an important element in achieving that goal and further supported with scientific research, education and cultural influences [6]. In 1996, China introduced the

*Correspondence: gchan@umac.mo; carolinaung@umac.mo
†Jiatong Li and Jianfan Zhu share co-first authorship
[1] State Key Laboratory of Quality Research in Chinese Medicine, Institute of Chinese Medical Sciences, University of Macau, Taipa, Macao
Full list of author information is available at the end of the article

concept of "internationalization of TCMs" which had two main objectives: (1) to achieve the sustainable development of TCMs through fostering international trade and expanding TCMs in the global pharmaceutical market; and (2) to facilitate the development of appropriate regulatory systems that allows reasonable market entry under the protection of the local laws and regulations [7].

In the past 2 decades, advancements in research technologies has enabled a substantial body of research in TCMs to be conducted [8]. Research of TCMs supported with advancement in technology has better informed our understanding of TCMs, through the identification of active constituents and mechanisms of actions, and the identifying the forms and doses required to achieve positive therapeutic outcomes and minimize side effects and toxicity [9]. Despite this progress in developing the evidence base, the internationalization of TCMs has faced both intrinsic and extrinsic challenges. Take Chinese patent medicines (CPMs, referring to any TCMs formulated into a finished dosage form) as an example. Like any other types of TCMs, CPMs have uniquely complicated features [10]. They are used based on Chinese Medicine theory which cannot be fully explained or comprehended within the language or context of modern science. Maintaining a consistent constituent profile for many CPMs is difficult due to the lability of some constituents during the production process [8]. The quality control of CPMs is also difficult to sustain with challenges in accurate plant identification, cultivation, harvesting and the processing of herbal materials. Extrinsic factors including pesticide residues, and contamination with heavy metal and other unwanted chemical are regularly encountered during the production of CPMs. To deal with some of these challenges, the development of specifications for quality control of end products is under development. In contrast to pharmaceutical drugs, CPMs are inherently more complex to evaluate due to the complexity of multiple constituents and diverse therapeutic actions, and being less commonly the subject of large randomized controlled trials (RCTs).

One of the biggest extrinsic challenges facing the internationalization of TCMs is the registration/policy barriers [3, 5, 10–12]. Firstly, the terms used to refer TCMs varies from country to country. Depending on the culture, TCMs may be known as traditional medicines or complementary medicines (referred to the broad set of health care practices that are not part of the country's own tradition or conventional medicine but used in additional to conventional medicine) [13]. More than 90 countries and regions have national polices, laws and regulations for the marketing approval of Traditional and Complementary Medicine (T&CM) products including TCMs [3]. However, depending on the national situation,

the criteria for marketing T&CM products varies across the countries indicating that regulatory authorities have different standards and/or interpret evidence for quality, safety (risk) and efficacy, therefore the possible risk of using such products differently.

Some countries, as reported by the World Health Organization (WHO), have national policies on T&CM products and measures to ensure the quality, safety and efficacy of the T&CM products with a respect for the uniqueness of the traditional modality [4]. For some other countries, the regulatory authorities may include T&CM products into the scope of drug regulation, requiring that T&CM products meet the same set of stringent registration requirement as for other pharmaceutical products for marketing approval [14]. In some cases, authorities have additional regulations and guidelines to supplement the drug legislations to address issues related to the safe and appropriate use of T&CM products. There are also cases where T&CM products, when deprived of certain health claims, may be marketed as "non-medicine" entities. As a result, eligible T&CM products may be marketed as "medicine" only in some countries and areas depending on the regulations [3, 14].

With due respect to the therapeutic values of T&CM products (particularly TCMs), the identity of "medicine" in any regulatory systems is sought after during the course of internationalization. Currently, little research has been conducted to systemically analyze the regulation standards of T&CM products as a "medicine" entity across the countries. Therefore, the objective of this study was to compare the regulatory process for T&CM products using CPMs as products of interests among selected countries and regions. Specifically, the requirements for assessing quality, safety and efficacy for T&CM products classified as 'medicine' were analyzed. The findings of this study will be useful to inform a global perspective on the regulations of T&CM products, and specifically the internationalization strategies for TCMs.

Countries and regions including Macau-China, Hong Kong-China, Singapore, Australia, Canada, the European countries and the United States (US) were selected for this study based on the following considerations: (1) they have established regulatory practices that assess T&CM products as medicine; and (2) they represents a range of regulatory systems for T&CM products. A systematic qualitative analysis was conducted and included the review and interpretation of official legal documents related to the marketing of T&CM products. The publicly available documents were identified from the official website of the respective governing authorities of the selected countries and regions: Health Bureau, The Government of the Macau SAR (http://www.ssm.gov.mo) [15], Chinese Medicine Council, The Government of the

Hong Kong SAR (http://www.cmchk.org.hk/) [16]; Chinese Medicine Division, Department of Health, The Government of the Hong Kong SAR (http://www.cmd.gov.hk/html/eng/index.html) [17], Health Sciences Authority of Singapore (http://www.hsa.gov.sg) [18], The Therapeutic Goods Administration of Australia (http://www.tga.gov.au) [19], Health Canada (https://www.canada.ca/en/health-canada/services/drugs-health-products/natural-non-prescription.html) [20], European Medicines Agency (http://www.ema.europa.eu/ema/) [21], Medicines and Healthcare Products Regulation Agency of the UK (https://www.gov.uk/government/organisations/medicines-and-healthcare-products-regulatory-agency) [22], Medicines Evaluation Board of the Netherlands (https://english.cbg-meb.nl/) [23], and US Food and Drug Administration (https://www.fda.gov/AboutFDA/default.htm) [24]. The terminology used to describe the regulatory framework for marketing T&CM products and evidence requirements for demonstrating quality, safety and efficacy of the product in each regulatory system was extracted, interpreted and analyzed.

Macau-China

Macau is one of the two special administrative regions (SAR) of the People's Republic of China, located on the western bank of the Pearl River Delta in the southern Guangdong Province. Macau had been a Portuguese colony since the mid-16th century until the handover to China in 1999 when it became a SAR. The city exercises a high degree of autonomy under the principle of "One country, two systems" and has a local regulatory system for TCMs which covers CPMs. Due to Macau's deep-rooted connections with Portuguese-speaking countries, Macau is strategically placed for the facilitation of TCMs internationalization.

The regulation of CPMs and other TCMs is overseen by the Department of Pharmaceutical Affairs, Health Bureau [15]. At the moment, Macau does not have a registration system for CPMs. However, an alternative process is in place that takes reference of the regulatory decision made by the authority of the country of origin. Therefore a "sales pre-approval system" is adopted and supported and supplemented by a number of legislations, regulations and technical instructions. *Decreta-Lei n 53/94/M*, enacted in 1994, is the main legislation governing the licensing and operating conditions of companies involved in the import, export and wholesale of TCMs, as well as the TCMs pharmacies. Although it does not cover the sales pre-approval requirements of TCMs, it gives the legal definition of TCMs which refers to any medicines, plant or animal ingredients, or any materials extracted from these ingredients, used according to Chinese Medicine and Chinese pharmacology for the

prevention or treatment of diseases, or the regulation of bodily functions.

In order to better inform the safety and efficacy of TCMs, a "List of Traditional Chinese Medicine Ingredients for consumption in Macao SAR" was developed by the Health Bureau, which consists of three sub-lists: (1) Part I—toxic traditional Chinese materials (30 types); (2) Part II—common therapeutic traditional Chinese materials (562 types); and (3) Part III—Chinese medicinal materials that are also used as food (112 types). According to *Technical Instruction No 02/2005*, CPMs refers to a product which has a definite pharmaceutical form and composes of (1) one or more ingredients from Part I and/or Part II; (2) one or more ingredients from Part III and carry claims about treating, alleviating or preventing a disease or symptoms on the product label; or (3) formulated with one or more natural medicinal ingredients from plants, animals, or minerals under the guidance of traditional Chinese Medicine theory, and are applied to the human body for the purpose of treating, alleviating, or preventing diseases or symptoms thereof. Sales of CPMs are exclusive to TCMs pharmacies. For products composing ingredients from Part III but without any claims of disease/symptom treatment, alleviation or prevention, they will not be considered as CPMs and not subject to sales restrictions.

The local manufacturing capacity of CPMs is very limited. Most of the CPMs available in the market are imported products. According to the "sales pre-approval system", prior to importation of CPMs by licensed importers, certain documents must be submitted which includes a Drug Registration Certificate issued by the governing authority in the country of origin, certificates of analysis (including microbial and heavy metal contamination) for each batch of CPMs and the manufacturer's license to demonstrate the minimal quality, safety and efficacy assurance. The adherence to GMP is recommended but not mandated. The maximum limits of heavy metal and toxic elements allowed in CPMs are specified in *Despacho No. 10/SS/2013*. *Technical Instruction 01/2004* outlines the microbiological limits for different dosage forms of TCMs. When the CPMs originate from a country with a registration system in place, test reports of microbiological limits, heavy metals and toxic element content may be exempted. Labelling requirements stipulated in *Technical Instruction 04/2005* apply to all TCMs.

Additional regulations and guidelines are in place for specific TCMs as a safeguard. For TCMs which contain high-risk Chinese medicinal materials, either a banning system or a restricted-use system is in place. For instance, *Radix Aconiti Lateralis Preparata*, which is an ingredient from Part II of the "List of Traditional Chinese Medicine Ingredients applied in the Macao SAR", is recommended to be processed and used according to specific instructions with precautions due to the potential risks of toxicity as indicated in the official document "Instructions of using *Radix Aconiti Lateralis Preparata*". Similar instructions are also in place for *Rhaponticum uniflorum* (L.) DC. Due to the high risk of toxicity, according to the *Health Bureau Director Decision No. 6/SS/2004*, utilization, manufacture, importation and sales of *Caulis Aristolochiae Manshuriensis* (Guanmutong), *Radix Aristolochiae Fangchi* (Guangfangji) and *Radix Aristolochiae* (Qingmuxiang) are prohibited in Macau. Additional document requirements are applicable to a special CPMs, Niuhuang Jiedu Tablets, as stipulated in the *Chief Executive Decision No. 132/2001*. In order to minimize the risks associated with bovine-derived drugs, additional production and importation requirements of bovine-derived drugs are listed in the *Chief Executive Decision No. 120/2005* and *Technical Instruction No. 02/2001*.

As stated by the Macau SAR Government, the draft regulations for the registration scheme for TCMs have been prepared by the Health Bureau, and the relevant legislative processes are underway.

Hong Kong-China

In Hong Kong, traditional Chinese Medicine is widely accepted as playing a substantial role in the public healthcare sector. To tighten the regulation of Chinese Medicine practice and Chinese herbal medicines, with a view to safeguarding the public, the Chinese Medicine Ordinance (Cap.549) was enacted in 1999, and officiated the legal status of TCMs. Accordingly, proprietary Chinese medicines (pCms) must be registered by the Chinese Medicines Board of the Chinese Medicine Council of Hong Kong (the Council) before they can be legally marketed [16]. The Council is a statutory body established under the Chinese Medicine Ordinance responsible for formulating and implementing regulatory measures of TCMs. The Council receives professional and administrative support from the Chinese Medicine Division of the Department of Health which is responsible for the enforcement of Chinese Medicine Ordinance [17].

By definition in the Chinese Medicine Ordinance [25], pCms refer to any proprietary product: (a) composed solely of the following as active ingredients: (i) any Chinese herbal medicines, (ii) any materials of herbal, animal or mineral origin customarily used by the Chinese; or (iii) any medicines and materials referred to in subparagraphs (i) and (ii) respectively; (b) formulated in a finished dosage form; and (c) known or claimed to be used for the diagnosis, treatment, prevention or alleviation of any disease or any symptom of a disease in human beings, or for the regulation of the functional states of the human body. For registration purposes [26], CPMs from China may

fall into one of the three categories for pCms in Hong Kong: Established Medicines (pCms that are formulated according to an ancient prescription, a modified ancient prescription, a pharmacopoeia prescription or other prescriptions originated from the National Drug Standards of the People's Republic of China), Non-established Medicines (pCms that are used for the purpose of regulating the functional states of the human body or Single Chinese medicine granules) and New Medicines (pCms that contain newly discovered Chinese herb or new ingredient, or have new indication, altered route of administration or altered dose form).

Any of these three categories may be subject to registration approval: Group I, Group II and Group III. Different registration groups mainly differ in the registration requirements and documents related to the safety and efficacy of the pCms. Group I and Group II registration groups have different documentary requirements for the mutagenicity, carcinogenicity and reproductive toxicity of the pCms. Group III registration requirements are the most stringent as they requirement full documentation to demonstrate safety and efficacy of the New Medicines.

Quality

The documentary requirements to demonstrate the quality of pCms are the same for Group I, Group II and Group III registration dossier. For the quality evaluation of pCms, manufacturing method, physicochemical properties of crude drugs, product specification, method, and certificate of analysis are assessed. As for stability of the pCms, Group I registration dossier composes of either an accelerated stability test report or general stability test report, but for Group II and Group III registration dossier, a real-time stability test report is essential. The manufacturers must be licensed to manufacture pCms. They are required to comply with all aspects of GMP as stipulated by the Hong Kong Good Manufacturing Practice Guidelines for Proprietary Chinese Medicines.

Safety

In order to demonstrate the safety of pCms, all of the three registration groups require the submission of a certificate of analysis that reports the test results for heavy metals and toxic chemicals, pesticide residues and microbes, acute toxicity data, long-term toxicity data and a summary report outlining the product safety. For pCms to be administered on the skin or mucous membrane, additional requirements including reporting on the topical application toxicity is required for all three registration groups. For Group II and Group III registration groups, a report on the mutagenicity, carcinogenicity and reproductive toxicity are required for pCms which contain established or new ingredients that are or suspected to be cytotoxic, carcinogenic or mutagenic, or relates to pregnancy or, proven to have toxic effects on reproductive system.

Efficacy

In order to demonstrate the efficacy the pCms, information about interpretation and principle of formulating a prescription (except for pCms are single Chinese medicine granules), as well as reference materials on the efficacy are needed. The major discrepancies in the requirements in the thee registration groups lie on the principal pharmacodynamic study reports, general pharmacological study reports, and the clinical trial protocol and summary report which are essential only to Group III registration. In other words, pCms which are not classified as New Medicines may have the health claims or indications supported with referencing materials only.

Singapore

The Health Science Authority (HSA) is responsible for the drug regulatory work, including the issuance of the licenses of the importers, wholesalers, manufactures and re-packers of Chinese proprietary medicines (Cpm) [18]. It is a statutory board of Singapore Ministry of Health that aims to protect and advance national health and safety. The Chinese Proprietary Medicines Unit is one of the divisions of HSA specifically responsible for the administration of regulatory control and approval of Cpm. Cpm that is intended to be imported and sold must be registered for product listing approval. In accordance with Medicines (Traditional Medicines, Homoeopathic Medicines and other Substances) (Exemption) Order in Medicine Act 1985 (CAP 176), Cpm refers to any medicinal product (a) which has been manufactured into a specific dosage form and contains one or more active substances derived wholly from any plant, animal and/or mineral using active substances that are listed in the current edition of "A Dictionary of Chinese Pharmacy" or "The Chinese Herbal Medicine Materia Medica". Injectable products or medicinal products containing chemically-defined isolated constituent of any plant, animal or mineral, or any combination thereof are not considered Cpm. The number of the approved Cpm increased considerably from 2076 in 2011 to over 10,000 in 2013.

Quality

Cpm in Singapore can be manufactured either locally or overseas. In order to ensure the Cpm are consistently produced with the quality standards, GMP guideline must be complied by all Cpm manufacturers and assemblers in Singapore in line with the Health Products Act 2007 and the Medicines Act 1985. Singapore is a member of PIC/S, thereby the PIC/S Guide (Guide to Good

Manufacturing Practice for Medicinal Products Part I and PIC/S GMP Guide (related annexes) are implemented for manufacturing or assembling Cpm to assure the quality of those products. When assessing registration application for Cpm, audits will be conducted to the Cpm manufacturers and assemblers to ensure adequate quality and safety. Overseas Cpm manufacturers and assemblers also need to provide the GMP certificate (if any). According to the Medicines (Prohibition of Sale and Supply) Order, Cpm in question also needs to undergo tests for toxic heavy metals, microbial contamination, TSE (only for products containing materials derived from ruminants) and fermented substances (only for products containing fermented substance such as Cordyceps, Red Yeast Rice). Extra requirements apply if the Cpm contain substances listed in the Endangered Species (Import & Export) Act 2008. The test parameters and methods of the finished Cpm should be developed in consultation of the latest edition of the British Pharmacopoeia, Chinese Pharmacopoeia, European Pharmacopoeia, United States Pharmacopoeia, etc. especially for the toxic metals and microbial contamination.

Safety

A declaration stating the absence of any poisons as defined in the Poisons Act 1999 (Cap. 234) (i.e. Amygdalin, pangamic acid or its salts, danthron, suprofen or its salts and rhodamine B) is required for the import of Cpm. According to the same Act, the naturally occurring poisons in Cpm, i.e. ephedra alkaloids, lovastatin, sodium borate, lobelia alkaloids and aconite alkaloids, and those substances considered as high-risk (e.g. those with slimming claims) must be tested and verified to be within the acceptable limits at local or overseas laboratories with accredited testing methods. Test reports must be compiled within 2 years from the evaluation date of the Cpm.

Efficacy

These market entry requirements focus on the safety and quality of the Cpm rather than efficacy as no clinical efficacy data is required for the registration application. The indications can be claimed in terms of TCMs system of therapeutics, historical records and traditional uses outlined in pharmacopeias or with reference to A Dictionary of Chinese Pharmacy and The Chinese Herbal Medicine Materia Medica. However, there are restrictions on the claims as the labels, packaging materials and package inserts of Cpm cannot indicate any of the 19 diseases/conditions in accordance with those specified in the First Schedule of the Medicines Act. These conditions include blindness, cancer, cataract, drug addiction, deafness, diabetes, epilepsy or fits, hypertension, insanity, kidney diseases, leprosy, menstrual disorders, paralysis, tuberculosis, sexual function, infertility, impotency, frigidity and conception and pregnancy.

Australia

In Australia, Chinese medicine herbal products (equivalent to CPMs in this study), together with other herbal medicines, vitamin and mineral supplements, nutritional supplements, and other traditional remedies, fall into the category of complementary medicines (Therapeutic Goods Act 1989) [19, 27]. 'Complementary medicines' are regulated by the Therapeutic Goods Administration (TGA) and are defined as 'therapeutic goods consisting wholly or principally of one or more designated active ingredients, each of which has a clearly established identity and (a) a traditional use or (b) any other use prescribed in the regulations.' The TGA has the responsibility for administering the federal Therapeutic Goods Act 1989, which provides the national framework for the regulation of therapeutic goods, including complementary medicines in Australia.

The regulatory framework for complementary medicines is based on a risk based system. The TGA currently takes a two-tiered approach based on risk: (1) Listed medicines or (2) Registered medicines. To be approved as a listed complementary medicine, the product is restricted to certain low risk ingredients in acceptable amounts that are permitted for use by the TGA and can only make indications for health maintenance and enhancement and/or for non-serious self-limiting conditions. Registered medicines can carry more specific therapeutic claims and/or contain a herb with a higher risk profile. In addition, registered medicines are independently assessed for quality, safety and efficacy. Registered CPMs on the Australian Register for Therapeutic Goods (ARTG) are currently outnumbered by listed CPMS. In 2016/2017, 1581 new complementary medicine products were listed on the ARTG as compared to 34 new registered complementary medicines. Listed medicines carry a unique AUST L number.

Quality

The same level of quality assurance mechanisms in terms of GMP requirements apply to all the products in the two-tiered regulatory system of Australia. As such, all the medicines regulated by the authority must be made in TGA approved manufacturing facilities. The TGA requires compliance with the Pharmaceutical Inspection Co-operation Scheme (PIC/s) Code of Good Manufacturing Practice for medicinal substances and provides interpretive guidelines for the particular requirements of complementary medicines on supplier qualification, stability testing, product quality reviews, sampling and testing, and process validation. Australian

and overseas manufacturers are assessed prior to supply of complementary medicines either through regular on-site inspections or, for manufacturers with evidence of GMP compliance available from recognized regulators, compliance verifications (paper-based assessments). Assessment conducted by the TGA includes, but is not limited to, information about the manufacturing process and controls. This requires evidence of the validation of processes, testing reference materials, test procedures and the results for the analysis of product strength, purity and stability. An application for a GMP clearance by an off-shore manufacturer may be made on the basis they are regulated by the manufacturing country's governing authority and are recognized by the Mutual Recognition Agreement.

Safety

Listed complementary medicines must only contain ingredients that have been approved by the TGA as being of low risk, with limits on quantities where relevant, and must not make high-level claims. For new and innovative ingredients, it is required to apply for the evaluation of the substance for its inclusion on the TGA's list of permissible ingredients. This process may take approximately 1–2 years for the application to be evaluated which is a significant investment of time and money. The number of new listed medicine ingredients in 2016/2017 was 79, most of which are ingredients that were made available for excipient use in specific circumstances in listed medicines [28]. The TGA makes an assessment about the safety of an ingredient as it relates to therapeutic claim being made and associated safety warnings.

Efficacy

The TGA regulates the claims about efficacy on the basis of the two tiered system as described above. For claims like "treats, cures or prevents a disease" or "treats vitamin/mineral deficiencies", it is considered a high level efficacy claim and the product would require being assessed for a registered status i.e. AUSTR#. Whereas lower level claims of efficacy like "health enhancement", "reduce the frequency of an event", "assists in management of a disease", "health maintenance", or "vitamin or mineral supplementation" are considered medium or general level. In this case, it is the responsibility of the sponsor to ensure they hold evidence to support such claims. There are no requirements for the sponsors to provide efficacy data to the TGA prior to or during the pre-marketing stage but the sponsors must certify that efficacy data is available on request. Traditional evidence is also taken into consideration for low risk claims of efficacy and is based on respected Pharmacopoeias, Materia Medica and herbal monographs documenting human use of over three generations, equating to approximately 75 years.

Recent development

It has been proposed that the current two-tiered regulatory framework is further developed to include a third or middle tier [29]. This will involve introducing a new product assessment pathway that will sit between the existing listed medicine (low risk) and registered medicine (high risk). Furthermore, a list of permitted indications which must be used by the lowest risk complementary medicines will be developed to further restrict the claims used and allowing sponsors to claim that their medicine has been independently assessed by the TGA for efficacy and that the product has undergone pre-market evaluation by the TGA. This regulatory reform aims to incentivize innovation within the complementary medicines sector. This presents an opportunity for data protection and market exclusivity if a product claims are based on new scientific evidence. In addition the proposed reform will improve transparency regarding the evidence for efficacy and allow consumers to make better informed decisions about the use of complementary medicines in their health care [27, 28].

Canada

In Canada, T&CM products may be considered and regulated as Natural Health Products (NHPs) and are regulated by the Health Canada (HC) according to the Food and Drugs Act and the Natural Health Product Regulations [20]. Although there is no implication of "medicine" nature by the name, NHPs, by definition, refers to herbal or medicines of traditional medicine practices intended for use in the diagnosis, treatment, mitigation or prevention of a disease, disorder, or abnormal physical state or the symptoms thereof. According to the Natural and Non-prescription Health Products Directorate (NNHPD), NHPs are restricted to oral, topical, or sublingual routes of administration. The intended uses of NHPs encompass a wide range of claims ranging from maintaining or promoting health to diagnosis, treatment, prevention, and symptomatic relief of some diseases. Compared to the regulatory systems mentioned above, the health claims for NHPs in Canada are allowed to a greater extent and yet overlaps with mild claims of other non-medicine entities such as dietary supplements.

There are two subcategories to the NHPs claims: traditional health claims and modern health claims. TCMs, for instance, which contain multiple ingredients and are used based on a single cultural system of traditional medicine, Chinese Medicine, are considered NHPs with traditional health claims. For other T&CM products whereby the intended uses are not based on any one

traditional medicine system, such claims are considered modern health claims. NHPs, when authorized for sale in Canada, are issued a product license and a Natural Product Number (NPN).

Quality

The quality of NHPs focus primarily on characterization, identification, quantification and purity. For this, quality requirements including specific standards for chemicals, processed ingredients and extracts; compliance with the Good Agricultural and Collections Practices Guidelines; assay of the botanical ingredients, isolates or synthetic duplicates, live microorganisms and enzymes; microbial contaminants testing; chemical contaminant testing such as heavy metals, mycotoxins, solvent residents, pesticides, antibiotics, etc. are mandated in the "Quality of Natural Health Products Guide" published by the HC. Sites responsible for conducting manufacturing, importing, packaging or other activities in Canada must comply with the Good Manufacturing Practice standards in order to obtain a site license.

Safety

The NNHPD has developed a collection monographs which can be used to support the safety and efficacy of a NHPs. These monographs are a comprehensive review of scientific data and information about a medicinal ingredient or multiple ingredients with certain health claims, containing all the information required for marketing approval. The "Traditional Chinse Medicine Ingredients" monograph, for instance, contains more than 300 TCM ingredients with indications of the specific conditions which the ingredients can be used for. NHPs conforming any of the monographs are likely to see expedition of the authorization process and consistency in the labeling of the products in the market. The evidence requirements for demonstrating safety depend greatly on the product's intended uses indicated in the product claims. For medicinal ingredients, "benefit to risk" assessment forms part of the registration dossier which listed out the potential risks of the products in terms of severity and seriousness, probability or frequency, and other inherent risks of each of the ingredients. For non-medicinal ingredients, safety evidence may also be required. In either cases, whenever uncertainties about the risks are noted, additional evidence may be requested to allow thorough assessment by the authority,

Efficacy

The therapeutic claims of NHPs must be supported with sufficient controlled clinical evidence of the ingredients generated from studies of which the protocols authorized by the Nonprescription and Natural Health Products

Directorate. While monographs may be used to support "traditional health claims" or "modern health claims", "traditional health claims" must be supported with evidence of at least 50 consecutive years of traditional use within a cultural health system or paradigm. Further to the safety document requirements, based on the three risk categories described in the "Management of Product Licence Applications (PLA) for Natural Health products" policy, different levels of evidence for premarket risk evaluation are required: Class I category refers to "low risk" products and attestation to a monograph is required to obtain marketing approval; Class II category refers to "medium risk" products and marketing application must be supported partly with the monograph and additional information such as phase 2 clinical trials to justify the novel features of the product; and Class III refers to "high risk" products whereby available information is limited and high level of evidence such as data from controlled clinical trials are required to obtain marketing approval. In cases of comparative therapeutic claims, head-to head clinical trials may also be required.

European countries

In European countries such as the UK and the Netherlands [22, 23, 30, 31], the marketing pathways of T&CM products can be either traditional herbal registration (THR) or marketing authorization (MA) via simplified registration for T&CM products as stipulated in the European Directive 2004/24/EC serving as an amendment of Directive 2001/83/EC. Either THR or MA mandates the marketing of T&CM products to be granted based on legislation applicable for all EU countries in the European Economic Area. However, the directive also sees slight variations when implemented in each country as an adaption to the country's own law [32–35].

The UK use the term herbal medicine to describe T&CM products including CPMs. According to the Human Medicines Regulation (2012), a herbal medicine refers to a product if the active ingredients are herbal substances (reduced or powdered, a tincture, an extract, an essential oil, an expressed juice or a processed exudate) and/or herbal preparations. On the other hand, T&CM products can be referred to herbal medicinal products in the Netherlands. By definition, herbal medicinal products, also referred to as phyto-therapeutic products, are medicinal products whose active ingredients contain exclusively plants, parts of plants or plant materials or combinations thereof, in a crude or processed form. Herbal medicines in the UK are regulated by the Medicines & Healthcare products Regulatory Agency (MHRA) whereas traditional herbal medicinal products in the Netherlands are regulated by the Medicines Evaluation Board.

Unlike the strict centralized marketing authorization applications of the medicines from European Medicines Agency, the decentralized simplified registration procedure which was officially promulgated in 2004 offers a simplified application pathway especially for the T&CM products with a longstanding historical use (used for at least 30 years, including at least 15 years within the EU), and hence provides an opportunity for T&CM products to enter the EU market in an expedited manner. The UK introduced the THR system for T&CM products relatively recently based on the EU Directives. In the Netherlands, presently only two traditional herbal medicinal products from China have been successfully licensed via these simplified procedures and marketed (*Diao Xin Xue Kang capsules* from Di Ao Group in 2012 and Sichuan, *and Danshen Capsules* from Tasly Holding Group in 2016) [36, 37]. In UK, the Phynova Cold and Flu Relief Powder for Oral Solution was the first CPMs approved to be marketed in the UK market as a herbal medicine to treat colds.

Quality

Quality of the medicinal products is considered the most important element in the simplified procedures of the application process. The authority requires the submission of evidence of GMP and QC tests for evidence of quality. The quality of the herbal substances, herbal preparations and finished product are required for inspection. For the quality of herbal substance, the Guideline on Good Agricultural and Collection Practice for Starting Materials of Herbal Origin (EMEA/HMPC/24618/2005) must be followed to assure the quality of the herbal substances from the cultivation in the wild, harvest and collection, to primary processing. In particular, detailed descriptions of the plants from which the herbal substances originate are required: botanical characteristics, phytochemical characteristics, toxic constituents, biological/geographical variation, cultivation/harvesting/ drying conditions, and pre/post-harvest chemical treatments. The manufacturing site and process must comply with the GMP standards. For the quality of finished products, the manufacturing process, in-process controls and linking specifications, water content, impurities, toxic (heavy) metals microbial limits, mycotoxins (aflatoxins, ochratoxin A), pesticide, fumigation agents will be carefully assessed. The test methods and parameters must be developed with reference to the European Pharmacopoeia or specific monographs. Assays for the contents of the constituents of known therapeutic activity or active markers of the herbal preparations should be determined. Quality tests specific to the dosage form are also applicable.

Safety

Unlike the full marketing authorization procedure, the simplified procedures do not require the submission of the full documentation on safety test and clinical trials to demonstrate safety and efficacy. Bibliographic data or toxicological tests to demonstrate safety may be acceptable. According to Article 16c (1) d of Directive 2001/83, safety should be justified by "a bibliographic review of safety data together with an expert report". The prerequisite of longstanding use of the products has substantiated the safety of the traditional herbal medicinal products without the need of safety test. However, in case there are concerns about the safety of a traditional herbal medicinal product, the marketing authorization holder will have to provide comprehensive data upon the request from the authority.

To provide further guidance on safety assurance of the traditional herbal medicinal products, a number of scientific guidelines have been introduced such as EMEA/HMPC/138139/2005 (allergenicity issues of soya and peanut protein containing products). The establishment of Community herbal monographs or entries to the Community "List of herbal substances, preparations or combinations thereof for use in traditional herbal medicinal products" can be used to identify the new safety aspects of the listed plants, and it has been advised to consult other guidance documents which describe chemical, toxicological, pharmacological and pharmacokinetic properties of the medicinal substances, and provide usage instructions for special products such as herbal medicinal products containing concerning ingredients such as asarone, estragole, methyleugenol, Aristolochia species, etc. To continuously monitor the safety of herbal medicine in UK, a doctor-directed statistical survey is in place to collect post-marketing data about the herbal medicines. Actions of product recall will be triggered should there be high level of safety risk detected.

Efficacy

As defined in the Directive 2001/83/EC, traditional use is justified by bibliographical or expert evidence showing that the medicinal product in question, or a corresponding product has been in medicinal use throughout a period of at least 30 years preceding the date of the application, including at least 15 years within the European Union countries. With the justification of traditional use, the registration procedure can be simpler and less costly without requiring the clinical efficacy data. The documentation of traditional use, if deemed sufficient, will be used as the primary evidence for its safety in specific conditions and plausible efficacy and pharmacological effects. The European herbal handbooks, sales figures and documented use in the Netherlands, as well as France,

Belgium and United Kingdom can be used as reference for indicated uses in EU. Moreover, due to inherent complexity of herbal active substance and lack of clinical data, indications for herbal medicines are restricted based on evidence of long standing use evidence in THR (Permitted indications under the Directive on Traditional Herbal Medicinal Products). More specifically, permitted claims of efficacy are only suitable for minor self-limit medical claim such as symptomatic relief cold, minor self-limiting bacterial infections, minor upper respiratory infections and other minor disease. The medical claims about treating more serious diseases such as cardiovascular disease that require proven medical treatments are restricted and require strong clinical data to support their safety and efficacy.

The US

In the US, there is no category established specifically for T&CM products. For products containing the same herbal ingredients, they may be regulated as drug, cosmetic or device depending on the route of administration, dosage form, formulation, evidence about the safety and the intended use. As a general rule, any product that contains plant materials, algae, macroscopic fungi, or combinations thereof, and is intended to be used as drug (to treat, prevent or mitigate a medical condition) is referred to botanical drug [24]. As far as structure functions claims are concerned, although these are allowed for drugs and dietary supplements, only drugs are allowed to have the structure function claims made specific to certain diseases or other medical conditions. According to the Dietary Supplement Health and Education Act (DSHEA), dietary supplements are not allowed to make any disease-related claims, neither explicitly not implicitly. Therefore, for the purpose of this study, DSHEA and other regulations bound to dietary supplements are not included for analysis.

T&CM products including TCMs containing herbal ingredients and carrying therapeutic claims are mostly considered as botanical drug product and may be marketed under either an over-the-counter drug monograph or an approved new drug application (NDA). For a botanical drug substance to be included in an OTC monograph, the safety and effectiveness must be well-established and supported with sufficient published data generated from adequate and well-controlled clinical studies. For T&CM products which do not have marketing history in the US or a foreign country, do not meet the criteria for inclusion in the OTC drug monograph based on available evidence of safety and effectiveness, nor carry a health claim appropriate for non-prescription use, the botanical drug product must undergo the NDA to obtain marketing approval from the FDA. NDA must be supported with substantial evidence of quality, safety and efficacy derived from adequate and well-controlled clinical studies. The recommendations on quality, non-clinical, clinical, and other unique aspects of botanical drug development are provided in the Guidance for Industry: Botanical Drug Development [38] and are summarized in the following.

Quality

Botanical raw material must confirm to Good Agricultural and Collection Practices (GACPs). In terms of compliance with pharmaceutical Good Manufacturing Practices, the same requirements hold for botanical drugs and other drug products in the US as required by the assessment process of NDA. Details information about the botanical raw material control (e.g., agricultural practice and collection), identification of the medicinal plants ingredients (e.g. morphology, macroscopic and microscopic analysis, chemical analysis, or DNA fingerprinting) may be required depending on the intended use. Demonstration of consistency in terms of identity, purity and impurities such as heavy metals, aflatoxins and pesticides) of the raw materials, ingredients, and products will also be assessed.

Safety

For non-prescription botanical drug, "absolute" safety is warranted meaning the benefits based on intended use outweighs any risks to the users despite in the absence of any professional guidance. For botanical drugs to be considered as "new" drugs, they are not generally recognized as safe and effective under the conditions prescribed, recommended, or suggested on the labeling. They are required to undergo the regulatory pathway of an Investigational New Drug (IND). Despite any long history of use, additional safety data from non-clinical and clinical stages, may be required to justify the proposed indication, route of administration or target populations. For the non-clinical safety assessment, the results of important in vitro assays in human and/or nonhuman animal tissue should be included when pharmacology/toxicology is evaluated, which includes carcinogenicity and reproductive toxicology studies. Clinical pharmacology trials are also needed to be included for ensuring the consistency of safety use, providing the findings from the pharmacokinetics and pharmacodynamics data, and exposure–response relationships which support dose selection and or dose modification. Overall exposure at appropriate doses/durations and demographics of target populations, explorations for dose response, special animal and/or in vitro testing, routine clinical testing, metabolic, clearance, and interaction workup and evaluation

for potential adverse events for similar drugs in drug class must also be accessed.

Efficacy

The evidence requirements demonstrating efficacy for botanical "new" drugs are the same as for other drugs. Substantial evidence consisting of adequate and well-controlled investigations including clinical investigations by qualified experts with scientific training and experiences is required. Consistency in safety and efficacy from batch to batch will also be assessed to address the inherent challenges of most botanical drugs. The FDA adopted a "totality-of-evidence" approach taking into consideration of the unique limitations of botanical drug products in terms of characterization of the ingredients and the end-products. Well-controlled raw materials, robust manufacturing process and quality controls including comprehensive fingerprints, clinically relevant bioassay, an multiple-dose and multiple batch clinical data are required to demonstrate the quality consistency, and thus therapeutic consistency of a botanical drug product from batch-to-batch. Up to date, the FDA has approved two NDAs for prescription botanical new drugs, both of which were complex botanical mixtures designed to become new therapies and yet met the legal requirements for drugs in the U.S.

Discussion

Policy standards regarding market entry of T&CM products vary greatly from one country/region to another [39, 40]. This is a significant factor determining the extent that these products can be internationalized. In this study, CPMs from China were used as the product of interest to systematically compare the market entry requirements of T&CM products in Macau-China, Hong Kong-China, Singapore, Australia, Canada, the European countries and the US. It has been shown that, across the countries and regions studied, the governing authorities' rulings on market entry of T&CM products including CPMs is primarily focused on the quality, safety and efficacy of the products. As presented in Table 1, substantial variations were identified among countries in the classification of the products, registration pathways and the document requirements for the registration dossier. This can be explained by the different interpretations of the risks and benefits of T&CM products, compounded by the unique features including complex composition and multiple mechanisms of actions [41–43].

With regards to quality, the minimal international consensus is that all T&CM products must meet certain quality standards that demonstrate authentication, identification and chemical composition of the products. All the countries/regions reviewed in this study require

Table 1 Regulation about Chinese patent medicines from China in selected countries and regions

| | Countries/regions | | | | | European countries | | |
	Macau SAR	Hong Kong SAR	Singapore	Australia	Canada	The Netherland	UK	US
Possible terminologies for CPMs from China in the country/region	Chinese patent medicines	Proprietary Chinese medicines	Chinese proprietary medicines	Complementary medicines (listed) Complementary medicines (registered)	Natural Health Products	Traditional herbal medicinal products	Herbal medicine	Botanical drug product
Definition	"A product which has a definite pharmaceutical form and composes of (1) one or more ingredients from Part I and/or Part II of "List of Traditional Chinese Medicine Ingredients for consumption in Macao SAR", or (2) one or more ingredients from Part III of "List of Traditional Chinese Medicine Ingredients for consumption in Macao SAR" and carry claims about treating, alleviating or preventing a disease or symptoms on the product label"	"Refer to any proprietary products: (a) composed solely of the following ingredients: (i) any Chinese herbal medicines, (ii) any materials of herbal, animal or mineral origin customarily used by the Chinese; or (iii) any medicines and materials referred to in sub-paragraphs (i) and (ii) respectively; (b) formulated in a finished dosage form; and (c) known or claimed to be used for the diagnosis, treatment, prevention or alleviation of any disease or any symptom of a disease in human beings, or for the regulation of the functional states of the human body	"Any medicinal product (a) which has been manufactured into a specific dosage forms and contains one or more active substances derived wholly from any plant, animal and/or mineral using active substances that are listed in the current edition of "A Dictionary of Chinese Pharmacy," or "The Chinese Herbal Medicine Materia Medica"	"Therapeutic goods consisting wholly or principally of one or more designated active ingredients, each of which has a clearly established identity and (a) a traditional use or (b) any other use prescribed in the regulations"	"Naturally occurring substances that are used to restore or maintain good health, often made from plants, but can also be made from animals, microorganisms and marine sources"	"Also referred to as phyto-therapeutic products, medicinal products whose active ingredients contain exclusively plants, parts of plants or plant materials or combinations thereof, in crude or processed form; used for at least 30 years, including at least 15 years within the EU"	"A product is a herbal medicine if the active ingredients are herbal substances and/or herbal preparations only"	"A botanical drug product is intended for use in the diagnosis, cure, mitigation, treatment or prevention of disease in humans, which consists of vegetable materials (plant materials, algae, macroscopic fungi, or combinations thereof)"

Table 1 (continued)

	Countries/regions					European countries		US
	Macau SAR	Hong Kong SAR	Singapore	Australia	Canada	The Netherland	UK	
Regulatory authority	Department of Pharmaceutical Affairs, Health Bureau	Chinese Medicine Council of Hong Kong (CMCHK) Chinese Medicine Division of the Department of Health	Health Science Authority (HSA)	Therapeutic Goods Administration (TGA)	Health Canada (HC)	Medicine Evaluation Board (MEB)	Medicines and Healthcare products Regulatory Agency (MHRA)	US Food & Drug Administration (FDA)
Major legal documents	Decreta-Lei n 53/94/M Decision No. 7/ SS/2004 Technical Instruction No. 02/2005	Chinese Medicine Ordinance July 1999 Section 119—registration 3rd Dec 2010	Medicine Act	Therapeutic Goods Act 1989	Natural Health Products Regulations of the Food and Drugs Act	Traditional Herbal Medicinal Products Directive (2004/24/EC); the Dutch Medicines Act; and relative guidelines	Directive 2004/24/EC for THR (Traditional Herbal Registration) Directive 2001/83/EC for MA conventional)	Federal Food, Drug, and Cosmetic Act
Requirements to demonstrate quality	Manufacturer's license, GMP standards recommended but not mandated	GMP standards and QC tests	GMP standards PIC/S guide	GMP standards PIC/S guide and QC tests	GMP standards and QC tests	GMP standards and QC tests	GMP standards and QC tests	GMP standards and QC tests
Requirements to demonstrate safety	Drug Registration Certificate issued by the competent authority in the country of manufacture or country of origin Limits of heavy metal content (Technical Instruction No. 2/2003) Microbiological limits (Technical Instruction No. 1/2004) Additional requirements for CPMs containing bovine-derived ingredients (Chief Executive Decision No. 120/2005 and Technical Instruction No. 02/2001)	Heavy metals and toxic elements test report, pesticide residues test report, microbial limit test report, acute toxicity test report, long-term toxicity test report, and the summary report on product safety documents	Declaration on the absence of any poisons as defined in the Poisons Act (Cap. 234); Endorsement by manufacturer that product does not contain any Western drugs or active synthetic substances; TSE undertaking for products containing materials derived from ruminants; Information about for fermented substance for products containing fermented substance(s)	Contains ingredients on the TGA's list of permissible ingredients only for listed complementary medicines Toxicological tests for registered complementary medicines	Conforming any of the monographs, "benefit to risk" assessment, additional evidence whenever needed	Bibliographic review of safety data together with an expert report"; no need for safety test; clinical safety data (supportive)	Bibliographic data for THR Toxicological tests for MA	Non-clinical safety assessment: pharmacology/toxicology tests; clinical pharmacology trials

Table 1 (continued)

Countries/regions	Macau SAR	Hong Kong SAR	Singapore	Australia	Canada	European countries		US
						The Netherland	UK	
Requirements to demonstrate efficacy		The materials of Interpretation and principle of formulating a prescription (excluding granules), reference materials on products efficacy and the summary report on product efficacy documents Extra documents (principal pharmacodynamic studies report, general pharmacological studies, clinical trial protocol and summary report) maybe required	TCM system of therapeutics, historical records and traditional uses in pharmacopeias or with reference to A Dictionary of Chinese Pharmacy and The Chinese Herbal Medicine Materia Medic	Traditional evidence and available efficacy data for listed complementary medicines Clinical studies for registered complementary medicines	Attestation to a monograph for Class I category (low risk); monograph and additional information such as phase 2 clinical trials for Class II category ("medium risk"); high level of evidence from controlled clinical trials for Class III category ("high risk")	Justification of traditional use [long tradition of use for at least 30 years (including 15 years in the EU)]; bibliographical or expert evidence Clinical studies for MA	Restricted indications and long tradition of use for at least 30 years (including 15 years in the EU) for THR Clinical studies for MA	Individual studies/clinical trials

manufacturing sites of T&CM products to follow GMP and/or PTC/s Guide, thereby, ensuring that the products are of consistent quality and are safe for use by consumers. Special emphasis on quality and therapeutic consistency from batch to batch was noted in some regulatory systems such as the FDA. The only exception to these quality requirements is Macau where there is no registration system for TCMs in place. In terms of safety, some countries/regions hold a list of ingredients considered safe for use, or require the attestation to the published monographs as a minimum, whilst others simply have a banned-for-use system. Most of the countries/regions in this study clearly specify the need for certificates of analysis that include tests for microbial, pesticide residues, and heavy metals and other harmful substances in all T&CM products. Respect and recognition of historical traditional use and knowledge is an important consideration adopted by most of the countries studied in their regulatory framework for supporting the efficacy and safety of T&CM products.

While marketing as "medicine" is important to preserve the therapeutic values of T&CM products, there is a growing trend to market eligible T&CM products as "non-medicine" products such as health care products, functional food or food supplements, depending on the terminology adopted in different countries. For TCMs supported with a long history and high prevalence of use, the international market potential and expansion into the non-drug category represents a promising route for TCMs to achieve sustainable development through internationalization. Criteria of market entry of T&CM products (with TCMs in particular) as non-drug entities will be worth exploring to further inform potential strategies for sustainable development of T&CM products and the internationalization of TCMs in future studies.

There were some limitations to this study. The sample size of the countries/regions included in this study is insufficient to fully demonstrate the possible variations of the current regulatory approach towards T&CM products around the world. However, the regulatory systems analyzed in this study does represent a wide spectrum of regulatory enforcement. The degree of variations observed in this study does raise awareness about one of the biggest challenges facing the internationalization of TCMs.

Conclusion

The market entry requirements for T&CM products for Macau-China, Hong Kong-China, Singapore, Australia, Canada, the European countries and the US were analyzed and compared with the major differences highlighted. The different evaluation standards adopted by these regulatory authorities pose a number of barriers

and opportunities for the internationalization of T&CM products and have great implications for internationalization of TCMs. In order to assure the quality, safety and efficacy of T&CM products, it is important for the sponsors and the regulators to follow closely the developments evolving around the regulation of these products.

Abbreviations
TCMs: traditional Chinese medicines; CPMs: Chinese patent medicines; RCTs: randomized controlled trials; T&CM: Traditional and Complementary Medicine; WHO: World Health Organization; SAR: special administrative region; pCms: Proprietary Chinese medicines; ARTG: Australian Register for Therapeutic Goods; HSA: Health Science Authority; Cpm: Chinese proprietary medicines; THR: traditional herbal registration; MA: marketing authorization; MHRA: Medicines & Healthcare products Regulatory Agency; MEB: Medicines Evaluation Board; GMP: Good Manufacturing Practices.

Authors' contributions
JTL, JFZ, HH, GC, COLU conceived, designed the study and drafted the manuscript. LCI, KYC and JH were major contributors in reviewing the manuscript. Based on the contributions, JTL and JFZ are listed as the first authors while GC and COLU are the correspondence. All authors read and approved the final manuscript.

Author details
[1] State Key Laboratory of Quality Research in Chinese Medicine, Institute of Chinese Medical Sciences, University of Macau, Taipa, Macao. [2] The University of Sydney School of Pharmacy, Faculty of Medicine and Health, The University of Sydney, Sydney, Australia. [3] Pharmaceutical Society of Macau, Taipa, Macau. [4] City University of Macau, Taipa, Macau.

Acknowledgements
Not applicable.

Competing interests
The authors declare that they have no competing interests.

Consent for publication
Not applicable.

Funding
Not applicable.

References
1. Zhong F. The current development status and prospect on Chinese medicine health foods. China Health Ind. 2014;11(10):187–8.
2. Nirali J, Shankar M. Global market analysis of herbal drug formulations. Int J Ayu Pharm Chem. 2016;4(1):59–65.
3. World Health Organization. Legal status of traditional medicine and complementary/alternative medicine: a worldwide review. 2001. http://apps.who.int/medicinedocs/pdf/h2943e/h2943e.pdf. Accessed 28 Jan 2018.
4. World Health Organization. WHO Traditional Medicine Strategy 2014–2023. 2013. http://apps.who.int/iris/bitstream/10665/92455/3/9789245506096_chi.pdf?ua=1. Accessed 28 Jan 2018.
5. Lin AX, Chan G, Hu Y, Ouyang D, Ung CO, Shi L, Hu H. Internationalization of traditional Chinese medicine: Current international market, internationalization challenges and prospective suggestions. Chin Med. 2018;13(1):9. https://doi.org/10.1186/s13020-018-0167-z.
6. The State Council, The People's Republic of China, The Health Care Plan in the 13th Five-Year Plan. 2017. http://www.gov.cn/zhengce/content/2017-01/10/content_5158488.htm. Assessed 16 Sept 2018.

7. Wu G. International opportunities and challenges of Chinese medicine. Co-op Econ Sci. 2015;11:83–4.

8. Wu WY, Hou JJ, Long HL, Yang WZ, Liang J, Guo DA. TCM-based new drug discovery and development in China. Chin J Nat Med. 2014;12(4):0241–50.

9. Jiang M, Yang J, Zhang C, Liu B, Chan K, Cao H, Lu A. Clinical studies with traditional Chinese medicine in the past decade and future research and development. Planta Med. 2010;76(17):2048–64.

10. Zhang H, Wang N, Zheng L. The influence of acceding to WTO on progress of modernization of Chinese materia medica in the 21st century. China Pharm. 2000;11(2):51–3.

11. Zhang L. Discuss on the export barriers and countermeasures of traditional Chinese medicine. Chin Bus Trade. 2011;7:204–5.

12. Alostad A, Steinke D, Schafheutle E. International comparison of five herbal medicine registration systems to inform regulation development: United Kingdom, Germany, United States of America, United Arab Emirates and Kingdom of Bahrain. Pharmaceut Med. 2018;32(1):39–49.

13. World Health Organization. Traditional, complementary and integrative medicine. 2018. http://www.who.int/traditional-complementary-integrative-medicine/about/en. Accessed 16 Sept 2018.

14. World Health Organization. National policy on traditional medicine and regulation of herbal medicines—report of a WHO Global Survey. 2005. http://apps.who.int/medicinedocs/en/d/Js7916e/. Accessed 16 Sept 2018.

15. Health Bureau, The Government of the Macau SAR. 2018. http://www.ssm.gov.mo. Accessed 16 Sept 2018.

16. Chinese Medicine Council of Hong Kong SAR Government. 2018. http://www.cmchk.org.hk/. Accessed 16 Sept 2018.

17. Chinese Medicine Division, Department of Health, The Government of the Hong Kong SAR. 2018. http://www.cmd.gov.hk/html/eng/index.html. Accessed 16 Sept 2018.

18. Health Sciences Authority of Singapore. 2018. http://www.hsa.gov.sg. Accessed 16 Sept 2018.

19. Therapeutic Goods Administration of Australia. 2018. http://www.tga.gov.au. Accessed 16 Sept 2018.

20. Health Canada. https://www.canada.ca/en/health-canada/services/drugs-health-products/natural-non-prescription.html. Accessed 16 Sept 2018.

21. European Medicines Agency. http://www.ema.europa.eu/ema/. Accessed 16 Sept 2018.

22. Medicines Evaluation Board of the Netherlands. 2018. https://english.cbg-meb.nl/. Accessed 16 Sept 2018.

23. Medicines and Healthcare Products Regulation Agency of the UK. 2018. https://www.gov.uk/government/organisations/medicines-and-healthcare-products-regulatory-agency. Accessed 16 Sept 2018.

24. US Food and Drug Administration. https://www.fda.gov/AboutFDA/default.htm. Accessed 16 Sept 2018.

25. Hong Kong e-Legislation. The Government of Hong Kong SAR Government. Chinese Medicine Ordinance 1999. 1999. https://www.elegislation.gov.hk/hk/cap549. Accessed 16 Sept 2018.

26. Chinese Medicine Council of The Government of Hong Kong SAR. Registration of proprietary Chinese Medicines Application Handbook. 2018. http://www.cmchk.org.hk/pcm/pdf/reg_handbook_e.pdf. Accessed 16 Sept 2018.

27. Graham D. Regulation of proprietary traditional Chinese medicines in Australia. Chin J Nat Med. 2017;15(1):12–4.

28. Therapeutic Goods Administration of Australia. Therapeutic Goods Administration Annual Performance Statistics Report July 2016 to June 2017. 2017. https://www.tga.gov.au/sites/default/files/annual-performance-statistics-report-july-2016-june-2017.pdf. Accessed 16 Sept 2018.

29. Therapeutic Goods Administration of Australia. Consultation: reforms to the regulatory framework for complementary medicines. 2017. https://www.tga.gov.au/sites/default/files/consultation-reforms-regulatory-framework-complementary-medicines-assessment-pathways.pdf. Accessed 16 Sept 2018.

30. European Medicines Agency. Human regulatory—herbal medicinal products. 2018. http://www.ema.europa.eu/ema/index.jsp?curl=pages/regulation/general/general_content_000208.jsp. Accessed 16 Sept 2018.

31. European Medicines Agency. Herbal products—multidisciplinary: herbal medicinal products. 2018. http://www.ema.europa.eu/ema/index.jsp?curl=pages/regulation/general/general_content_000497.jsp&mid=WC0b01ac0580033a9b. Accessed 16 Sept 2018.

32. Kroes B. The legal framework governing the quality of (traditional) herbal medicinal products in the European Union. Eur J Integr Med. 2014;6(6):701.

33. van Galen E. Traditional herbal medicines worldwide, from reappraisal to assessment in Europe. J Ethnopharmacol. 2014;158:498–502.

34. Cranz H, Anquez-Traxler C. TradReg 2013: regulation of herbal and traditional medicinal products—European and global strategies—international symposium. J Ethnopharmacol. 2014;158:495–7.

35. Wiesener S, Falkenberg T, Hegyi G, Hök J, di Sarsina PR, Fønnebø V. Legal status and regulation of complementary and alternative medicine in Europe. Forsch Komplementmed. 2012;19(Suppl. 2):29–36.

36. Medicine Evaluation Board, The Netherlands. Diao Xin Xue Kang, capsules for oral use SU BioMedicine B.V., The Netherlands. 2012. https://db.cbg-meb.nl/Pars/h102142.pdf. Accessed 16 Sept 2018.

37. Tasly Phar. International Co., Ltd. Tasly Danshen Capsule was certified by CBG-MEB as a herbal drug. 2016. https://www.taslyint.com/show-86-506-1.html. Accessed 16 Sept 2018.

38. US Food and Drug Administration. Guidance for industry: botanical drug development. https://www.fda.gov/downloads/Drugs/GuidanceComplianceRegulatoryInformation/Guidances/UCM458484.pdf. Accessed 16 Sept 2018.

39. Fan TP, Deal G, Koo HL, et al. Future development of global regulations of Chinese herbal products. J Ethnopharmacol. 2012;140:568–86.

40. Wiesner J, Knöss W. Future visions for traditional and herbal medicinal products—a global practice for evaluation and regulation? J Ethnopharmacol. 2014;158:516–8.

41. Shen J, Wang K, Hu Q, Su J, Zhang W. Establishment quality control method of traditional Chinese medicine based on efficacy and safety. Modernization Trad Chin Med Materia Med. 2014;3:502–5.

42. Fleischer T, Su Y, Lin S. How do government regulations influence the ability to practice Chinese herbal medicine in western countries. J Ethnopharmacol. 2017;196:104–9.

43. Ajazuddin SS. Legal regulations of complementary and alternative medicines in different countries. Pharmacogn Rev. 2012;6(12):154.

8

Pharmacokinetics of Chinese medicines: strategies and perspectives

Ru Yan[1,2*], Ying Yang[1] and Yijia Chen[1]

Abstract

The modernization and internationalization of Chinese medicines (CMs) are hampered by increasing concerns on the safety and the efficacy. Pharmacokinetic (PK) study is indispensable to establish concentration-activity/toxicity relationship and facilitate target identification and new drug discovery from CMs. To cope with tremendous challenges rooted from chemical complexity of CMs, the classic PK strategies have evolved rapidly from PK study focusing on marker/main drug components to PK-PD correlation study adopting metabolomics approaches to characterize associations between disposition of global drug-related components and host metabolic network shifts. However, the majority of PK studies of CMs have adopted the approaches tailored for western medicines and focused on the systemic exposures of drug-related components, most of which were found to be too low to account for the holistic benefits of CMs. With an area under concentration-time curve- or activity-weighted approach, integral PK attempts to understand the PK–PD relevance with the integrated PK profile of multiple co-existing structural analogs (prototyes/metabolites). Cellular PK–PD complements traditional PK–PD when drug targets localize inside the cells, instead of at the surface of cell membrane or extracellular space. Considering the validated clinical benefits of CMs, reverse pharmacology-based reverse PK strategy was proposed to facilitate target identification and new drug discovery. Recently, gut microbiota have demonstrated multifaceted roles in drug efficacy/toxicity. In traditional oral intake, the presystemic interactions of CMs with gut microbiota seem inevitable, which can contribute to the holistic benefits of CMs through biotransforming CMs components, acting as the peripheral target, and regulating host drug disposition. Hence, we propose a global PK–PD approach which includes the presystemic interaction of CMs with gut microbiota and combines omics with physiologically based pharmacokinetic modeling to offer a comprehensive understanding of the PK–PD relationship of CMs. Moreover, validated clinical benefits of CMs and poor translational potential of animal PK data urge more research efforts in human PK study.

Keywords: Chinese medicines, Pharmacokinetic strategy, Pharmacokinetics–pharmacodynamics relevance, Gut microbiota, Global pharmacokinetics–pharmacodynamics

Background

Pharmacokinetics (PK) characterizes drug disposition in the body by studying the time-course of drug concentrations in biofluids and cell/tissue/organ samples and factors governing its absorption, distribution, metabolism and excretion (ADME) processes. PK study is a prerequisite to establish relevance of the activities/clinical benefits to the chemical contents. The information obtained is crucial for lead identification and optimization in drug discovery and dosage regimen design and adjustment in clinical practice. Comparing to the PK study of western drugs which are generally single ingredient with known target, PK characterization of Chinese medicines (CMs) is fraught with tremendous challenges rooted from their chemical complexity (over hundreds ingredients of diverse chemical types in a single constituent herb or a compound formula, wide concentration ranges, distinct physiochemical properties, etc.), undefined targets (multi-target), and unclear mechanisms of actions. These difficulties are further superimposed by interactions with biological systems (different ADME profiles) as well as

*Correspondence: rl-1003@163.com
[1] State Key Laboratory of Quality Research in Chinese Medicine, Institute of Chinese Medical Sciences, University of Macau, Taipa, Macao, China
Full list of author information is available at the end of the article

those among co-existing ingredients. Unraveling PK profiles of CMs requires adopting strategies distinct from that for western medicines, not only coping with the chemical complexity but also treating the CMs and the compound formula as a whole to provide a holistic and mechanistic understanding of the therapeutic benefits of CMs. Recent rapid development in analytical techniques, systems biology, biochemical pharmacology, as well as multivariate data analysis approaches has promoted the evolution of PK strategies to deal with these challenges.

The fascination of CMs lies in the art of constructing a prescription with multiple CMs which act as "monarch", "minister", "assistant" and "messenger", respectively, to enhance efficacy or reduce toxicity in the intended disease therapy. Mechanistic understanding of the compatibility in this ancient combination therapy guided by the traditional Chinese medicine (TCM) principles is another focus and challenge and has been attempted from pharmaceutical, pharmacodynamic (PD) and pharmacokinetic perspectives [1–3]. The PK interactions among constitute herbs of herb pairs or compound formulas were recently reviewed somewhere else [2, 3]. Majority of the work evaluated the toxicity-reducing [4] or efficacy-enhancing [5] effects of combinatorial use through comparing the PK parameters of a few marker compounds or main components of main constitute herbs in the formula with those dosed in the single herb or pure form. Due to the chemical complexity, complex interactions with biological systems as well as the unavailability of authentic compounds and suitable analytical platform in many laboratories, studies on global chemical changes and kinetic shifts are scarce. It was found that absorptive interactions account for two-thirds (32 from 48 reports) of the PK interactions of CMs [2]. This may be ascribed to the oral intake tradition of CMs which makes intestinal absorption the obligatory path for the constituents to reach the blood circulation. P-glycoprotein (P-gp), the major efflux transporter expressed along the intestine, is the major contributor of the absorptive interactions. For example, Schisandra lignans extract is a strong P-gp inhibitor. Single-dose and multi-dose of this extract could increase the plasma exposure (AUC value) of ginsenoside Rb2, Rc and Rd significantly without affecting terminal elimination half-time [6].

PK study is also imperative to predict interactions of CMs with concomitantly dosed western medicines, unravel the PK interactions among co-existing components, validate the different processing methods, as well as guide formulation design. Co-prescription of western medicines and CMs is very common in China. Herbal products are also increasingly incorporated into western health care owing to an increasing awareness of their health-promoting effects and perceived less side effects.

Concomitant use of CMs may mimic, magnify, oppose the effect or even cause toxicity of drugs through PD and/or PK mechanisms. Herb-drug interactions (HDI) have received wide attentions in the past decades. For examples, Radix *Puerariae lobatae* (Gegen), not *Salvia miltiorrhiza* radix (Danshen), offsets the anticoagulant effects of warfarin by accelerating cytochrome P450 (CYP)-mediated metabolism of warfarin, increasing activity and expression of vitamin K epoxide reductase while decreasing those of thrombomodulin in rats [7]. Rhein, the major bioactive anthraquinone of many CMs including rhubarb and *Polygonum multiflorum*, could influence the PK and PD of clozapine to alleviate clozapine-induced constipation [8]. Rhein acyl glucuronide, the major metabolite of rhein in human, significantly decreased the transport of methotrexate mediated by human organic anion transporters (hOAT1, hOAT3) in vitro and inhibited excretion and hence increased methotrexate exposure in rats [9]. Non-toxic dosage of ginsenoside Rh2 enhanced the antibacterial effect of ciprofloxacin towards *Staphylococcus aureus* strains through inhibiting NorA-mediated efflux and promoting ciprofloxacin accumulation in the bacteria [10]. Saikosaponin D did not alter the plasma PK of doxorubicin but enhanced the anticancer efficacy by inhibiting tumor growth and P-gp expression [11]. Recent reviews summarized pharmacokinetic HDI studies and offered insights into the mechanisms, consequences, conflicting results and reasons [12, 13]. So far, majority HDI data were obtained from in vitro studies or animal models, requiring extensive efforts to strengthen the translational potential.

The increasing applications of CMs in disease therapy, the tremendous interests in drug discovery from CMs and the growing concerns on the clinical outcome consistency and safety urgently need the development of suitable PK strategies to dissect the multi-component multi-target holistic clinical effects of CMs. This review offers an overview of the evolving PK strategies and provides a perspective on the future PK study of CMs.

Strategies for PK study of CMs

People believe that, similar to western medicines, CMs also need to meet the following two requirements to elicit effects: significant exposure and suitable retention time in the target organ or tissue. The chemical complexity, unknown targets, combinatorial use tradition guided by esoteric principles (TCM theory), long history of clinical applications of CMs make them distinguishable from western medicines which are usually chemically simple and have definite targets, requesting distinct PK strategies that can establish concentration-activity/toxicity relevance to allow mechanistic insights into the efficacy/toxicity of CMs. However, despite these inherent differences, the majority of previous PK studies of CMs adopted the same strategy tailored for western medicines which usually focus on the systemic exposure (drug levels in blood) of drugs. To cope with the chemical complexity of CMs, major efforts of the PK study of CMs have been laid on selecting representative components as well as improving sensitivity of analytical methods for PK measurement. Thus, considerable research efforts have been devoted to identify or predict in vivo available components of CMs using in silico, in vitro or in vivo approaches and describe their plasma PK profiles [14]. The strategies have evolved from single PK study to PK–PD correlation study, with analytes spanning from quality control chemical marker, major herbal components, selected PK markers, multi-components, to global drug-related components profiling together with host metabolic network shifts adopting metabolomics approaches [15, 16].

Chemical marker/major component/multi-component PK using classic strategy

The diverse chemical types and the wide concentration ranges of the components in CMs demand excellent analytical capability in both accurate structural identification and sensitive quantitation. Relying on the availability of analytical instruments and standard compounds, earlier PK study of CMs usually investigate the in vivo fates of single components (in pure or mixed form), and gradually assemble the findings into a whole picture. Quality control marker compounds documented in China Pharmacopoeia and/or major components in the herbs were usually chosen for PK studies because the authentic compounds were more easily obtained. They were either dosed as pure compound or in mixed form (extract or fraction) or both to obtain the PK parameters and identify PK interactions with co-existing components. For example, PK of ferulic acid was depicted in normal and blood-deficiency-syndrome rats receiving Fo-Shou-San which is composed of Danggui and Chuanxiong [17]. PK of Z-butylidenephthalide, a bioactive phthalide present in a significantly low quantity in medicinal herb Chuanxiong Rhizoma, was investigated in rats using a Chuanxiong extract, a fraction containing Z-butylidenephthalide and the standard compound, and found that the major compound coexisting in the herb ligustilide can form Z-butylidenephthalide, making the latter one of the major circulating components after oral intake of the herbal extract [18]. However, each CM usually contains hundreds of components of a variety of chemical types which possess diverse physiochemical properties, and as consequences, the PK profile of a single or a few compounds may not describe the PK profiles well or show good relevance to PD measurements of the CMs. Moreover, the

chemical markers documented for quality control may not be the abundant or specific in the herb. For example, tetramethylpyrazine and ferulic acid, the two marker compounds used for Chuanxiong Rhizoma and related products, are traceful (< 0.1 μg/g crude drug) [19] and ubiquitously distributed in plant kingdom [20], respectively. Moreover, the major component in the herb may show low systemic exposure due to poor absorption or extensive elimination [21]. The rapid advances in analytical techniques, in particular the LC–MS/MS techniques (Qtrap, QqQ, QTOF, etc.) allow simultaneously identifying and/or monitoring dynamics of multiple components using classic strategy which generally requires prior knowledge of herbal chemistry and is time-consuming [22]. Simultaneously monitoring PK of multiple parent compounds and metabolites (i.e., poly-PK) has only been reported in a handful of studies [23, 24]. For examples, 142 metabolites were identified from bile and plasma samples from rats receiving Danggui Buxue Decoction [25]; more than 60 metabolites were identified and PK profiles of 55 were obtained for metabolites of licorice [26, 27].

Identification of surrogate PK markers

Simultaneous determination of PK of multiple components in herbal medicines is technically challenging due to the wide concentration ranges, complex interactions with the body/among the co-existing components in ADME processes, as well as diverse elimination dynamics in vivo. Although poly-PK using classic strategy allows simultaneous determination of multi-components, most of the in vivo available components may not show ideal PK properties due to the following reasons: (1) too low systemic exposures in blood to contribute to the efficacy of CMs (PK–PD disconnection), (2) poor dose-exposure relevance (blood exposure does not change proportionally with dose), (3) the metabolites, not the prototypes from CMs, reaching considerable exposure, (4) exposure not relevant to efficacy/safety, (5) unclear targeting tissues/organs/molecules and mechanisms of actions. Moreover, it usually has poor high-throughput (time-consuming), relies on availability of analytical instrument and chemical standards, thus, is not practicable to be applied in other laboratories or readily translated to industry or clinical practice to improve the efficacy, safety, and quality consistency of CMs. In the past decade, Chuan Li's group has carried out poly-PK studies of many CMs using integrated in vivo–in vitro–in silico approaches [14, 28–30]. The authors advocated the use of surrogate "pharmacokinetic markers" to describe PK profiles of CMs. The surrogate PK markers (prototypes and/or metabolites) of CMs should meet the following requirements at the same time [31]: (1) exhibit significant exposure, (2) show good dose-exposure correlation, (3) exhibit good correlation or prediction of drug efficacy, safety, or factors that affect exposure. For examples, tanshinol from Danshen showed dose-dependent systemic exposure (as judged from the area under concentration–time (AUC) value) and significant correlation between the urinary recovery and its plasma AUC. Oral or sublingual intake of cardiotonic pills which contain Danshen as the major constitute herb showed no differences in absorption and bioavailability of tanshinol. As such, tanshinol was proposed as a promising PK marker for the cardiotonic pills [28]. In rats receiving oral administration of *Panax notoginseng* (Sanqi) extract in rats, ginsenosides Ra3, Rb1 and Rd were identified as PK markers for systemic exposure of the herb due to long-circulating and high exposure levels of the three ginsenosides resulted from their slow biliary excretion, low metabolism, and slow renal excretion [29]. However, in healthy volunteers taking Sanqi extract orally, plasma 20(*S*)-protopanaxadiol (PPD) and 20(*S*)-protopanaxatriol (PPT) were considered as more suitable PK markers which reflect the individual microbial activity, dynamics and inter-individual differences in plasma exposures of respective oxidized metabolites, the major circulating forms of ginsenosides in the blood circulation [30]. Very interestingly, poly-PK study of Danhong injection [Danshen and Carthami Flos (Honghua)] suggested that a combination of the daily dosage with the elimination half-life determines whether a component can serve as an appropriate PK marker to reflect systemic exposure of CM injections [30]. When given alone, berberine showed very low concentration in blood and failed to prevent anaphylaxis reactions in peanut allergic mice, while the intestinal absorption of berberine was significantly enhanced by co-existing components in an herbal formula, leading to remarkable increase of berberine bioavailability and consequent the prevention of peanut anaphylaxis. Thus, berberine was identified as the chemical and PK marker of the compound formula [32].

Integrated PK of CMs

The chemical components of CMs usually fall into several main different chemical types, each containing tens of compounds bearing a same skeleton with varied substituents/conformations. In vivo metabolism of these structural analogs will produce even more metabolites keeping the same skeleton. Owing to the structural similarity, compounds and their metabolites of the same chemical type possibly exhibit similar biological activities with potency varied to different extents. For each single compound, it may not be detectable or the exposure is too low to allow significant contribution to the clinical outcomes. However, when administered together in a mixture (the CM fraction or extract), these components

may produce additive/synergistic effect, contributing significantly to the holistic actions of CMs. Thus, comparing to PK of single compound or individual PK data of multiple effective components, integrated PK property of CMs can offer more comprehensive understanding of the exposure-efficacy/toxicity relevance. Cai's team detected 191 metabolites of taxifolinb, a ubiquitous bioactive constituent of foods and herbs, in rats receiving 3-day consecutive oral dosing of the compound. These metabolites exhibited a wide distribution in the body and more than 60 metabolites were predicted to have similar targets as the prototype does, suggesting that these metabolites which keep the same pharmacophore as the bioactive parent compound may act on the same targets in vivo and hence produce additive effects [33]. An AUC-weighting integral PK approach was proposed for evaluating the holistic PK characteristics of multiple components bearing the same core structure. Xie et al. found that the integral PK of Schisandra lignans obtained using an AUC-weighting approach correlated well with their hepatoprotective effect and the hepatic injury biomarkers [34]. Considering that different substituents of structural analogs may affect efficacy/toxicity to different extents, Wang and colleagues compared the integrated toxicokinetics of major diosbulbins after oral administration of *Dioscorea bulbifera* rhizome extract using AUC- and IC50-weighting approaches, respectively. The IC50-weighting integrated plasma concentration–time profile showed better correlation with the hepatic injury measurement total bile acids [35], suggesting bioactivity of structural analogs as weighting coefficient offer better integrated kinetics than the exposure data.

Classic PK–PD study of CMs

Many CMs have well-documented therapeutic benefits and multiple pharmacological activities but elusive targets and mechanisms. The PK profiles of CMs and the PK–PD relationship are key to identify real active components (prototype or metabolite), unravel efficacy/toxicity mechanism of CMs and reveal PK compatibility in a compound formula and predict HDI. An increasing number of studies have included both PK and PD measurements into the efficacy/safety assessment of CMs. Ren et al. found that three chemical types (flavonoids, iridoids, alkaloids) of Huang-Lian-Jie-Du decoction, a compound formula consisting of Coptidis Rhizoma, Scutellaria Radix, Phellodendri Cortex, Gardenia Fruit, and notable for heat-dispersing and detoxifying effects, showed distinct modes of anti-inflammatory activity by determining the concentration-effect relevance between the plasma PK profiles of 41 drug-related components (prototypes and metabolites) and the levels of 7 cytokines in lipid polysaccharides-induced rat inflammation model

[36]. A transdermal patch containing glycyrrhetinic acid and paeoniflorin, two primary active compounds in peony-liquorice decoction, exerted a synergistic constant analgesic effect (number of writhes) on dysmenorrhea model mice with a single dose. The pharmacological response versus plasma concentration plot of glycyrrhetinic acid revealed a counterclockwise hysteresis loop [37]. Ginsenoside Rb1 coupled with schisandrin delayed the elimination of ginsenoside Rg1 and the three compounds in a mixture displayed a synergistic effect on NO release [38]. Blood–brain barrier opening property of borneol was well explained by measuring the expression and function of efflux transporters (Mdr1a, Mdr1b and Mrp1) and the distribution of borneol in different brain regions (cortex, hippocampus, hypothalamus and striatum) [39]. These classic PK–PD studies usually focus on one or a few main prototypes/metabolites of the CMs and determined limited biochemical measurements or clinical endpoints which may be not relevant to the biological responses directly elicited at the target organ/tissue. The multi-component multi-target working mode of CMs requires a comprehensive insight into the mechanisms through global analysis of the dynamic changes of CMs and biological responses.

Metabolomics is a technology originally developed to inform what did happen to a biological system (organism, organ, cell, etc.) through comprehensive unbias analysis of small molecules in a biofluid, cell, organ or organism. It is a promising approach to address the challenges in poly-PK and classic PK–PD of CMs when coupled with multivariate statistical tools. Metabolomics can not only decode biological network perturbation to a stimulus by identifying the most significantly affected endogenous metabolites and their metabolic pathways, but also resolve the relationships between endogenous and xenobiotic metabolic processes [40]. Metabolomics has been successfully applied to numerous xenobiotic metabolism studies and to predict drug efficacy and drug-related side effect through the knowledge of metabotype (known as pharmacometabolomics) [41]. Wei Jia and co-workers proposed a poly-PK strategy using metabolomics approach [15], which was recently applied to a study of Huangqi Decoction (consisting of Astragali Radix and Glycyrrhizae Radix) in healthy Chinese volunteers [16]. A total of 56 prototypes of Huangqi Decoction and 292 metabolites were identified and the concentrations of the herbal metabolites were correlated with 166 endogenous metabolites [16], providing an unprecedented level of insight into the mechanism of action for Huangqi Decoction. Undoubtedly, the tremendous analytical capability enables metabolomics a powerful tool in unraveling the mechanisms under the efficacy/toxicity of CMs through analysis of the metabolome to ascertain the perturbations resulting from CMs intervention.

Cellular PK–PD to address PK–PD disconnection of CMs

Poor plasma concentration-efficacy/toxicity relevance is a common issue for CMs. Most drug-related components (prototype or metabolite) showed poor blood exposure owing to low abundance in the original herb or unsatisfactory in vivo ADME property, thus is believed to be impossible to contribute to efficacy/toxicity of CMs. For instances, ginsenoside Rb1 and Rg1 showed extremely low oral bioavailability due to poor absorption, extensive microbial deglycosylation, biliary excretion, acidic degradation [29, 42]. They showed definite neuroprotective effects, while were hardly detected in brain [43]. The cerebral exposure levels to flavonols and terpene lactones in rats receiving oral administration of GBE50 (a standardized extract of *Ginkgo biloba* leaves) are much lower than the concentrations required to elicit neuroprotective effects in vitro [44]. Although showing a very low systemic exposure (< 10 ng/mL), berberine has demonstrated remarkable anti-diabetic effects in vivo in animals and human which could not be explained by activity observed in vitro at a much higher concentration. To address the PK–PD disconnection of CMs, a cellular PK–PD strategy was proposed which determines the cellular drug accumulation and intracellular drug distribution and correlates the cellular dynamic drug disposition with its intracellular target binding and efficacy [45]. Cellular drug exposure is believed to be more relevant to drug efficacy than plasma drug exposure when drug targets localize inside the cells, instead of at the surface of cell membrane or extracellular space, and hence, cellular PK–PD is complementary to traditional PK in unraveling the action mechanisms of CMs. Cellular PK–PD of some compounds originated from CMs have been summarized in a recent review article [45]. Acidotropic trapping, binding to intracellular sites and carrier-mediated import and export transport systems, contribute to steady-state intracellular of accumulation quinine, an antimalarial component from Cinchona Bark [46]. Comparison of the localization signals of the fluorescent artemisinin derivative with organelle specific dyes revealed that endoplasmic reticulum is the main site of artemisinin accumulation [47]. Anti-oxidation effects of herbal flavonoids kaempferol, galangin correlated to stronger autofluorescence in the nucleus than cytoplasm in hepatocytes visualized by confocal laser scanning fluorescence microscope [48]. In H_2O_2 treated neuronal culture, quercetin pretreatment prevented neuronal death from the oxidant exposure although intracellular quercetin or related metabolites were undetectable, suggesting alternative mechanisms of quercetin neuroprotection beyond its long-established ROS scavenging properties [49]. The cellular PK has also been successfully applied to explain the anti-cancer effects of paclitaxel from *Taxus brevifolia* and camptothecin from *Camptotheca acuminate*. Comparing to imaging techniques, in particular fluorescence imaging, cell fraction approach provides an alternative method for drugs having no fluorescence, offering not only intracellular distribution but also accurate drug concentrations [50]. The determinants of drug subcellular distribution include active transport, metabolic inactivation, pH partitioning, electrochemical gradient, and target binding. Among these factors, drug transporters and enzymes are still the key determinants that govern the amount of drugs entering the target intracellular organelle and the corresponding drug efficacy. Particle size is one of the determinants for formulations. Anti-cancer potency and cellular uptake of curcumin micellar nanoparticles are directly correlated to particle size and the smaller nanoparticles are more potent and localized in both nucleus and cytoplasm [51].

Reverse pharmacokinetics to aid target identification and drug discovery

Acknowledgement of the multifactorial property in the etiology of many chronic diseases has facilitated multi-target drug discovery [52]. A recent review of new molecular entities (NMEs) approved by the US FDA between 2000 and 2015 revealed an increasing number of multi-target NME [53]. Multi-target therapy can be achieved through combinatorial use of existing drugs with known different targets. On the other hand, CMs have shown validated clinical benefits from a long history of use. Many compounds from CMs, such as berberine, curcumin, ginsenosides, and baicalein, have been confirmed to possess diverse pharmacological activities in vivo. Thus, CMs offer an attractive and promising source for discovery of pleiotropic single molecule or multi-component preparations for multi-target therapy. However, the targeting tissues, organs or molecules and mechanisms of CMs are largely unclear. The pleiotropic compounds from CMs generally have low oral bioavailability and could not provide significant exposure and sufficient retention time at the diseased sites which are considered as prerequisites to elicit the pharmacological effects in modern drug discovery. To cope with these challenges in reverse pharmacology guided drug discovery from CMs, a new concept 'reverse pharmacokinetics' was comprehensively introduced by Hao et al. [54]. Comparing to conventional drug discovery which evaluate PK desirability of compounds with a definite target to assess their druggability, reverse PK assesses metabolism and PK of CMs and

integrate these knowledge with validated clinical benefits/pharmacological activities to aid target identification and mechanistic understanding of the holistic outcomes (efficacy or toxicity), define exposure-efficacy/toxicity relevance, and facilitate discovery of NMEs or multi-target multi-component drugs. Increasing evidence support complex manifestations of many chronic diseases via multiple signaling pathways at remote sites other than directly targeting on the pathological nodes. For example, the neuroprotective effect of ginsenosides could not be well explained by a direct action due to their extremely low brain exposure, rather, it can be attributed to their immunomodulatory and anti-inflammatory activities in the periphery which can interplay with central nervous system and is functionally implicated in the pathogenic development of many brain diseases [43]. Promising evidence suggests that berberine can boost intestinal health partially through balancing gut microbial structure [55], which is in line with its poor plasma exposure, but high exposure and long retention in gut. In contrast, the high hepatic extraction and distribution (70-fold increase in liver) [56] correlates well with the hypolipidemic effect of berberine probably through targeting hepatic low density lipoprotein receptors. Moreover, the reverse PK information can also help design and selection of physiologically relevant in vitro models to evaluate the molecular mechanisms, facilitate efficient drug discovery from CMs, as well as justify personalized medicine in TCM practice.

Perspectives

In the past decades, numerous PK studies of CMs have been reported owning to a wider recognition of the crucial roles of PK in mechanistic understanding of the multi-component, multi-target holistic benefits of CMs and new drug discovery from CMs. The PK strategies for CMs also evolve faster to meet the growing demands. The ultimate goal is to establish PK–PD relevance of CMs to ensure suitable quality control, pertinent pharmacological evaluation and consistent clinical output, which undoubtedly is crucial but tremendously challenging due to chemical complexity by nature, undefined targets, complex interactions among co-existing compounds and combinatorial use tradition guided by obscure TCM theory, disconnection between disease site and target site, etc. The rapid advances in systems biology, omics, multivariate data analysis approaches allow us to translate the holistic clinical benefits into modern scientific data and bring our understanding of the mystery of the old tradition to unprecedented depths. The future research efforts may consider improving the PK–PD relevance study in the following two aspects.

Global PK–PD to address presystemic interplay of CMs with gut microbiota

The recent rapid advancement of our knowledge in the physiological, pathological and pharmacological roles of gut microbiota in human also promote an in-depth understanding of its multifaceted roles in drug metabolism, efficacy and toxicity [57] and the holistic therapeutic benefits of CMs [58]. The enormous gut microbial metabolic capability has been well recognized from numerous reports in the past decades, which is demonstrated to be complementary to host drug metabolizing system by generating more permeable metabolites to facilitate intestinal absorption/enterohepatic recirculation, leading to enhanced systemic exposure [59]. Gut microbiota catalyze a variety of reactions of structurally diverse compounds, in particular hydrolysis of glycosides from natural products [60, 61]. The typical example is ginsenosides which undergo stepwise deglycosylation in gut lumen [42] and the more permeable secondary metabolites or aglycones showed higher exposures [14, 29] and were believed to mainly account for the pharmacological activities of ginseng. The chemical complexity and the traditional oral route also favor manipulation of intestinal homeostasis by some ingredients of CMs. An increasing evidence support the beneficial effects of CMs on gut microbiota structure, intestinal inflammation, intestinal epithelial barrier function (P-gp, tight junction, etc.). For instances, Mori Cortex extract can alleviate colitis-like symptoms in dextran sulfate sodium-induced colitis rat model through reinstating microbial balance, regulating inflammatory responses, and up-regulating intestinal P-gp which involved a direct effect and a gut microbiota-mediated mechanisms [22]. It has been well recognized that gut microbiota play a pivotal role in shaping host intestinal immune responses [62]. Recent reports on the crosstalk between gut and other organs, such as the gut- brain, liver, kidney, lung axes [63–65] revealed tight connections between gut microbiota and many diseases, implying gut microbiota as an important potential peripheral target of drug therapy. This may provide another explanation for the disconnection between the therapeutic benefits of CMs in many chronic diseases [66] and undesirable PK profile. The last, scattering data pointed to a third role of gut microbiota in manipulating host drug disposition. Comparative analysis of hepatic gene expression from germ-free and conventionally-raised mice revealed a cluster of 112 differentially expressed target genes predominantly connected to xenobiotic metabolism and pathways inhibiting retinoid X receptor function [67]. A number of gut microbiota derived metabolites, bacterial strains, bacterial components such as outer membrane vesicles, or fecal microbiota transplantation could regulate

transporters and drug-metabolizing enzymes or their up-stream regulator nuclear receptors PXR, CAR, PPARs etc. [68–71]. The PK and PD study of calycosin-7-O-β-D-glucoside suggested the contributions of gut microbiota to both disposition and efficacy of CMs. We conceived that the holistic health benefits of CMs should be attributed to components that can interact with gut microbiota to manipulate intestinal hemeostasis and those, either prototypes or the metabolites formed by gut microbial metabolism, which can reach the blood circulation to elicit effects [72]. Therefore, it is imperative to include the presystemic interactions with gut microbiota into the PK–PD study of CMs.

Physiologically based pharmacokinetic (PBPK) modeling is a powerful mathematical modeling technique for predicting drug ADME in humans and other animal species through integrating anatomical, physiological, physical, and chemical descriptions [73]. It offers mechanistic insights into the factors determining drug disposition in specifically designated compartment (predefined organs or tissues) and enables personalized medicine by providing precisely characterized individual variability. Including individual gut microbiota information (structure, metabolic activity, etc.) into a physiologically based pharmacokinetic and pharmacodynamic (PBPK/PD) model is a challenging task but will be a promising approach to allow more precise prediction of inter-individual variability in drug disposition and response and assessment of the contributions of gut microbiota to the holistic therapeutic benefits of CMs. Thus, here we propose a global PK/PD strategy which will combine classic PK–PD which measures systemic drug exposure and extracellular and/or membrane targets, cellular PK–PD which examines cellular drug distribution and intracellular targets, with presystemic PK–PD which determines relevance between gut drug exposure and microbial targets, for examples, gut microbiota composition or specific microbial drug-metabolizing activity (Fig. 1). The advantages and disadvantages of classic PK-PD, cellular PK–PD and the newly proposed global PK–PD are summarized in Table 1.

Clinical PK–PD study of CMs in patients

So far, majority of the PK knowledge of CMs was obtained from animal models. Advances in molecular biology and pharmacogenetics enable a more comprehensive view of interspecies differences in drug disposition and the underlying physiological and pathophysiological mechanisms. Big differences have been reported between humans and animals commonly used (rat, mouse) for preclinical PK study [74]. Although allometric approaches do allow successful extrapolations of PK data of many western medicines from animals to humans [75], species differences are not only numerous

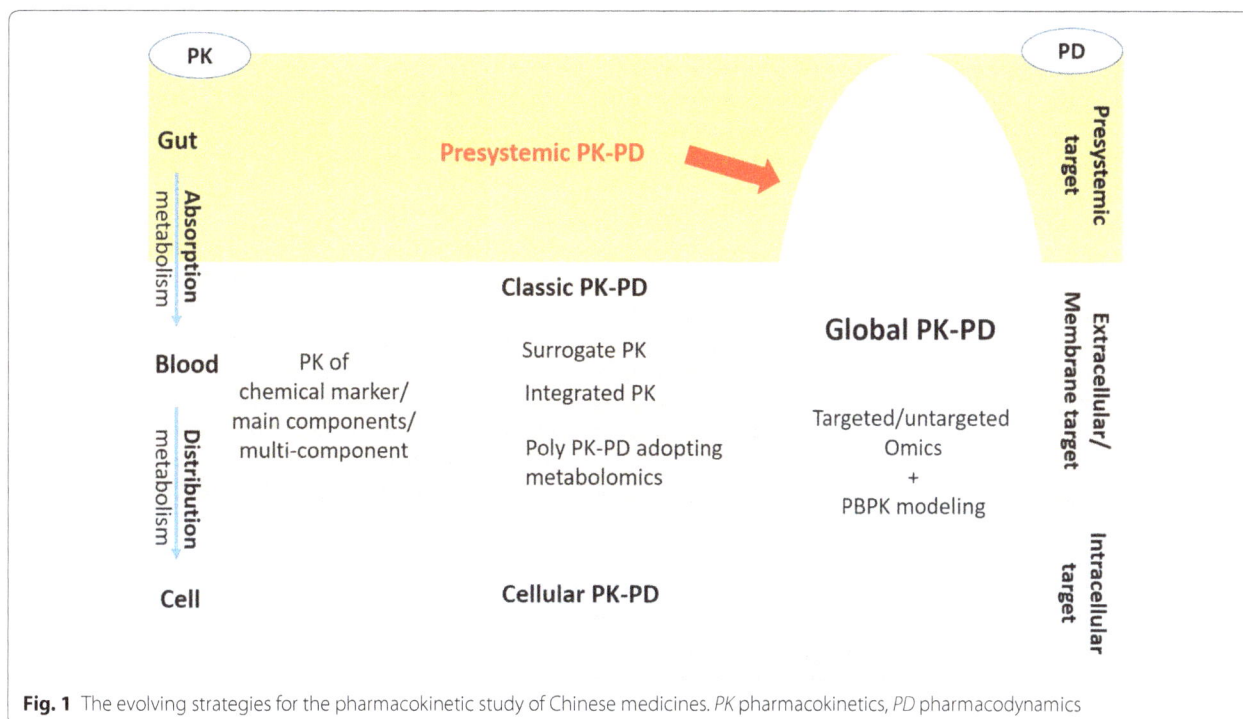

Fig. 1 The evolving strategies for the pharmacokinetic study of Chinese medicines. *PK* pharmacokinetics, *PD* pharmacodynamics

but also sometimes unpredictable, not allowing generalisation. For PK of CMs, the chemical complexity and other factors rooted from it superimpose the species differences, thus preclinical PK data of CMs generally have less translational potential and poorer clinical implications than western medicines.

An increasing number of human PK studies of CMs were reported. Most studied widely prescribed single herbs or famous compound formulas in healthy volunteers at one single oral dose, with single or a few marker/main compounds measured. The impact of inflammation on host drug metabolizing enzymes has been well documented [76, 77]. Changes of drug transporters in diseases accounted for PK alterations of many drugs [78]. Diseases and drug/nutrients interventions cause gut microbiota structure shifts, leading to the microbial metabolic activity changes [79], and as consequences, have impacts on host immune status, drug disposition and efficacy, which will be finally converged to affect the holistic clinical outcomes of CMs. Comparing to the 'laboratory to clinic' discovery process of western medicines, CMs have demonstrated to be effective in long history of clinical applications with undefined targets. The 'clinic to laboratory' paradigm allows mechanistic insights into the holistic benefits of CMs at clinical relevant dosages with less ethical hurdle in clinical PK study in patients. In a recently released guidance for industry on botanical drug development, the US Food and Drug Administration also

requested the sponsor to 'measure the blood levels of known active constituents or major chemical constituents in a botanical drug product using a sensitive analytical method to achieve the same objectives of Phase 1 and 2 clinical pharmacology studies for non-botanical drugs [80]. Collective efforts from relevant parties (clinic practitioners, pharmacokineticists, pharmacologists, and bioanalysts) are needed for establishing PK–PD relevance to unravel holistic mechanisms under the efficacy/toxicity of CMs in human.

Conclusion

The chemical complexity undoubtedly is the basis of the multi-target holistic action mode of CMs which makes them attractive, in particular, in an era when more diseases are found to be multifactorial and demand combination drug therapy, while on the other hand, it hampers the mechanistic understanding of their holistic therapeutic benefits. The validated clinical benefits/pharmacological activities, the elusive targets and mechanisms, the undesirable ADME properties and the PK–PD disconnection, appeal for a PK strategy that follows a distinct paradigm from the one tailored for western medicines to address these challenges. The rapid advancement of the analytical techniques, systems biology, and multivariate analysis methods have promoted the development of several PK strategies, allowing the study of PK–PD relevance between the disposition of multiple/global drug-related

Table 1 The advantages and disadvantages of strategies/approaches for the pharmacokinetic study of Chinese medicines

Strategy	Advantages	Disadvantages
Classic PK-PD	PK study adopts the same strategy tailored for western medicines which focuses on systemic exposures PD study usually measures limited pharmacological parameters/clinical endpoints, except for poly PK-PD Can identify bioactive components with ideal PK property for new drug discovery from CMs	PK–PD profiles of limited number of components may not describe the complex dose-exposure-efficacy/toxicity relationship and explain the multi-component multi-target action mode rooted from the chemical complexity of the herb/compound formulas Systemic exposures of most components are too low to account for the holistic benefits of CMs The interactions with gut microbiota prior to intestinal absorption were ignored Components targeting at cellular components show poor PK–PD relevance
PK of chemical marker/main component/multi-component	Obtains individual PK profile of chemical marker/main components/multi-component of CMs	Restricted by herbal chemistry knowledge, availability of authentic compounds and analytical technology Chemical markers documented for quality control may not be the abundant or specific in the herb Main compounds may not show ideal PK property and be main circulating components
Surrogate PK	Describes pharmacokinetic profiles of CMs using surrogate PK markers (prototypes and/or metabolites) which exhibit significant exposure, show good dose-exposure correlation, and exhibit good correlation or prediction of drug efficacy, safety, or factors that affect exposure Less time-consuming, more readily be translated to industry or clinical practice	It's difficult to find compounds which show both high exposure and good dose-exposure and efficacy correlation The PK profiles of the surrogate marker may subject to changes when the amounts/compositions of co-exiting components vary
Integrated PK	Describe the holistic PK characteristics of CMs using the integral PK of components bearing the same core structure Establish dose-exposure and efficacy relationship for a group of, not individual, bioactive components Bioactivity/toxicity-weighting integral PK approach correlated better with efficiency/toxicity	Establishment of structure–activity relationship is limited by the availability of authentic compounds The metabolites of the components which are bioactive and the main circulating form should be included for calculating integral PK Bioactivity/toxicity-weighting integral PK will change with specific bioactivity/toxicity tested
Poly PK-PD	Applies metabolomics for PK and PD profiling Allows the correlation of the perturbations of endogenous metabolic network with the disposition of the drug-related components Monitors global/specific metabolic shifts using untargeted/targeted metabolomics approaches	The analyte coverage and detection sensitivity rely on the analytical techniques Only those gut microbial metabolites and host-microbial co-metabolites entering the circulating system are possibly detected
Cellular PK-PD	Determines the cellular drug accumulation and intracellular drug distribution and correlates the cellular dynamic drug disposition with its intracellular target binding and efficacy Be more relevant to drug efficacy than plasma drug exposure when drug targets localize inside the cells	Drugs entering cell are limited by transporters and drug-metabolizing enzymes Intracellular drug concentrations are generally low Relies on the specificity and sensitivity of imaging techniques Performed in vitro, complementary to traditional PK to establish PK–PD relevance
Global PK-PD	Combines classic PK–PD which measures systemic drug exposure and extracellular and/or membrane targets, cellular PK–PD which examines cellular drug distribution and intracellular targets, with presystemic PK–PD which determines relevance between gut drug exposure and microbial targets The association study of gut microbial alterations and host metabolic shifts allows estimating the contribution of gut microbiota to the health benefits of CMs Adding a compartment describing individual microbial structure/function data into the PBPK modeling allows more precise prediction of inter-individual variability in drug disposition and response	Requires powerful instrumental platform and multivariate statistical tools to deal with very complex sample analysis and data analysis and interpretation

components and the extracellular/membrane targets and intracellular targets. The emerging enormous evidence support the close connections of gut microbiota with many diseases and its multifaceted role in drug disposition, efficacy, and toxicity. The presystemic interactions of gut microbiota are believed to constitute a significant contribution to the holistic therapeutic benefits of CMs.

A presystemic PK–PD focusing on gut drug exposure and gut-originated targets should be included into a global PK–PD strategy to complement the current PK–PD strategies to provide a comprehensive mechanistic understanding of the multicomponent multitarget holistic clinical outcomes of CMs.

Abbreviations
PK: pharmacokinetics; PD: pharmacodynamics; CMs: Chinese medicines; TCM: traditional Chinese medicine; AUC: area under concentration–time curve; ADME: absorption, distribution, metabolism and excretion; P-gp: *P*-glycoprotein; HDI: herb-drug interactions; NMEs: new molecular entities; PBPK: physiologically based pharmacokinetics.

Authors' contributions
RY conceived and designed the study and responsible for the published work. YY and CYJ collected and analyzed relevant literature. All authors read and approved the final manuscript.

Author details
[1] State Key Laboratory of Quality Research in Chinese Medicine, Institute of Chinese Medical Sciences, University of Macau, Taipa, Macao, China. [2] Zhuhai UM Science & Technology Research Institute, Zhuhai 519080, China.

Acknowledgements
Not applicable.

Competing interests
The authors declare that they have no competing interests.

Consent for publication
Not applicable.

Funding
This work is financially supported by the National Natural Science Foundation (Ref. Nos: 81473281), the Science and Technology Development Fund of Macao SAR (Ref. Nos 043/2011/A2, 029/2015/A1), the National Basic Research Program of China 973 program (Grant No. 2009CB522707), and the Research Committee of University of Macau (Ref. Nos MYRG207-ICMS11-YR, MYRG 2015-00220-ICMS-QRCM, MYRG 2015-00207-ICMS-QRCM).

References
1. Wang L, Zhou GB, Liu P, Song JH, Liang Y, Yan XJ, et al. Dissection of mechanisms of Chinese medicinal formula Realgar-Indigo natural is as an effective treatment for promyelocytic leukemia. Proc Natl Acad Sci USA. 2008;105:4826–31.
2. Zhou M, Hong Y, Lin X, Shen L, Feng Y. Recent pharmaceutical evidence on the compatibility rationality of traditional Chinese medicine. J Ethnopharmacol. 2017;206:363–75.
3. Zhang KM, Yan GL, Zhang AH, Sun H, Wang XJ. Recent advances in pharmacokinetics approach for herbal medicine. Rsc Adv. 2017;7:28876–88.
4. Shi L, Tang XL, Dang XL, Wang QH, Wang XR, He P, et al. Investigating herb-herb interactions: the potential attenuated toxicity mechanism of the combined use of Glycyrrhizae radix et rhizoma (Gancao) and *Sophorae flavescentis* radix (Kushen). J Ethnopharmacol. 2015;165:243–50.
5. Xiao BX, Wang Q, Fan LQ, Kong LT, Guo SR, Chang Q. Pharmacokinetic mechanism of enhancement by Radix Pueraria flavonoids on the hyperglycemic effects of Cortex Mori extract in rats. J Ethnopharmacol. 2014;151:846–51.
6. Liang Y, Zhou Y, Zhang J, Rao T, Zhou L, Xing R, et al. Pharmacokinetic compatibility of ginsenosides and Schisandra Lignans in Shengmai-san: from the perspective of *p*-glycoprotein. PLoS ONE. 2014;9:e98717.
7. Ge BK, Zhang Z, Zuo Z. Radix *Puerariae lobatae* (Gegen) suppresses the anticoagulation effect of warfarin: a pharmacokinetic and pharmacodynamics study. Chin Med. 2016;11:7.
8. Hou ML, Lin CH, Lin LC, Tsai TH. The drug-drug effects of rhein on the pharmacokinetics and pharmacodynamics of clozapine in rat brain extracellular fluid by in vivo microdialysis. J Pharmacol Exp Ther. 2015;355:125–34.
9. Yuan Y, Yang H, Kong LH, Li Y, Li P, Zhang HJ, et al. Interaction between rhein acyl glucuronide and methotrexate based on human organic anion transporters. Chem Biol Interact. 2017;277:79–84.
10. Zhang JW, Sun Y, Wang YY, Lu M, He JC, Liu JL, et al. Non-antibiotic agent ginsenoside 20(*S*)-Rh2 enhanced the antibacterial effects of ciprofloxacin in vitro and in vivo as a potential NorA inhibitor. Eur J Pharmacol. 2014;740:277–84.
11. Li C, Xue HG, Feng LJ, Wang ML, Wang P, Gai XD. The effect of saikosaponin D on doxorubicin pharmacokinetics and its MDR reversal in MCF-7/adr cell xenografts. Eur Rev Med Pharmacol Sci. 2017;21:4437–45.
12. Oga EF, Sekine S, Shitara Y, Horie T. Pharmacokinetic herb-drug interactions: insight into mechanisms and consequences. Eur J Drug Metab Pharmacokinet. 2016;41:93–108.
13. Ma BL, Ma YM. Pharmacokinetic herb-drug interactions with traditional Chinese medicine: progress, causes of conflicting results and suggestions for future research. Drug Metab Rev. 2016;48:1–26.
14. Liu H, Yang J, Du F, Gao X, Ma X, Huang Y, et al. Absorption and disposition of ginsenosides after oral administration of *Panax notoginseng* extract to rats. Drug Metab Dispos. 2009;37:2290–8.
15. Lan K, Xie GX, Jia W. Towards polypharmacokinetics: pharmacokinetics of multicomponent drugs and herbal medicines using a metabolomics approach. Evid-Based Compl Alt. 2013;2013:819147. https://doi.org/10.1155/2013/819147.
16. Xie G, Wang S, Zhang H, Zhao A, Liu J, Ma Y, et al. Poly-pharmacokinetic study of a multicomponent herbal medicine in healthy Chinese volunteers. Clin Pharmacol Ther. 2017;103:784. https://doi.org/10.1002/cpt.784.
17. Li W, Guo J, Tang Y, Wang H, Huang M, Qian D, et al. Pharmacokinetic comparison of ferulic acid in normal and blood deficiency rats after oral administration of *Angelica sinensis*, *Ligusticum chuanxiong* and their combination. Int J Mol Sci. 2012;13:3583–97.
18. Yan R, Ko NL, Ma B, Tam YK, Lin G. Metabolic conversion from co-existing ingredient leading to significant systemic exposure of Z-butylidenephthalide, a minor ingredient in Chuanxiong Rhizoma in rats. Curr Drug Metab. 2012;13:524–34.
19. Yan R, Li SL, Chung HS, Tam YK, Lin G. Simultaneous quantification of 12 bioactive components of *Ligusticum chuanxiong* Hort. by high-performance liquid chromatography. J Pharmaceut Biomed. 2005;37:87–95.

20. Tsao R. Chemistry and biochemistry of dietary polyphenols. Nutrients. 2010;2:1231–46.

21. Yan R, Ko NL, Lin G, Tam YK. Pharmacokinetics and metabolism of ligustilide, a major bioactive component in Rhizoma Chuanxiong, in the rat. Drug Metab Dispos. 2008;36:400–8.

22. Jing W, et al. Mori Cortex regulates *P*-glycoprotein in Caco-2 cells and colons from rats with experimental colitis via direct and gut microbiota-mediated mechanisms. RSC Adv. 2017;7:2594–605.

23. He SM, Chan E, Zhou SF. ADME properties of herbal medicines in humans: evidence, challenges and strategies. Curr Pharm Des. 2011;17:357–407.

24. Xie GX, Zhao AH, Zhao LJ, Chen TL, Chen HY, Qi X, et al. Metabolic fate of tea polyphenols in humans. J Proteome Res. 2012;11:3449–57.

25. Li CY, Qi LW, Li P. Correlative analysis of metabolite profiling of Dang-gui Buxue Tang in rat biological fluids by rapid resolution LC-TOF/MS. J Pharmaceut Biomed. 2011;55:146–60.

26. Xiang C, Qiao X, Wang Q, Li R, Miao WJ, Guo DA, et al. From single compounds to herbal extract: a strategy to systematically characterize the metabolites of licorice in rats. Drug Metab Dispos. 2011;39:1597–608.

27. Qiao X, Ye M, Xiang C, Wang Q, Liu CF, Miao WJ, et al. Analytical strategy to reveal the in vivo process of multi-component herbal medicine: a pharmacokinetic study of licorice using liquid chromatography coupled with triple quadrupole mass spectrometry. J Chromatogr A. 2012;1258:84–93.

28. Lu T, Yang J, Gao X, Chen P, Du F, Sun Y, et al. Plasma and urinary tanshinol from Salvia miltiorrhiza (Danshen) can be used as pharmacokinetic markers for cardiotonic pills, a cardiovascular herbal medicine. Drug Metab Dispos. 2008;36:1578–86.

29. Hu ZY, Yang JL, Cheng C, Huang YH, Du FF, Wang FQ, et al. Combinatorial metabolism notably affects human systemic exposure to ginsenosides from orally administered extract of *Panax notoginseng* roots (Sanqi). Drug Metab Dispos. 2013;41:1457–69.

30. Li MJ, Wang FQ, Huang YH, Du FF, Zhong CC, Olaleye OE, et al. Systemic exposure to and disposition of catechols derived from Salvia miltiorrhiza Roots (Danshen) after intravenous dosing DanHong injection in human subjects, rats, and dogs. Drug Metab Dispos. 2015;43:679–90.

31. Li C. Multi-compound pharmacokinetic research on Chinese herbal medicines: approach and methodology. China J Chin Materia Medica. 2017;42:607–17.

32. Yang N, Srivastava K, Song Y, Liu CD, Cho S, Chen YJ, et al. Berberine as a chemical and pharmacokinetic marker of the butanol-extracted food allergy herbal formula-2. Int Immunopharmacol. 2017;45:120–7.

33. Yang P, Xu F, Li HF, Wang Y, Li FC, Shang MY, et al. Detection of 191 taxifolin metabolites and their distribution in rats using HPLC-ESI-IT-TOF-MS[n]. Molecules. 2016;21:1209. https://doi.org/10.3390/molecules21091209.

34. Xie YA, Hao HP, Kang A, Liang Y, Xie T, Sun SQ, et al. Integral pharmacokinetics of multiple lignan components in normal, CCl4-induced hepatic injury and hepatoprotective agents pretreated rats and correlations with hepatic injury biomarkers. J Ethnopharmacol. 2010;131:290–9.

35. Wang LL, Zhao DS, Shi W, Li ZQ, Wu ZT, Li P, et al. Describing the holistic toxicokinetics of hepatotoxic Chinese herbal medicines by a novel integrated strategy: *Dioscorea bulbifera* rhizome as a case study. J Chromatogr B Analyt Technol Biomed Life Sci. 2017;1064:40–8.

36. Ren W, Zuo R, Wang YN, Wang HJ, Yang J, Xin SK, et al. Pharmacokinetic–pharmacodynamic analysis on inflammation rat model after oral administration of Huang Lian Jie Du decoction. PLoS ONE. 2016;11:e0156256.

37. Ding X, Sun YM, Wang Q, Pu TT, Li XH, Pan YQ, et al. Pharmacokinetics and pharmacodynamics of glycyrrhetinic acid with Paeoniflorin after transdermal administration in dysmenorrhea model mice. Phytomedicine. 2016;23:864–71.

38. Zhan SY, Guo WJ, Shao Q, Fan XH, Li Z, Cheng YY. A pharmacokinetic and pharmacodynamic study of drug-drug interaction between ginsenoside Rg1, ginsenoside Rb1 and schizandrin after intravenous administration to rats. J Ethnopharmacol. 2014;152:333–9.

39. Yu B, Ruan M, Dong XP, Yu Y, Cheng HB. The mechanism of the opening of the blood–brain barrier by borneol: a pharmacodynamics and pharmacokinetics combination study. J Ethnopharmacol. 2013;150:1096–108.

40. Nicholson JK, Wilson ID. Understanding 'global' systems biology: metabonomics and the continuum of metabolism. Nat Rev Drug Discov. 2003;2:668–76.

41. Johnson CH, Patterson AD, Idle JR, Gonzalez FJ. Xenobiotic metabolomics: major impact on the metabolome. Annu Rev Pharmacol Toxicol. 2012;52:37–56.

42. Shen H, Leung WI, Ruan JQ, Li SL, Lei JP, Wang YT, et al. Biotransformation of ginsenoside Rb1 via the gypenoside pathway by human gut bacteria. Chin Med. 2013;8:22.

43. Kang A, Hao HP, Zheng X, Liang Y, Xie Y, Xie T, et al. Peripheral anti-inflammatory effects explain the ginsenosides paradox between poor brain distribution and anti-depression efficacy. J Neuroinflammation. 2011;8:100.

44. Chen F, Li L, Xu F, Sun Y, Du F, Ma X, Zhong C, Li X, Wang F, Zhang N, Li C. Systemic and cerebral exposure to and pharmacokinetics of flavonols and terpene lactones after dosing standardized Ginkgo biloba leaf extracts to rats via different routes of administration. Br J Pharmacol. 2013;170:440–57.

45. Zhang JW, Zhou F, Lu M, Ji W, Niu F, Zha WB, et al. Pharmacokinetics–pharmacology disconnection of herbal medicines and its potential solutions with cellular pharmacokinetic–pharmacodynamic strategy. Curr Drug Metab. 2012;13:558–76.

46. Sanchez CP, Stein WD, Lanzer M. Dissecting the components of quinine accumulation in Plasmodium falciparum. Mol Microbiol. 2008;67:1081–93.

47. Liu Y, Lok CN, Ko BC, Shum TY, Wong MK, Che CM. Subcellular localization of a fluorescent artemisinin derivative to endoplasmic reticulum. Org Lett. 2010;12:1420–3.

48. Mukai R, Shirai Y, Saito N, Yoshida K, Ashida H. Subcellular localization of flavonol aglycone in hepatocytes visualized by confocal laser scanning fluorescence microscope. Cytotechnology. 2009;59:177–82.

49. Arredondo F, Echeverry C, Abin-Carriquiry JA, Blasina F, Antunez K, Jones DP, Go YM. Liang YL, Dajas F. After cellular internalization, quercetin causes Nrf2 nuclear translocation, increases glutathione levels, and prevents neuronal death against an oxidative insult. Free Radic Biol Med. 2010;49:738–47.

50. Duvvuri M, Feng W, Mathis A, Krise JP. A cell fractionation approach for the quantitative analysis of subcellular drug disposition. Pharm Res. 2004;21:26–32.

51. Lee WH, Bebawy M, Loo CY, Luk F, Mason RS, Rohanizadeh R. Fabrication of curcumin micellar nanoparticles with enhanced anti-cancer activity. J Biomed Nanotechnol. 2015;11:1093–105.

52. Lu JJ, Pan W, Hu YJ, Wang YT. Multi-target drugs: the trend of drug research and development. PLoS ONE. 2012;7:e40262.

53. Lin HH, Zhang LL, Yan R, Lu JJ, Hu YJ. Network analysis of drug-target interactions: a study on FDA-approved new molecular entities between 2000 and 2015. Sci Rep. 2017;7:12230. https://doi.org/10.1038/s41598-017-12061-8.

54. Hao HP, Zheng X, Wang GJ. Insights into drug discovery from natural medicines using reverse pharmacokinetics. Trends Pharmacol Sci. 2014;35:168–77.

55. Zhang X, Zhao YF, Xu J, Xue ZS, Zhang MH, Pang XY, et al. Modulation of gut microbiota by berberine and metformin during the treatment of high-fat diet-induced obesity in rats. Sci Rep. 2015;5:14405. https://doi.org/10.1038/srep14405.

56. Liu YT, Hao HP, Xie HG, Lai L, Wang QO, Liu CX, et al. Extensive intestinal first-pass elimination and predominant hepatic distribution of berberine explain its low plasma levels in rats. Drug Metab Dispos. 2010;38:1779–84.

57. Wilson ID, Nicholson JK. Gut microbiome interactions with drug metabolism, efficacy, and toxicity. Transl Res. 2017;179:204–22.

58. Li H, Zhou M, Zhao A, Jia W. Traditional Chinese medicine: balancing the gut ecosystem. Phytother Res. 2009;23:1332–5.

59. Spanogiannopoulos P, Bess EN, Carmody RN, Turnbaugh PJ. The microbial pharmacists within us: a metagenomic view of xenobiotic metabolism. Nat Rev Microbiol. 2016;14:273–87.

60. Zhou RN, Song YL, Ruan JQ, Wang YT, Yan R. Pharmacokinetic evidence on contribution of intestinal bacterial conversion to beneficial actions of astragaloside IV, a marker compound of Astragali Radix, in traditional oral use of the herb. DMPK. 2012;27(6):586–97.

61. Mei M, Ruan JQ, Wu WJ, Zhou RN, Lei JP, Yan R, Zhao HY, Wang YT. In Vitro pharmacokinetic characterization of mulberroside A, the Main polyhydroxylated stilbene in mulberry (*Morus alba* L.), and its bacterial metabolite oxyresveratrol in traditional oral use. J Agric Food Chem. 2012;60(9):2299–308.

62. Round JL, Mazmanian SK. The gut microbiome shapes intestinal immune responses during health and disease. Nat Rev Immunol. 2009;9:313–23.

63. Foster JA, KaM Neufeld. Gut-brain: how the microbiome influences anxiety and depression. Trends Neurosci. 2013;36:305–12.
64. Ma JL, Zhou QH, Li HK. Gut microbiota and nonalcoholic fatty liver disease: insights on mechanisms and therapy. Nutrients. 2017;9:1124. https ://doi.org/10.3390/nu9101124.
65. Tulic MK, Piche T, Verhasselt V. Lung-gut cross-talk: evidence, mechanisms and implications for the mucosal inflammatory diseases. Clin Exp Allergy. 2016;46:519–28.
66. Jiang M, Zhang C, Cao HX, Chan K, Lu AP. The role of Chinese medicine in the treatment of chronic diseases in China. Planta Med. 2011;77:873–81.
67. Bjorkholm B, Bok CM, Lundin A, Rafter J, Hibberd ML, Pettersson S. Intestinal microbiota regulate xenobiotic metabolism in the liver. PLoS ONE. 2009;4:e6958.
68. Matsumoto J, Dohgu S, Takata F, Nishioku T, Sumi N, Machida T, et al. Lipopolysaccharide-activated microglia lower *P*-glycoprotein function in brain microvascular endothelial cells. Neurosci Lett. 2012;524:45–8.
69. Inan MS, Rasoulpour RJ, Yin L, Hubbard AK, Rosenberg DW, Giardina C. The luminal short-chain fatty acid butyrate modulates NF-kappaB activity in a human colonic epithelial cell line. Gastroenterology. 2000;118:724–34.
70. Gao XJ, Li T, Wei B, Yan ZX, Yan R. Regulatory mechanisms of gut microbiota on intestinal CYP3A4 and P-gp in rats with dextran sulfate sodium-induced colitis. Acta Pharmaceutica Sinica. 2017;52:34–43.
71. Gao XJ, Li T, Wei B, Yan ZX, Hu N, Huang YJ, Han BL, Wai TS, Yang W, Yan R. Bacterial outer membrane vesicles from dextran sulfate sodium-induced colitis differentially regulate intestinal UDP-glucuronosyltransferase 1A1 partially through TLR4/MAPK/PI3K pathway. Drug Metab Dispos. 2018. https://doi.org/10.1124/dmd.117.079046.
72. Ruan JQ, Li S, Li YP, Wu WJ, Lee MY, Yan R. The presystemic interplay between gut microbiota and orally administered calycosin-7-*O*-β-D-Glucoside. Drug Metab Dispos. 2015;43:1601–11.
73. Jones HM, Rowland-Yeo K. Basic concepts in physiologically based pharmacokinetic modeling in drug discovery and development. CPT Pharmacometrics Syst Pharmacol. 2013;2(8):e63.
74. Daublain P, Feng KI, Altman MD, Martin I, Mukherjee S, Nofsinger R, Northrup AB, Tschirret-Guth R, Cartwright M, McGregor C. Analyzing the potential root causes of variability of pharmacokinetics in preclinical species. Mol Pharm. 2017;14:1634–45.
75. Evans CA, Jolivette LJ, Nagilla R, Ward KW. Extrapolation of preclinical pharmacokinetics and molecular feature analysis of "discovery-like" molecules to predict human pharmacokinetics. Drug Metab Dispos. 2006;34:1255–65.
76. Morgan ET, Goralski KB, Piquette-Miller M, Renton KW, Robertson GR, Chaluvadi MR, et al. Regulation of drug-metabolizing enzymes and transporters in infection, inflammation, and cancer. Drug Metab Dispos. 2008;36:205–16.
77. Nan Hu, Huang Yanjuan, Gao Xuejiao, Li Sai, Yan Zhixiang, Wei B, Yan R. Effects of dextran sulfate sodium induced experimental colitis on cytochrome P450 activity in rat liver, kidney and intestine. Chem Biol Interact. 2017;271:48–58.
78. Chu X, Bleasby K, Evers R. Species differences in drug transporters and implications for translating preclinical findings to humans. Expert Opin Drug Metab Toxicol. 2013;9:237–52.
79. Wu WJ, Yan R, Li T, Li YP, Zhou RN, Wang YT. Pharmacokinetic alterations of rhubarb anthraquinones in experimental colitis induced by dextran sulfate sodium in the rat. J Ethnopharmacol. 2017;198:600–7.
80. The Food and Drug Administration. Botanical drug development guidance for industry, vol. 30. Silver Spring: The Food and Drug Administration; 2015.

9

Predicting the potential global distribution of diosgenin-contained *Dioscorea* species

Liang Shen[†], Jiang Xu[†], Lu Luo, Haoyu Hu, Xiangxiao Meng, Xiwen Li[*] and Shilin Chen[*]

Abstract

Background: Diosgenin, mainly extracted from wild diosgenin-contained *Dioscorea* species, is a well-known starting material of steroidal and contraceptive drugs. However, due to large market demand and increasingly ecological damage, wild *Dioscorea* species resources available have been gradually declining. Therefore, identification of new potential ecological distribution of diosgenin-contained *Dioscorea* species is necessary for diosgenin production.

Methods: In this study, a large occurrence dataset (1808 data points) of diosgenin-contained *Dioscorea* species was obtained from Eastern Asia, Southern North America and Southern Africa. Along with the data for six critical environmental parameters and one soil factor, Geographic Information System for Global Medicinal Plant was applied to predict the potential suitable distribution of *Dioscorea* species.

Results: The results showed that the potential distribution of these *Dioscorea* species covered a wide field, and that new ecological suitability areas were mainly distributed in the central region of South America, the southern part of the European and coastal region of Oceania. Jackknife test indicated that annual precipitation and annual mean radiation were the important climatic factors controlling the distribution of *Dioscorea* species.

Conclusions: The suitable areas and critical climatic factors will serve as a useful guide for diosgenin-contained *Dioscorea* species conservation and cultivation in ecological suitable areas.

Keywords: *Dioscorea* species, Diosgenin material, GMPGIS, Potentially suitable areas, Climate characteristics

Background

Diosgenin is a versatile starting material for the manufacture of steroidal drugs, and it is mainly extracted from *Dioscorea* species [1]. Steroidal has strong anti-infection, anti-allergic and other pharmacological effects which plays an important role in the treatment of rheumatoid arthritis, heart disease, peptic ulcer disease, etc. [2]. Diosgenin has also been prescribed as an oral contraceptive with large market demands in recent years. There are 137 kinds of *Dioscorea* species containing diosgenin, 41 kinds of which contain over 1% diosgenin with great utilization value [3]. However, their resources have been declining

quickly due to excessive harvesting, and some species are even getting nearly extinct. Nevertheless *Dioscorea* became a major source to produce steroid hormone due to the failure of accomplishing chemical synthesis of steroids [4]. In India, approximate 100% production of steroidal drugs is based on diosgenin material from *Dioscorea* species [5]. Therefore, it is necessarily needed to explore approaches in conservation and cultivation of diosgenin-contained *Dioscorea* species to obtain diosgenin materials.

Recently, booming market demands boosted the expansion of introduction and cultivation of *Dioscorea* species worldwide. China and Mexico are the two main production countries, which account for 67% of diosgenin yield with the richest *Dioscorea* resource in the world [1]. However, the yield and quality of diosgenin was declined due to the lack of high-quality germplasm, unknown

*Correspondence: xwli@icmm.ac.cn; slchen@icmm.ac.cn
[†]Liang Shen and Jiang Xu contributed equally to this work
Institute of Chinese Materia Medica, China Academy of Chinese Medical Sciences, Beijing 100700, China

suitable plant region and shortage of useful technology [6]. As far as we are concerned, there still exist some *Dioscorea* species cultivated in rural China, what remains confusing to us is that whether they can be used as diosgenin source or not has not been testified yet [7]. Understanding the requirements of habitat conditions of these *Dioscorea* species may be useful for managing population recovery and plantation, as well as promoting economic growth. The cultivation methods for *Dioscorea* species, such as breeding, management, and planting have been discussed by previous reports [8, 9]. Nevertheless, suitable distribution and ecological requirements of these *Dioscorea* species remain unknown. Quite a limited number of studies have assessed the distribution patterns of the *Dioscorea* species, and there was an article about habitats across Bangladesh by the species distribution modeling (SDM) [10]. Additionally, the *D. nipponica* potential distribution was assessed across Jilin province in China by the MaxEnt. High fitness suitable areas were also identified to concentrate at the central and southern regions of Jilin [11]. Hence, it is essential to conduct conservation and cultivation study on a global scale for *Dioscorea* species which analyzes ecological factor similarities include climate, soil between the origin and introduction sites and to draw an accurate global cultivation region map.

With the development of network technology, the geographic information system (GIS) is just an ideally digital mapping tool adopted for geospatial database creation, data integration and modeling [12]. GMPGIS can predict the impact of climate on medicinal plants potential distribution model, and the model is verified successfully in predicting the distribution of *Panax* species [13–15]. It is of great significance to predict the potential suitable distribution of *Dioscorea* species by GMPGIS with primary ecological factors for their protection and utilization. In this study, we analyzed the potential global suitable habitats of diosgenin-contained *Dioscorea* species by means of GMPGIS based on six climate variables and soil factor, and mapped the key environmental variables that constrain the geographical distribution of those *Dioscorea* species by Jackknife test. These results will provide a valuable reference for conservation, introduction and cultivation of diosgenin-contained *Dioscorea* species worldwide.

Materials and methods

Species data

In this study, ten *Dioscorea* species were selected in accordance with the principle of higher diosgenin content, crop yield and industrialized application [4, 16–18]. Samples points of *Dioscorea* species were drawn from main producing areas, wild distribution and historical growing region [13]. Data on the distribution of *Dioscorea* species were obtained from the following sources: (1) the Global Biodiversity Information Facility Data Portal (GBIF, http://www.gbif.org/); (2) Royal Botanic Gardens, Kew (Kew, http://www.kew.org/); (3) the Chinese Virtual Herbarium (CVH: http://www.cvh.org.cn/); (4) relevant literature and field investigation. Additionally, sampling bias were reduced with regard to environmental conditions, only one sample was kept when replicated. Each sampling site was converted into geographic coordinates (World Geodetic System 1984 data) by ArcGIS (ver. 10.2) (http://www.esri.com/). Finally, a total of 1808 points were valid, and the samples points were mainly from China, Mexico, United States and South Africa, etc. (Fig. 1; Additional file 1: Table S1) [16–26].

Environmental variables

Following the main controlling factors of the distribution and characteristics of medicinal plants, the prediction of model selection of variables should reflect the coldest and warmest temperatures, moisture, radiation and precipitation of species, and the most influential variables associated with diosgenin yield are considered as well [15]. In this study, the selection of mainly used variables was based on the biological characteristics of medicinal plants, references and the data analysis [13–15, 27, 28]. A total of six related ecological factors for medicinal plants were selected and down from the Worldclim database (http://www.worldclim.org/) (Period 1970–2000) (Additional file 1: Table S2) [29, 30], with a resolution of 2.5 arcmin-seconds, and availability of data of 10 *Dioscorea* species were in supply files (Additional file 2). The soil variables were obtained from Harmonized World Soil Database (http://www.iiasa.ac.at/). For region measurements, the layers were projected into UTM coordinates with the original data in WGS84. Global administrative areas come from the GADM database, and the version is 2.8 (http://www.gadm.org/).

Species distribution modeling

GMPGIS was a model using global geographic information system for medicinal plant distribution prediction, and it was self-developed by the Institute of Chinese Materia Medica, China Academy of Chinese Medical Sciences (CACMS) based on GIS technology. GMPGIS climate database was adopted from the World Clim-Global Climate Data [29] and CliMond (https://www.climond.org/), and the soil database was obtained from Harmonized World Soil Database (HWSD) [13–15]. In GMPGIS, the occurrences of plant species with known distributions are related to climate data by using improved k-means method in Euclidean distances algorithms, and the accuracy of GMPGIS model has been

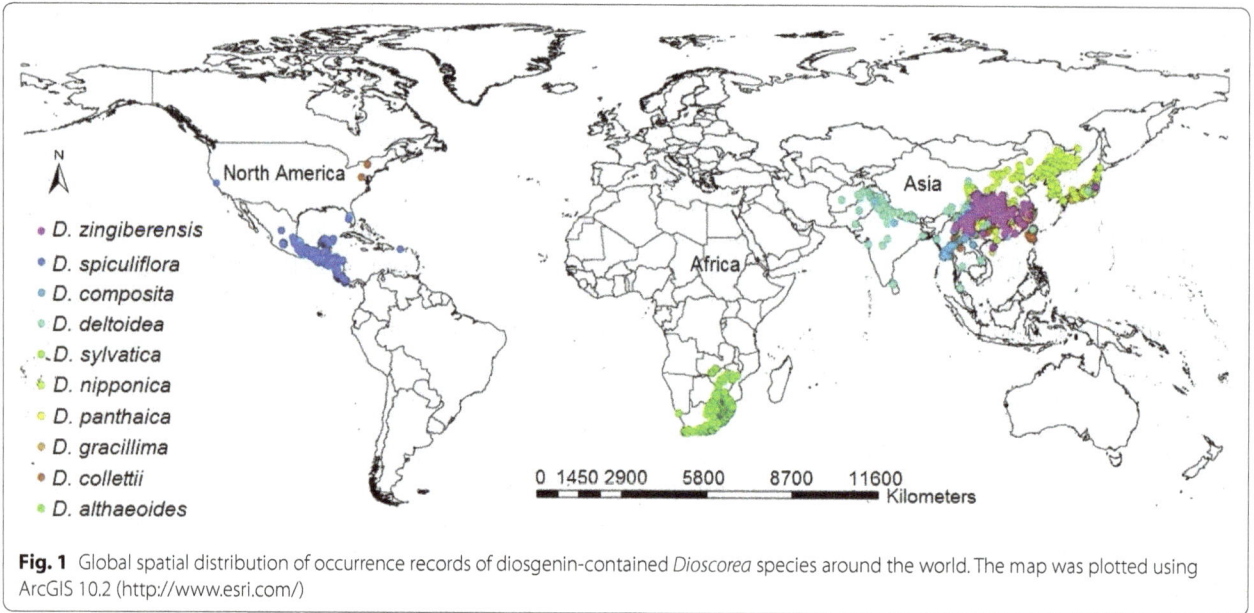

Fig. 1 Global spatial distribution of occurrence records of diosgenin-contained *Dioscorea* species around the world. The map was plotted using ArcGIS 10.2 (http://www.esri.com/)

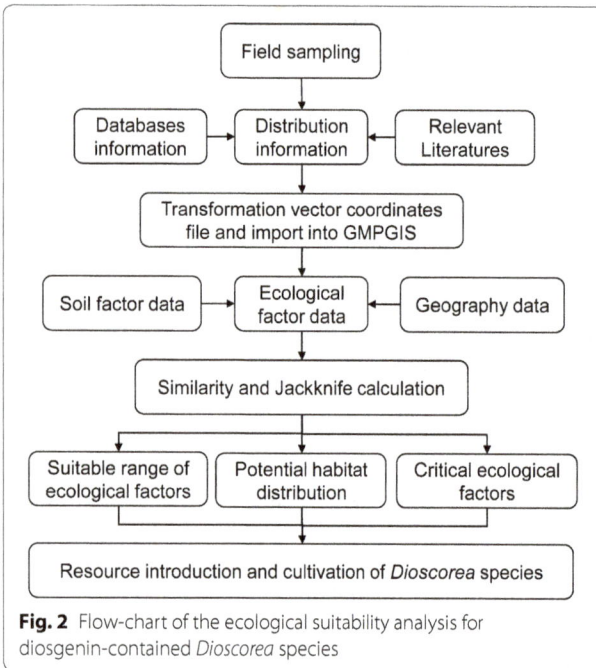

Fig. 2 Flow-chart of the ecological suitability analysis for diosgenin-contained *Dioscorea* species

(0 = unsuitable to 0.999 = best habitat) was presented by the model logistic outcomes [31].

$$v'_i = \frac{v_i - min_A}{max_A - min_A} \times 100, \tag{a}$$

$$E = \sum_{i=1}^{k} \sum_{p \in D_i} dist(p, d_i)^2, \tag{b}$$

$$dist(p, d_i) = \text{IF}[min \leq v_i \leq max, 0,$$
$$\min(|v'_i - newmin_A|, |v'_i - newmax_A|)]. \tag{c}$$

where (*vi*), the *vi* of *A* to *vi* in the range [*newminA*, *newmaxA*], and *di* is the scope of cluster *Di*, *newminA* is the minimum value after normalizing the layer, *newmaxA* is the maximum value after normalizing the layer.

In this research, analysis of the key environmental variables which constrained the geographical distribution of *Dioscorea* species were conducted by jackknife testing in MaxEnt version 3.3.3 k [32]. Parameter setting of modeling was as follows: The training set was 75% of the sampling data points. For the test set, 25% residual was used to examine the predictive ability of the MaxEnt, and the jackknife was used to test the weight. In order to prevent over-fitting of the test data, the regularization multiplier value was set as 1, and convergence threshold 0.00001 [33]. All other settings were kept as default value and output format settings [34].

successfully verified by six *Panax* plants [14, 15]. A suitable habitat map for *Dioscorea* species was established according to the following four main steps: linear normalization (a), grid-based spatial clustering, vector-based overlaying and suitable region analysis (b and c). The suitable soil layer and climatic factors in the Euclidean distance layer were intersected, and the predicted map was drawn [13, 15] (Fig. 2). A natural probabilistic explanation representing degrees of ecology suitability

Phylogenetic relationship among *Dioscorea* species

The chloroplast genomes *matK* and *rbcL* sequence possessed highly interspecific differences and were capable of distinguishing medicinal plants at the species level [35]. In the present study, *matK* and *rbcL* sequences of ten diosgenin of *Dioscorea* species were downloaded from the GenBank database. Consensus sequences and coting generation were obtained by the software CondonCode Aligner V3.7.1 (CodonCode Co., USA). The sequences of *Dioscorea* species were aligned by Muscle, and the genetic distance was computed with MEGA6.0 software (http://www.megasoftware.net) by using K2P model [36]. A phylogenetic tree based on *matK* and *rbcL* was constructed by employing the neighbor-joining (NJ) tree method, and bootstrap tests were calculated with 1000 resamples to assess the statistical confidence in phylogenetic analysis. Accordance with the phylogenetically related genetic information inferred from APGIV, and same sequence of *Tacca chantieri* Andre and *Alisma plantago-aquatica* Linn downloaded from GenBank were chosen as our group when the NJ tree was built [37–39] (Additional file 1: Table S3). The Minimum Standards of Reporting Checklist contains details of the experimental design, and statistics, and resources used in this study (Additional file 3).

Results

Model performance and contribution of environmental variables

D. deltoidea and *D. nipponica* showed a significantly different performance in regions and climatic factors comparing to all the other species (Table 1, Additional file 4: Figure S1). *D. deltoidea* and *D. composita* variation of climatic factors were the maximum and minimum, respectively. In six climatic factors, the maximal variation factor was T-warm, while the minimal change factor was T-cold. Soil types of ten *Dioscorea* species were mainly in Acrisols, Alisols, Andosols, Anthrosols, Cambisols, Fluvisols, and so on. Thus, the results indicated that these ecological conditions were optimal for the growth of diosgenin-contained *Dioscorea* species.

The contributions of each ecological factor were revealed by Jackknife test (Fig. 3). According to the result, annual precipitation and annual mean radiation were the key factors driving the modelled distribution of most of the ten *Dioscorea* species. For four of the taxa (*D. zingiberensis*, *D. sylvatica*, *D. spiculiflora* and *D. nipponica*), radiation emerged as an important contributor to the modelled distribution, as well as precipitation probability for other three taxa (*D. composita*, *D. deltoidea* and *D. panthaica*), humidity for *D. gracillima* and T-cold for *D.*

Table 1 Range values (minimum–maximum) of the ecological factors for ten diosgenin-contained *Dioscorea* species

Species	T-aver (°C)	T-warm (°C)	T-cold (°C)	Precipitation (mm)	Radiation (W m⁻²)	Humidity (%)
D. althaeoides	4.80 to 21.50	12.00 to 28.50	− 4.10 to 14.20	347 to 1736	125.58 to 153.30	41.90 to 76.40
	Soil types: Acrisols, Alisols, Andosols, Anthrosols, Chernozems etc.					
D. collettii	4.40 to 27.20	10.90 to 29.30	− 4.10 to 26.20	543 to 4854	119.08 to 168.05	50.20 to 77.00
	Soil types: Acrisols, Alisols, Anthrosols, Cambisols, Fluvisols etc.					
D. composita	12.40 to 27.20	13.30 to 32.80	4.80 to 25.20	785 to 4143	136.80 to 198.97	51.60 to 78.10
	Soil types: Acrisols, Andosols, Arenosols, Cambisols, Fluvisols etc.					
D. deltoidea	− 6.70 to 28.10	4.20 to 34.10	− 18.20 to 26.1	142 to 3774	122.83 to 228.01	38.40 to 76.50
	Soil types: Acrisols, Andosols, Arenosols, Cambisols, Fluvisols etc.					
D. gracillima	2.00 to 19.50	13.20 to 28.70	− 18.70 to 10.3	543 to 2821	116.73 to 144.76	56.80 to 76.40
	Soil types: Acrisols, Alisols, Andosols, Anthrosols, Cambisols etc.					
D. nipponica	− 1.70 to 25.90	5.60 to 28.80	− 20.30 to 220	295 to 3338	113.89 to 165.42	47.60 to 76.80
	Soil types: Acrisols, Alisols, Andosols, Arenosols, Anthrosols etc.					
D. panthaica	6.20 to 20.30	13.20 to 27.50	− 3.50 to 15.10	543 to 1743	122.15 to 154.77	50.20 to 75.70
	Soil types: Acrisols, Alisols, Anthrosols, Cambisols, Fluvisols, etc.					
D. spiculiflora	11.20 to 27.10	13.10 to 29.30	9.00 to 26.30	344 to 4296	150.92 to 207.56	46.50 to 80.50
	Soil types: Acrisols, Andosols, Cambisols, Gleysols, Kastanozems etc.					
D. sylvatica	6.20 to 24.00	10.40 to 26.40	1.20 to 20.20	68 to 1600	161.28 to 206.69	46.00 to 73.80
	Soil types: Acrisols, Arenosols, Calcisols, Cambisols, Fluvisols etc.					
D. zingiberensis	7.40 to 24.20	16.60 to 28.70	− 3.50 to 18.80	543 to 1849	117.70 to 150.39	52.90 to 76.00
	Soil types: Acrisols, Alisols, Andosols, Anthrosols, Cambisols etc.					

T-aver annual mean temperature, *T-warm* mean temperature of warmest quarter, *T-cold* mean temperature of coldest quarter, *Precipitation* annual precipitation, *Radiation* annual radiation, *Humidity* annual relative humidity

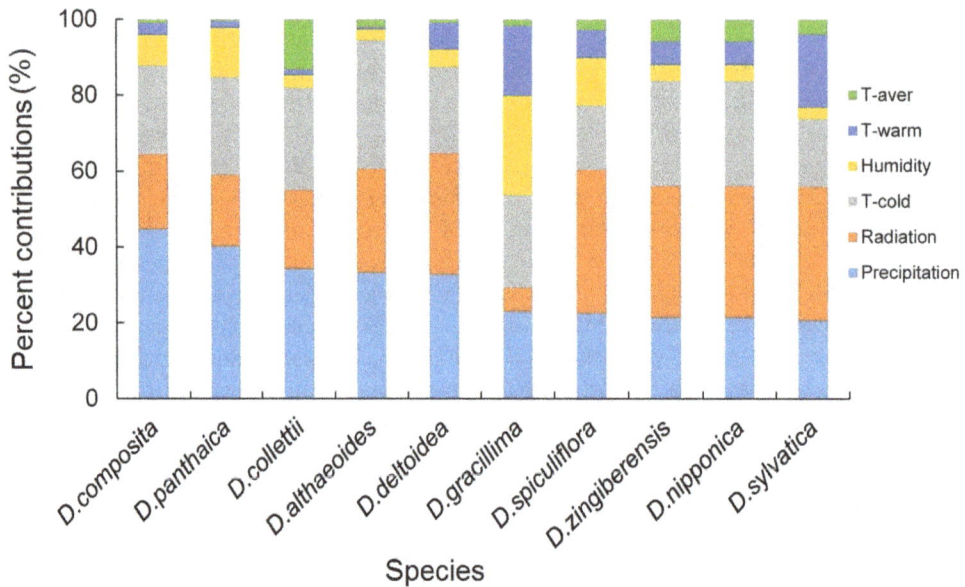

Fig. 3 Contribution of individual variable to habitat suitability allowing the diosgenin-contained *Dioscorea* species

althaeoides. The T-cold was also an important contributor to the modelled distribution in whole species, except for the *D. spiculiflora*, *D. deltoidea* and *D. sylvatica*. None of the species was strongly constrained by T-aver or T-warm. The range of suitable environmental factors provided a useful reference for the cultivation of those ten *Dioscorea* species.

Potential global distribution

According to ecological similarity growth of *Dioscorea* species, the results showed that the potential distribution areas of ten *Dioscorea* species stretched a rather wide area (Fig. 4, Additional file 1: Table S4). Ecological range of *D. deltoidea*, *D. collettii*, *D. composita* and *D. spiculiflora* covered a wide field, and the potential areas were more than $(158.16–465.91) \times 10^5$ km^2, mainly distributed in the central region of South America, southern part of Africa and Asia (Fig. 4a, c–e). *D. nipponica* was potentially distributed in most parts of the earth, but mainly in most parts of North America, southern part of Europe and the eastern part of Asia, and suitable areas were 262.33×10^5 km^2 (Fig. 4b). *D. sylvatica* was mainly potentially distributed in southern part of Africa, South America and Asia, and potentially suitable areas are 107.40×10^5 km^2 (Fig. 4f). In contrast, the potential areas of *D. althaeoides*, *D. zingiberensis*, *D. gracillima* and *D. panthaica* areas were within the scope of $(59.02–68.37) \times 10^5$ km^2, and mainly distributed in the eastern part of North America, southern part of European and Asia (Fig. 4g–j). Based on the area of producing

district, there were some countries suitable for promoting planting such as China, Mexico, United States, Brazil, France, Japan, North Korea, Indonesia, India, Australia and so on (Additional file 4: Figure S2). The results indicated that *D. deltoidea*, *D. nipponica* and *D. collettii* were proper plantations in Eastern Asia; *D. deltoidea*, *D. composita* and *D. spiculiflora* were proper plantation in North America; the proper plantation species in Southern Africa contained *D. deltoidea* and *D. sylvatica*, and *D. spiculiflora* were suitable cultivation in North America (Fig. 5). The suitable areas in Southern Europe and Oceania seemed limited, and the proper species were *D. deltoidea* and *D. nipponica*. Asia was found to be the largest planting area, and Oceania, the smallest.

Phylogenetic relationships among ten *Dioscorea* species

Phylogenetic trees of ten diosgenin-contained species from *Dioscorea* were created by the NJ method. The result of the analysis on the bootstrap values above 50% is given (Fig. 6). The tree was derived by alignment of concatenation *matK* and *rbcL* sequences. The moderately and strongly supported groups of phylogenetic trees were clearly shown to be two trees. Among ten *Dioscorea* species, two North America species of *D. spiculiflora* and *D. composita* and one African species *D. sylvatica* belonged to the same cluster (Cluster I), six Asian species such as *D. gracillima*, *D. althaeoides*, *D. panthaica*, *D. deltoidea*, *D. zingiberensis* and *D. nipponica* formed a moderate support to the same cluster (Cluster II). As expected,

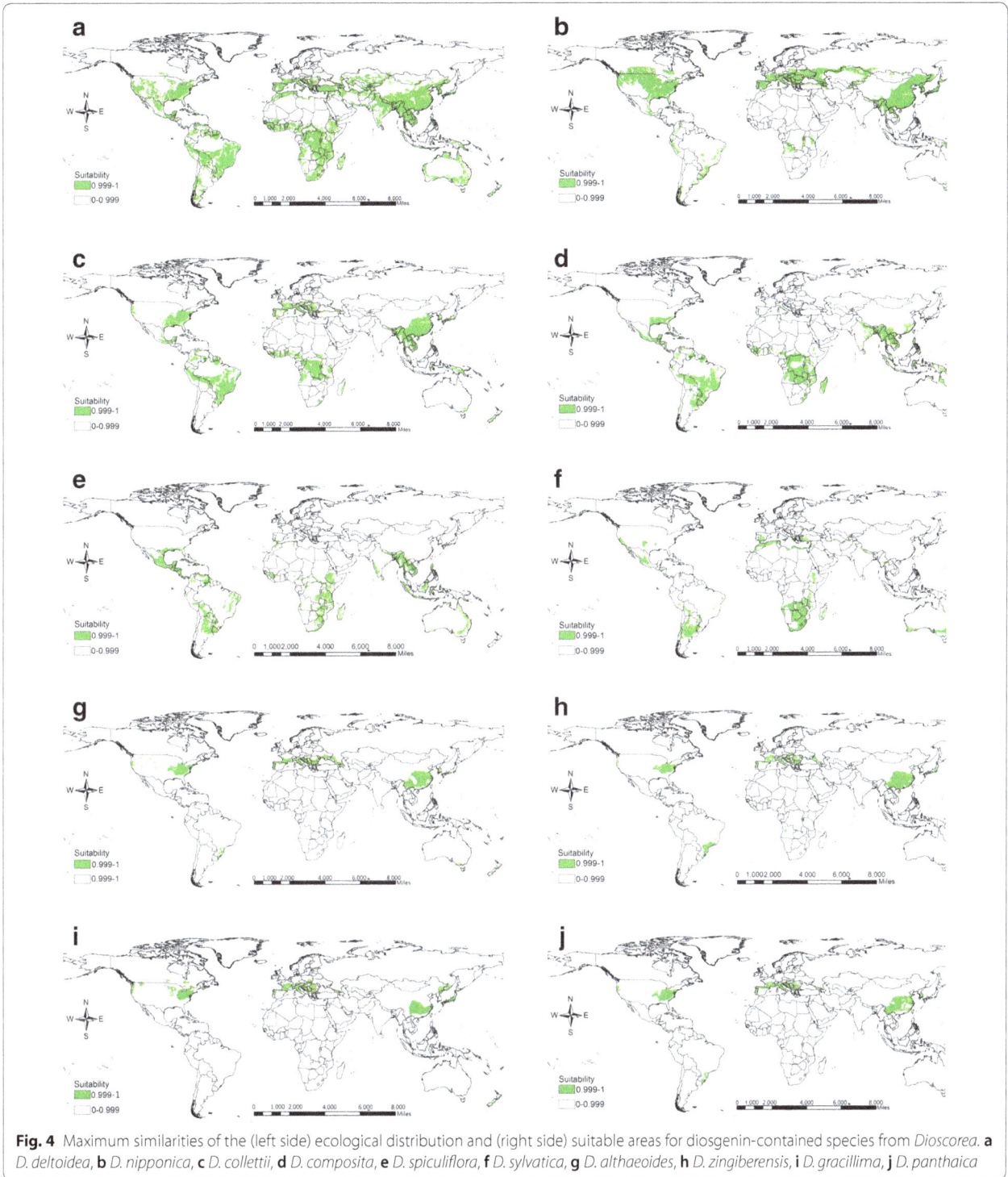

Fig. 4 Maximum similarities of the (left side) ecological distribution and (right side) suitable areas for diosgenin-contained species from *Dioscorea*. **a** *D. deltoidea*, **b** *D. nipponica*, **c** *D. collettii*, **d** *D. composita*, **e** *D. spiculiflora*, **f** *D. sylvatica*, **g** *D. althaeoides*, **h** *D. zingiberensis*, **i** *D. gracillima*, **j** *D. panthaica*

D. collettii and the six species above were in one group together. As can be evaluated from the branch length, the evolutionary divergence between two groups was significant, the outgroup were *Tacca chantieri* Andre and *Alisma plantago-aquatica* Linn.

Discussion

In recent years, species distribution models (SDMs) developed to be a significant tool to estimate the impact of climate change on plant distribution [40, 41]. These models formed a correlation between species

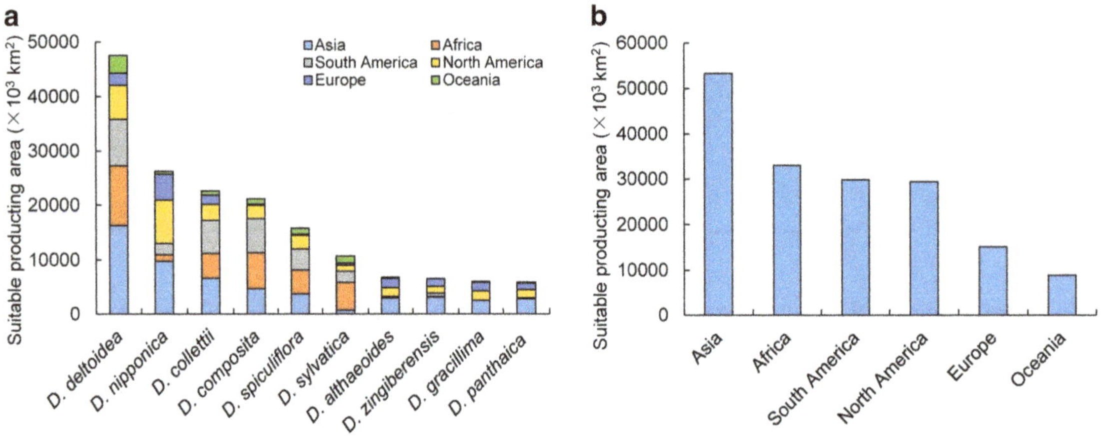

Fig. 5 Results of diosgenin-contained plants of ten *Dioscorea* species for suitable regions area in continents worldwide based on GMPGIS. **a** Suitable producing area of species, **b** suitable producing area of each continent

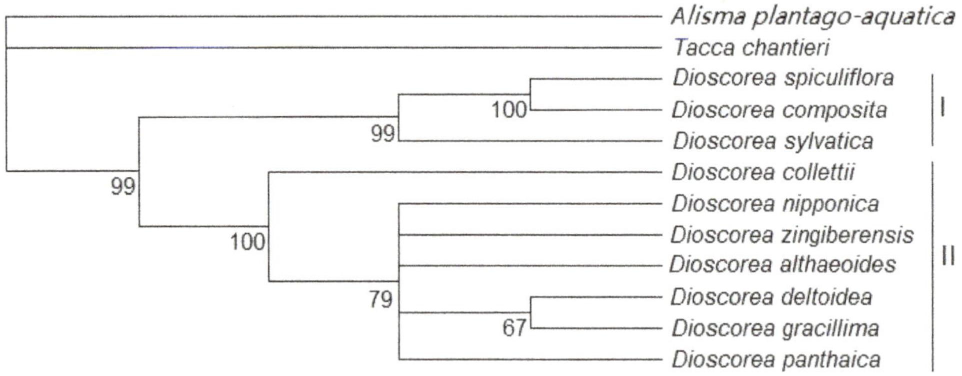

Fig. 6 Neighbor-joining tree of the *matK* and *rbcL* genes from accessions belonged to *Dioscorea* Numbers at the nodes indicate bootstrap values (% over 1000 replicates). I (African and North America species) II (Asia species)

existence and its geophysical environment to predict the current potential distribution of species [42, 43]. GMPGIS is a model capable of indicating the range of ecological factors and the suitable potential ecological areas simply by running a relatively small number of present data, presenting accuracy in predicting suitable region of plants, such as *Panax ginseng, Panax japonicas* [14, 15]. In this study, sample points from 108 to 274 of ten higher diosgenin-contained *Dioscorea* species were used in GMPGIS, the model suggested that the potentially suitable areas of *Dioscorea* species shared similarity distribution with occurrence dataset of ten species [21, 22], and some unknown potential areas were predicted in our study. Those data reiterated the conclusion of GMPGIS, which indicated that it was a viable accuracy method for modelling plant distributions. Consequently, the combination of GMPGIS and jackknife test will play a dominate role in the prediction

of suitable areas for medicinal species protection and cultivation.

Generally, environmental factors are the ones to blame for the driving forces of changes in *Dioscorea* species distribution and various ecological factors contribute to the growth of different species [15]. Most researches declared that *Dioscorea* species should be cultivated in high-temperature and fertile soil sandy loam, and its growth was determined by water shortage, strong light radiation and cold injury [44–46]. Therefore, summarizing the suitable climate factor of *Dioscorea* species distribution could provide a scientific basis for high-quality plants cultivation. This study found that the annual precipitation and annual mean radiation were the key factors driving the *Dioscorea* species distribution according to environment variable contributions. These results were confirmed by the results from current ecological feature study on *Dioscorea* species distribution. Seven *Dioscorea* species are distributed in Sichuan basin, China, and those plant species require a relatively damp habitat with low radiation to grow [45]. Previous studies on the relationship between effective constituent and ecological factors suggested that precipitation and radiation were the principal ecological factors affecting the diosgenin accumulated from *Dioscorea* species [47], and similarities or differences in growth habits could lead to different yields and qualities. Besides, the variety in annual mean radiation could also influence photosynthesis, and further affect the grow stage of diosgenin-contained *Dioscorea* species [48]. The results of this study proved a similar correlation between ecological factors and cultivation. In conclusion, during the process of introduction and cultivation of diosgenin plants, it is necessarily needed to make scientific plant management according to various suitable environmental conditions of *Dioscorea* species.

It seems fundamental to detect the potential distribution regions for the conservation and plantation of medicinal plants [49]. In this study, the modelled ecological niches and geographic distributions of these ten diosgenin-contained *Dioscorea* species showed a high degree of differentiation. The potential suitable areas of three Asia *Dioscorea* species (*D. deltoidea*, *D. nipponica* and *D. collettii*) were mainly located in the mideast region of North America and South America, southern part of Africa and eastern part of Asia, and the potential global distributions were within the scope of $(226.23–465.91) \times 10^5$ km^2. However, the other four Asia *Dioscorea* species (*D. zingiberensis*, *D. panthaica*, *D. althaeoides* and *D. gracillima*) were mainly potentially distributed in China, the United States and southern areas of Europe, and the potential suitable areas were within the scope of $(59.02–68.37) \times 10^5$ km^2. It indicated that some of *Dioscorea* species were distributed within a very narrow region, whereas other taxa were widely distributed in the world. Perhaps genetic information is one of the most significant causes to determine the distribution of *Dioscorea* species. Consequently, to select "where to plant or grow" the primary thing to do before the introduction and cultivation of diosgenin plant.

Our model results indicated that diosgenin-contained *Dioscorea* species could be introduced to many undiscovered potential areas, such as south of Europe and central north of America, except for the original production regions of *Dioscorea* above. According to the diosgenin contents and potential distribution, *D. deltoidea* and *D. nipponica* were recommended plants in the Asia. *D. deltoidea* and *D. sylvatica* were suggested being planted in Africa, *D. composita* and *D. spiculiflora* were suitable to be cultivated in North America. Potential suitable regions prediction in this study could provide a scientific basis for *Dioscorea* species selection, as well as the

introduction and cultivation worldwide. However, a field test is necessary before *Dioscorea* species cultivation in large areas, since the production would be affected by many other factors, such as local transport, natural disaster, and so on.

Phylogenetic trees of ten *Dioscorea* species were created by NJ methods. Among those species, seven from Asia formed a moderately supported group belonging to the same cluster. Three species of *D. spiculiflora*, *D. composita* and *D. sylvatica* belonged to another cluster, which came from Africa and North America. Previous studies showed that the Hengduan Mountains of China was a distributing center of *Dioscorea* species, and it also demonstrated a suitable potential area for *Dioscorea* species introduction and cultivation in this research [3]. Shen et al. reported seed traits character of *Haloxylon ammodendron* was strongly affected by climatic and geographical factors, and were moderately correlated with genetic diversity [50]. This study indicated that distribution region of species was correlated to its genetics and environment, and these potential suitable regions could introduce and cultivate *Dioscorea* species in the future.

Containing diosgenin, *Dioscorea* species owns a fine cultivated character and high reproduction, so the plantation scale of *Dioscorea* species in recent years has expanded constantly. However, cultivation distribution and ecological requirements of *Dioscorea* species remain chaotic and is in need of universal unification globally, yet confusion in its introduction and cultivation has led to a decline in yield and quality of diosgenin [7]. Our research result will provide a practical reference for the production of diosgenin in different areas worldwide. Combining with the research result, the plantation development directions of diosgenin-contained *Dioscorea* species in the future are (1) selecting suitable diosgenin species in accordance with the research results to conduct plantation; (2) strengthening ecological study on the quality of *Dioscorea* species, studying ecological characteristics of main cultivated species, and analyzing the influencing mechanism of environmental factors, such as light, temperature and water on the content and yield of diosgenin; (3) to develop a new variety of high-quality and stress-resistant *Dioscorea* species in the future.

Conclusions

In this study, a large occurrence dataset of diosgenin-contained *Dioscorea* species were obtained from Eastern Asia, Southern North America and Southern Africa. Results showed the potential distribution of these *Dioscorea* species presented a higher degree of differentiation, and that new ecological suitability areas were mainly distributed in the central region of South America, the southern part of the European and coastal region of Oceania. The annual precipitation and annual mean radiation were the important climatic factors controlling the distribution of those *Dioscorea* species. The suitable areas and assessment of climatic factors will serve as a useful reference for the conservation, introduction and cultivation of diosgenin *Dioscorea* plants in ecological suitable areas.

Additional files

Additional file 1: Table S1. Sample points and numbers of ten diosgenin-contained *Dioscorea* species. **Table S2.** Bioclimatic variables used as predictors in this study. **Table S3.** GenBank accessions of *matK* and *rbcL* sequences from *Dioscorea* and outgroup species. **Table S4.** Potential distribution sites and areas of diosgenin-contained *Dioscorea* species around the world ($\times 10^5$ km^2).

Additional file 2. Bioclimatic variables of 10 diosgenin-contained *Dioscorea* species.

Additional file 3. Minimum standards of reporting checklist.

Additional file 4: Figure S1. Boxplots are showing the percentage of stable habitat data of diosgenin-contained *Dioscorea* species under climate change models. **Figure S2.** Suitable areas for diosgenin-contained species from *Dioscorea*.

Authors' contributions
LXW and CSL conceived and designed the study. SL and XJ collected and performed the data analysis. SL, XJ, LL, HHY and MXX wrote the manuscript. All authors are responsible for reviewing data. All authors read and approved the final manuscript.

Acknowledgements
This study is supported and sponsored by the National Science-technology Support Plan Project (Grant No. 2015BAI05B02), Project supported by the China Postdoctoral Science Foundation (Grant No. 2017M611128).

Competing interests
The authors declare that they have no conflict of interest.

Consent for publication
All of authors consent to publication of this study in Journal of Chinese Medicine.

Funding
Project supported by the National Science-technology Support Plan Project (Grant No. 2015BAI05B02), Project supported by the China Postdoctoral Science Foundation (Grant No. 2017M611128).

References
1. Li X, Ma JZ, Shi YD. Research progress and prospects of dioscorea and diosgenin. Chem Ind For Prod. 2010;30(2):107–12.
2. Nie LH, Lin SZ, Ning ZY. Research progress of diosgenin from *Dioscorea* plants. Chin J Biochem Pharm. 2004;25(5):318–20.
3. Wan JR, Ding ZZ, Qin HZ. A phytogeographical study on the family Dioscoreaceae. Acta Bot Boreal-Occident Sin. 1994;14(2):128–35.
4. Yi T, Fan LL, Chen HL, Zhu GY, Suen HM, Tang YN, Zhu L, Chu C, Zhao ZZ, Chen HB. Comparative analysis of diosgenin in *Dioscorea* species and related medicinal plants by UPLC-DAD-MS. BMC Biochem. 2014;15:19.
5. Chaturvedi HC, Jain M, Kidwai NR. Cloning of medicinal plants through tissue culture-a review. Indian J Exp Biol. 2007;45(11):937–48.
6. Sautour M, Mitaine-Offer AC, Lacaille-Dubois MA. The *Dioscorea* genus, a review of bioactive steroid saponins. J Nat Med. 2007;61(2):91–101.
7. Liu P, Guo SL, Lv HF, Xie XW, Wu XY. A summary of the study on Chinese Dioscorea. J Zhejiang Nornal Univ (Nat. Sci). 1993;16(4):100–6.
8. Dansi A, Mignouna HD, Zoundjihekpon J, Sangare A, Asiedu R, Quin FM. Morphological diversity cultivar groups and possible descent in the cultivated yams *Dioscorea cayenensis, D. rotundata*) complex in Benin Republic. Genet Resour Crop Ev. 1999;46(4):371–88.
9. Ondo ovono P, Kevers C, Dommes J. Effects of planting methods and tuber weights on growth and yield of yam cultivars (*Dioscorea rotundata* Poir.) in Gabon. Int Res J Agr Sci. Soil Sci. 2016;6(3):32–42.
10. Viruel J, Catalán P, Segarra-Moragues JG. Latitudinal environmental niches and riverine barriers shaped the phylogeography of the central Chilean endemic *Dioscorea humilis* Dioscoreaceae). PLoS ONE. 2014;9(10):e110029.
11. Wang Z, Li B, Xiao JL, Jiang DC. Regionalization study of *Dioscorea nipponica* in Jilin province based on MaxEnt and ArcGIS. China J Chin Mater Med. 2017;42(22):4373–7.
12. Irfan-Ullah M, Amarnath G, Murthy MSR, Peterson AT. Mapping the geographic distribution of *Aglaia bourdillonii* Gamble (Meliaceae) an endemic and threatened plant using ecological niche modeling. Biodivers Conserv. 2006;16(6):1917–25.
13. Chen SL. Analysis on ecological suitability and regionalization of traditional Chinese medicinal material. 2nd ed. Beijing: Science Press; 2017.
14. Shen L, Wu J, Li XW, Xu J, Dong LL, Sang MC, Sun CZ, Fujiharas L, Chen SL. A study of global ecological adaptability and field selection practices of *Panax ginseng*. China J Chin Mater Med. 2016;41(18):3314–22.
15. Du ZX, Wu J, Meng XX, Li JH, Huang LF. Predicting the global potential distribution of four endangered *Panax* species in middle-and low-latitude regions of china by the geographic information system for global medicinal plants (GMPGIS). Molecules. 2017;22(10):1630.
16. Li BG. Research and industrial development of Chinese medicinal plant resources of Dioscorea. Beijing: Science press; 2006.
17. Singh KN, Kaushal R. Comprehensive notes on commercial utilization characteristics and status of steroid yielding plants in India. Ethnobot Leaflets. 2007;11:45–51.
18. Avula B, Wang YH, Ali Z, Smillie TJ, Khan IA. Chemical fingerprint analysis and quantitative determination of steroidal compounds from *Dioscorea villosa*, *Dioscorea* species and dietary supplements using UHPLC-ELSD. Biomed Chromatogr. 2014;28(2):281–94.
19. Viruel J, Segarra-Moragues JG, Raz L, Forest F, Wilkin P, Sanmartin I, Catalan P. Late cretaceous-early eocene origin of yams (*Dioscorea Dioscoreaceae*) in the Laurasian Palaearctic and their subsequent Oligocene-Miocene diversification. J Biogeogr. 2016;43(4):750–62.
20. Thapyai C, Wilkin P, Chayamarit K. The *Dioscorea* species of Doi Chiang Dao with particular reference to *Dioscorea collettii* Hook. f. Dioscoreaceae) a new record for northern Thailand. Thai Fort Bull Bot. 2005;33:213-9.
21. Tang SR, Yang RT, Pan FS, Zhao AM, Pang ZJ. Steroidal saponin and steroidal sapogenin in Chinese *Dioscorea* L. J Plant Resour Environ. 2007;16(2):64–72.
22. Hsu KM, Tsai JL, Chen MY, Ku HM, Liu SC. Molecular phylogeny of *Dioscorea* (Dioscoreaceae) in East and Southeast Asia. Blumea-Biodivers Evol Biogeogr Plant. 2013;58(1):21–7.
23. Yang LY, Xu ZZ, Chen C, Lv LF, Zhao Q, Yuan LC. A preliminary report on the domesitic cultivation experiment of *Dioscorea deltoidea*. Southwest China J Agr Sci. 2006;19(Suppl 1):218–21.
24. Cho J, Choi H, Lee J, Kim MS, Sohn HY, Lee DG. The antifungal activity and membrane-disruptive action of dioscin extracted from *Dioscorea nipponica*. BBA-Biomembranes. 2013;1828(3):1153–8.
25. Sun HQ, Luo K, Zou WJ, PsbA-trnH Deng SY. Fragment Sequence Analysis of *Dioscorea nipponica D. panthaica* and *D. zingiberensis*. Chin J Appl Environ Biol. 2006;12(6):792–7.
26. Blunden G, Hardman R, Hind FJ. The comparative morphology and anatomy of *Dioscorea sylvatica* Eckl. from Natal and the Transvaal. Bot J Linn Soc. 2008;64(4):431–46.
27. Pan RZ. Plant physiology. 7th ed. Beijing: Higher Education Press; 2012.

28. Zhang X, Meng XX, Wu J, Huang LF, Chen SL. Global ecological region-alization of 15 Illicium species: nature sources of shikimic acid. CHIN MED-UK. 2018;13(1):31.

29. Hijmans RJ, Cameron SE, Parra JL, Jones PG, Jarvis A. Very high resolution interpolated climate surfaces for global land areas. Int J Climatol. 2005;25:1965–78.

30. Kriticos DJ, Webber BL, Leriche A, Ota N, Macadam I, Bathols J, Scott JK. CliMond: global high-resolution historical and future scenario climate surfaces for bioclimatic modelling. Methods Ecol Evol. 2012;3(1):53–64.

31. Pearson RG, Raxworthy CJ, Nakamura M, Peterson AT. Predicting species distributions from small numbers of occurrence records, a test case using cryptic geckos in Madagascar. J Biogeogr. 2010;34(1):102–17.

32. Phillips SJ, Dudík M. Modeling of species distributions with Max-ent, new extensions and a comprehensive evaluation. Ecography. 2008;31(2):161–75.

33. Elith J, Phillips SJ, Hastie T, Dudík M, Chee YE, Yates CJ. A statistical expla-nation of MaxEnt for ecologists. Divers Distrib. 2011;17(1):43–57.

34. Phillips SJ, Anderson RP, Schapire RE. Maximum entropy modeling of spe-cies geographic distributions. Ecol Model. 2006;190(3):231–59.

35. Uchoi A, Malik SK, Choudhary R, Kumar S, Rohini MR, Pal D, Ercisli S, Chaudhury R. Inferring phylogenetic relationships of indian Citron Citrus medica L.) based on rbcL and matK sequences of chloroplast DNA. Biochem Genet. 2016;54(3):249–69.

36. Zinger L, Philippe H. Coalescing molecular evolution and DNA barcoding. Mol Ecol. 2016;25(9):1908–10.

37. Li DZ, Gao LM, Li HT, Wang H, Ge XJ, Liu JQ, et al. Comparative analysis of a large dataset indicates that internal transcribed spacer (ITS) should be incorporated into the core barcode for seed plants. Proc Natl Acad Sci USA. 2011;108(49):19641–6.

38. Chen ZD, Yang T, Lin L, Lu LM, Li HL, Sun M, et al. Tree of life for the genera of Chinese vascular plants. J Syst Evol. 2016;54(4):277–306.

39. Chase MW, Soltis DE, Olmstead RG, Morgan D, Les DH, Mishler BD, et al.

Phylogenetics of seed plants: an analysis of nucleotide sequences from the plastid gene rbcL. Ann Mo Bot Gard. 1993;80(3):528–80.

40. Thomas CD, Cameron A, Green RE, Bakkenes M, Beaumont LJ, Collingham YC, et al. Extinction risk from climate change. Nature. 2004;427:114–45.

41. Thuiller W, Lavorel S, Araujo MB, Sykes MT, Prentice IC. Climate change threats to plant diversity in Europe. Proc Natl Acad Sci USA. 2005;102(23):8245–50.

42. Kumar S, Stohlgren TJ. MaxEnt modeling for predicting suitable habitat for threatened and endangered tree Canacomyrica monticola in New Caledonia. J Ecol Nat Environ. 2009;1(1):94–8.

43. Elith J, Graham CH, Anderson RP, Dudik M, Ferrier S, Guisan A, et al. Ecological niche and species distribution modelling of sea stars along the Pacific Northwest continental shelf. Divers Distrib. 2016;22(12):1314–27.

44. Zhang SX, Zhou LY, Yu YJ. Study progress of Dioscorea nipponica Makino. Mol Plant Breed. 2005;3(1):107–11.

45. Xu XD, Hu P, Wu H. Planting situation of Dioscorea Zingiberensis C.H Wright in Sichuan and strategy of industrialized development. Resour Devel Market. 2005;21(5):447–8.

46. Sun J, Li XM, Zhang J. Preliminary studies on the influence of light inten-sity on growth and saponin contents of Dioscorea zingiberensis. Acta Bot Boreal-Occident Sin. 2011;31(3):536–42.

47. Akula R, Ravishankar GA. Influence of abiotic stress signals on secondary metabolites in plants. Plant Signal Behav. 2011;6(11):1720–31.

48. Srivastava AK, Gaiser T, Paeth H, Ewert F. The impact of climate change on Yam (Dioscorea alata) yield in the savanna zone of West Africa. Agric Ecosyst Environ. 2012;153(24):57–64.

49. Qin AL, Liu B, Guo QS, Bussmann RW, Ma FQ, Jian Z, Xu GX, Pei SX. Maxent modeling for predicting impacts of climate change on the potential dis-tribution of Thuja sutchuenensis Franch. An extremely endangered conifer from southwestern, China. Glob Ecol Conserv. 2017;10(C):139–46.

50. Shen L, Xu R, Liu S, Chen J, Xu CQ, Xie CX, Liu TN. Phenotypic variation of seed traits of Haloxylon ammodendron and its affecting factors. Biochem Syst Ecol. 2015;60:81–7.

10

A concise classification of *bencao* (*materia medica*)

Zhongzhen Zhao*, Ping Guo* and Eric Brand

Abstract

Books that record the sources and applications of medicinal materials are commonly known as *bencao* (*materia medica*) in China. *Bencao* (*materia medica*) literature review is the very first step in the standard authentication procedure of Chinese medicinals. As an important part of China's cultural heritage, these various *bencao* (*materia medica*) texts represent centuries of accumulated wisdom in combating disease and preserving health. In this short review, *bencao* (*materia medica*) classics of China are broadly divided into three major categories in our routine practice: mainstream *bencao* (*materia medica*), thematic *bencao* (*materia medica*) and regional *bencao* (*materia medica*). The overall significance and current situation of exploration of *bencao* (*materia medica*) literature are summarized as well.

Keywords: *Bencao* (*materia medica*), Chinese medicinal authentication, Traditional Chinese medicine

Background

China is a large country with diverse ecological conditions and abundant botanical, zoological and mineral resources. Among them, some are of medicinal value and have been used medicinally since ancient times. In China, books that record the sources and applications of medicinal materials are commonly known as *bencao* (*materia medica*). The Chinese term "*bencao*", which literally means "rooted in herbs", reflects the fact that most medicinal materials are derived from botanical sources. *Bencao* (*materia medica*) texts of past dynasties primarily describe three aspects of Chinese medicinals: medicinal materials, medicinal properties, and medicinal principles. As an important part of China's cultural heritage, these various *bencao* (*materia medica*) texts represent centuries of accumulated wisdom in combating disease and preserving health. *The Complete Collection of Traditional Texts on Chinese Materia Medica*, a 410-volume and 246,000-page collection complied by the Association of Chinese Culture Research, includes more than 800 *bencao* (*materia medica*) classics from 220 BC to 1911 AD. This collection highlights the value of traditional

Chinese medicine (TCM) as a rich source for knowledge-based medical rediscovery due to its documentation of clinical experiences over thousands of years, and also illustrates the monumental challenge of selecting the best parts of TCM for modern innovation ([1–3], Fig. 1).

The genre of *bencao* (*materia medica*) literature is uniquely developed in Chinese medicine, and represents a tremendous historical and cultural resource as well as an important reference point for clinicians, medical historians, and scientists in disciplines such as new drug discovery and Chinese medicinal authentication. Authentication is fundamental for Chinese medicinal standardization, and *bencao* (*materia medica*) literature review is the very first step in the standard authentication procedure of Chinese medicinals ([4], Fig. 2).

In practice, *bencao* (*materia medica*) classics of China are broadly divided into three major categories: (a) mainstream *bencao* (*materia medica*): the most influential *bencao* (*materia medica*) classics from key historical periods, (b) thematic *bencao* (*materia medica*): specialized *bencao* (*materia medica*) texts dedicated to specific topics, and c) regional *bencao* (*materia medica*): *bencao* (*materia medica*) texts focused on medicinal materials from specific regions.

*Correspondence: zzzhao@hkbu.edu.hk; s193231@hkbu.edu.hk
School of Chinese Medicine, Hong Kong Baptist University, Kowloon
Tong, Hong Kong, China

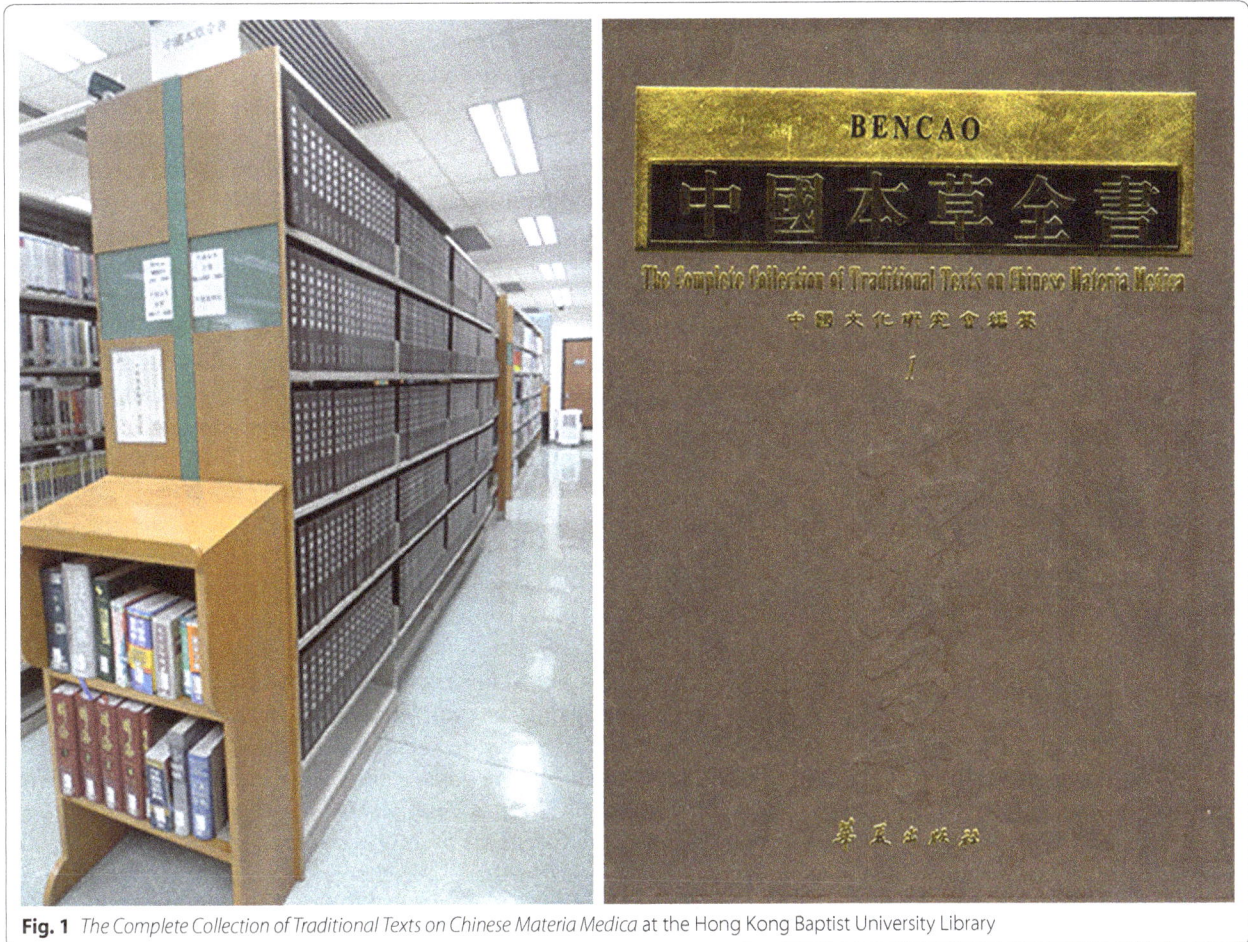

Fig. 1 *The Complete Collection of Traditional Texts on Chinese Materia Medica* at the Hong Kong Baptist University Library

Mainstream *bencao* (*materia medica*)

Over the past 2000 years, five monumental works stand out in the genre of *bencao* (*materia medica*) literature. They are the most influential classics from key historical periods.

(1) *The Divine Husbandman's Classic of Materia Medica* (*Shen Nong Ben Cao Jing*) This is the earliest extant *bencao* (*materia medica*) text, compiled in the Eastern Han Dynasty (25–220 AD). This text records 365 medicinals and summarizes medicinal experiences up to the Han Dynasty. Medicinals are classified into three categories (high-grade, medium-grade and low-grade) based on their medicinal effects and toxicity. Entries for each medicinal substance include nomenclature, properties, compatibilities, and medical applications. Descriptions of production regions and the ecological environment of some medicinal plants are also recorded briefly.

(2) *Collection of Commentaries on the Classic of the Materia Medica* (*Ben Cao Jing Ji Zhu*) Tao Hongjing, a physician of the North and South Kingdoms period (420–589 AD), compiled this text by preserving and annotating *The Divine Husbandman's Classic of Materia Medica* (*Shen Nong Ben Cao Jing*) and adding another 365 medicinals. It records 730 medicinals and established the framework of *bencao* (*materia medica*) compilations adopted by later generations. In this book, medicinal substances are further classified into seven categories based on their natural properties: jades/stones, herbs, trees, insects/beasts, fruits/vegetables, crops, and medicinals with names but without actual applications.

(3) *Newly Revised Materia Medica* (*Xin Xiu Ben Cao*) In 659 AD, commissioned by the government of the Tang Dynasty (618–907 AD), this text records 850 medicinals and is considered to be the earliest national pharmacopoeia in China.

(4) *Materia Medica Arranged According to Pattern* (*Zheng Lei Ben Cao*) Compiled by a physician named Tang Shenwei and published in 1108 AD, this is the most praiseworthy *bencao* (*materia medica*) of the Song Dynasty (960–1279 AD) as it comprehensively summarizes herbal knowledge up

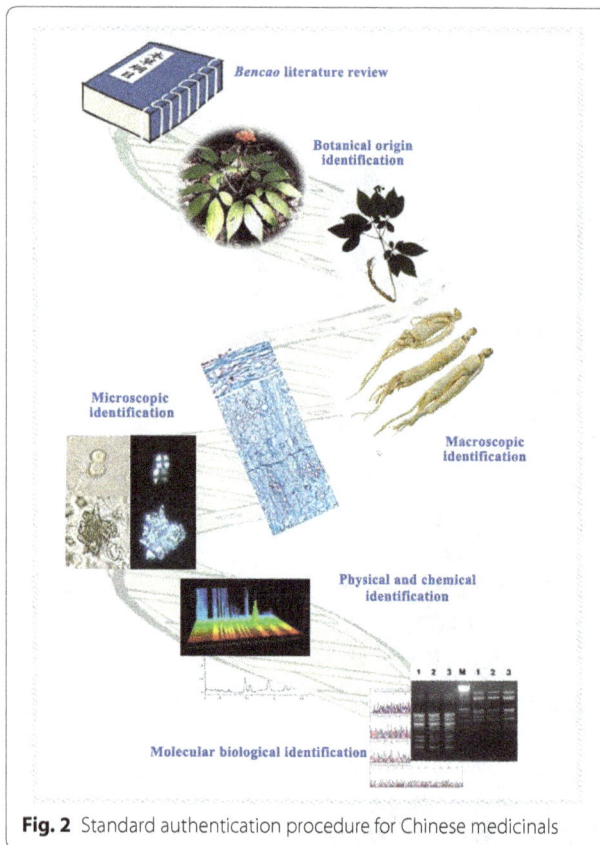

Fig. 2 Standard authentication procedure for Chinese medicinals

to that time. There are three versions of this book ("*Da Guan*", "*Zheng He*" and "*Shao Xing*") currently in circulation. It records 1746 medicinals and is the only *bencao* (*materia medica*) text from the Song and previous dynastic periods that survived intact. It features clearly preserved quotations from previous works and stands out as an important reference point for *bencao* (*materia medica*) knowledge leading up to the Song Dynasty.

(5) *Compendium of Materia Medica* (*Ben Cao Gang Mu*) Written by Li Shizhen, a physician of the Ming Dynasty (1368–1644 AD), this text was first published in 1596. It records 1892 medicinal substances. This massive and influential compilation represents the highest academic achievement among all the ancient Chinese *bencao* (*materia medica*). It not only comprehensively summarized medical knowledge up to the sixteenth century in China, but also contributed greatly to the development of natural sciences in the world.

Thematic *bencao* (*materia medica*)

Thematic *bencao* (*materia medica*) refer to specialized *bencao* (*materia medica*) texts dedicated to specific topics, such as medicinal processing, authentication, dietary

therapy, and medicinal properties. Examples include *Grandfather Lei's Treatise on Herbal Processing* (*Lei Gong Pao Zhi Lun*) and *Origins of the Materia Medica* (*Ben Cao Yuan Shi*). The former is the first monograph on Chinese medicinal processing, written in about 500 AD in the North and South Kingdoms period; it summarizes the literature and experiences of the ancient practice of processing. The latter stands out in the history of *bencao* (*materia medica*) as an outstanding monograph on macroscopic identification, written by Li Zhongli in the Ming Dynasty (1368–1644 AD). It is characterized by detailed illustrations and descriptions of diagnostic features of raw medicinal materials. Other examples of thematic *bencao* texts include the *Materia Medica of Dietary Therapy* (*Shi Liao Ben Cao*) of the Tang Dynasty and the *Materia Medica for Decoctions* (*Tang Ye Ben Cao*) of the Yuan Dynasty (1279–1368 AD). The former was dedicated to the theory and practice of dietary therapy, and the latter to the theory of medicinal properties and clinical experience.

Regional *bencao* (*materia medica*)

Regional *bencao* (*materia medica*) texts record knowledge related to medicinal substances derived from specific local regions. Examples include the *Materia Medica from Steep Mountainsides* (*Lu Chan Yan Ben Cao*) and the *Essentials of Raw Herbs in Lingnan* (*Sheng Cao Yao Xing Bei Yao*). The former was the first regional *bencao* (*materia medica*) with color illustrations dedicated to local medicinal plants; compiled in 1220 AD in the Song Dynasty, it focused on the area around modern-day Hangzhou. The latter was compiled in 1711 AD in the Qing Dynasty (1644–1911 AD); it records botanical medicinals used in the Lingnan region, a geographic area located in the southern part of China.

Conclusion

Bencao (*materia medica*) tradition provides a rich record of knowledge that has been gradually refined for centuries, opening a window into the cultural tradition of scholarship and textual research that defines TCM. *Bencao* (*materia medica*) literature such as the *Compendium of Materia Medica* (*Ben Cao Gang Mu*) illustrates important developments in the broader history of natural sciences in China, and this text has been translated into European languages since 1735 AD. In recent decades, exploration of *bencao* (*materia medica*) literature has facilitated dramatic medical discoveries, such as the antimalarial drug artemisinin from sweet wormwood (*qinghao*, Artemisiae Annuae Herba) [5].

However, at present, the overall significance of *bencao* (*materia medica*) literature remains underestimated outside of the TCM community. Therefore, in addition to other aspects of TCM, attention is needed to preserve the cultural resources that lie at the heart of *bencao* (*materia medica*).

Although our research efforts related to *daodi* medicinal materials, medicinal authentication and Chinese medicinal processing are closely connected to *bencao* (*materia medica*) literature [6–9], the future of *bencao* (*materia medica*) research depends upon a multidisciplinary approach that protects the past while embracing the future.

Abbreviation
TCM: traditional Chinese medicine.

Authors' contributions
ZZ and PG designed the study. ZZ, PG and EB drafted and revised the manuscript. All authors read and approved the final manuscript.

Acknowledgements
Not applicable.

Competing interests
The authors declare that they have no competing interests.

Consent for publication
Not applicable.

Funding
Not applicable.

References
1. Lu J, editor. The complete collection of traditional texts on Chinese materia medica. Beijing: Huaxia Publishing House; 1999.
2. Zhao ZZ, Liang ZT, Guo P, Chen HB. Medicinal plants of China. In: Singh RJ, editor. Genetic resources, chromosome engineering, and crop improvement: medicinal plants, vol. 6. Boca Raton: CRC Press; 2012. p. 123–62.
3. Xu QH, Bauer R, Hendry BM, Fan TP, Zhao ZZ, Duez P, Simmonds MSJ, Witt CM, Lu AP, Robinson N, Guo DA, Hylands PJ. The quest for modernisation of traditional Chinese medicine. BMC Complement Altern Med. 2013;13:132.
4. Zhao ZZ, Hu YN, Liang ZT, Yuen JPS, Jiang ZH, Leung KSY. Authentication is fundamental for standardization of Chinese medicines. Planta Med. 2006;72:865–74.
5. Tu YY. The discovery of artemisinin (qinghaosu) and gifts from Chinese medicine. Nat Med. 2011;17:1217–20.
6. Zhao ZZ, Guo P, Brand E. The formation of daodi medicinal materials. J Ethnopharmacol. 2012;140:476–81.
7. Zhao ZZ, Liang ZT, Guo P. Macroscopic identification of Chinese medicinal materials: traditional experiences and modern understanding. J Ethnopharmacol. 2011;134:556–64.
8. Zhao ZZ, Chen HB, Guo P, Brand E. Chinese medicinal identification: an illustrated approach. Taos: Paradigm Publications; 2014.
9. Guo P, Brand E, Zhao ZZ. Chinese medicinal processing: a characteristic aspect of ethnopharmacology of traditional Chinese medicine. In: Heinrich M, Jager AK, editors. ethnopharmacology. Chichester: Wiley; 2015. p. 303–16.

11

The neuroprotective effects of *Tao-Ren-Cheng-Qi Tang* against embolic stroke in rats

Ling-Wei Hsu[1†], Wei-Cheng Shiao[1,2†], Nen-Chung Chang[3], Meng-Che Yu[1], Ting-Lin Yen[1], Philip Aloysius Thomas[4], Thanasekaran Jayakumar[1*] and Joen-Rong Sheu[1,5*]

Abstract

Background: Combinations of the traditional Chinese and Western medicines have been used to treat numerous diseases throughout the world, and there is a growing body of evidence showing that some of the herbs used in traditional Chinese medicine elicit significant pharmacological effects. The aim of this study was to demonstrate the neuroprotective effects of *Tao-Ren-Cheng-Qi Tang* (TRCQT) in combination with aspirin following middle cerebral artery occlusion (MCAO)—induced embolic stroke in rats.

Methods: A blood clot was embolized into the middle cerebral artery of rats to induce focal ischemic brain injury. After 24 h of MCAO occlusion, the rats were arbitrarily separated into five groups and subjected to different oral treatment processes with TRCQT and aspirin for 30 days before being evaluated in terms of their neurological behavior using a four-point system. The rats were sacrificed at 30 days after drug treatment and the infarct volumes were measured using a 2,3,5-triphenyltetrazolium chloride staining method. Tumor necrosis factor-α (TNF-α), c-Jun N-terminal kinases (JNK), activated caspase-3 and Bax were detected by western blot analysis. The apoptotic cells were identified by Terminal deoxynucleotidyl transferase dUTP nick end labeling (TUNEL) staining. ROS generation was also measured by electron spin resonance spectrometry.

Results: Rats treated with TRCQT alone or in combination with aspirin showed a significantly reduced infarct volume ($P < 0.001$) and improved neurological outcome compared with those treated with distilled water. Rats treated with TRCQT alone ($P = 0.021$) or in combination with aspirin ($P = 0.02$) also showed significantly reduced MCAO-induced expression levels of TNF-α and pJNK ($P < 0.001$) in their ischemic regions. Rats treated with TRCQT alone or in combination with aspirin showed decreased apoptosis by a reduction in the number of TUNEL positive cells, which inhibited the expression of activated caspase-3 ($P = 0.038$) and Bax ($P = 0.004$; $P = 0.003$). TRCQT also led to a significant concentration-dependent reduction in the formation of hydroxyl radicals ($P < 0.001$).

Conclusions: TRCQT reduced brain infarct volume and improved neurological outcomes by reducing apoptosis, attenuating the expression of TNF-α and p-JNK, and reducing the formation of hydroxyl radicals in MCAO-induced embolic stroke of rats.

Background

The incidence of stroke has markedly increased in developing countries over the past four decades [1]. Most strokes are caused by a thromboembolism, which disrupts cerebral blood flow, leading to oxygen and glucose deprivation in cells [2]. Secondary strokes who the individuals have a stroke history often have a higher rate of death and disability because of existing damage to the parts of the brain injured by the original stroke. Aspirin has been used to prevent secondary stroke. The incidence of cerebral hemorrhage and other bleeding events

*Correspondence: tjaya_2002@yahoo.co.in; sheujr@tmu.edu.tw
†Ling-Wei Hsu and Wei-Cheng Shiao contributed equally to this work
[1] Graduate Institute of Medical Sciences, College of Medicine, Taipei Medical University, Taipei, Taiwan
Full list of author information is available at the end of the article

is higher in China than it is in people from other high-income countries [3]. Ischemic brain tissue can be partially prevented from sprouting into infarction by several neuroprotective drugs [4]. It is noteworthy however, that numerous experimentally effective neuroprotective drugs have failed in clinical trials in human because of serious side effects [5].

Chinese medicines (CMs) usually contain a large number of compounds, which can affect multiple targets [6, 7], and several CMs have been used to treat stroke [8]. Previous studies have reported that the well-known Chinese formula *Tao-Hong-Si-Wu Tang* can be used to treat type 2 diabetes [9], as well as several mental disorders, including periodic psychosis, mania, neurosis, menopausal syndrome and involutional depression [10]. However, *Tao-Ren-Cheng-Qi Tang* (TRCQT) has not been clinically or experimentally used to treat stroke. In this study, we have used TRCQT, which consists of *Tao Ren* (*Prunus persica* (L.) Batsch., 5.0 g), *Gui Zhi* (*Cinnamon Twig.*, 5.0 g), *Mang Xiao* (*Natrii Sulfas*, 5.0 g), *Zhi Gan Cao* (*Radix Glycyrrhizae Preparata.*, 5.0 g) and *Da Huang* (*Radix et Rhizoma Rhei.*,10 g), to treat ischemic stroke in a rat animal model. The aim of this study was to demonstrate the neuroprotective effects of TRCQT in combination with aspirin following a middle cerebral artery occlusion (MCAO)-induced embolic stroke in rats.

Methods
Tao-Ren-Cheng-Qi Tang
A dried powder sample of TRCQT (Batch Number, 161342) was purchased from the Sun Ten Pharma. Co. (Taichung, Taiwan). The composition of a 30-g portion of this material was as follows: *Tao Ren* 5.0 g, *Gui Zhi* 5.0 g, *Mang Xiao* 5.0 g, *Da Huang* 10 g, *Zhi Gan Cao* 5.0 g. Thirty grams of this herbal mixture was extracted with water, yielding 7.0 g of dry extract (30.0:7.0 = 4.3:1). This material was mixed with 5 g of corn starch to give 12 g of final product. For sample preparation, the dried extract of TRCQT was dissolved in sterilized saline water (0.9% NaCl) at a concentration of 0.5 g/kg.

Reagents
3-(4,5-Dimethylthiazol-2-yl)-2,5-diphenyltetrazolium bromide (MTT) and propidium iodide (PI) were purchased from Sigma-Aldrich (St. Louis, MO, USA). TNF-α, JNK, Bax and activated caspase-3 antibodies were purchased from Cell Signaling Technology (Beverly, MA, USA). The anti-α-tubulin mAb was purchased from Neo Markers (Fremont, CA, USA). The Hybond-P polyvinylidene difluoride membrane, enhanced chemiluminescence (ECL) western blotting detection reagent and analysis system, horseradish peroxidase (HRP)-conjugated donkey anti-rabbit immunoglobulin G (IgG) and

sheep anti-mouse IgG were purchased from Amersham (Buckinghamshire, UK).

MCAO-induced ischemia rat model
Healthy male Wistar rats (250–300 g) were used in this study. All of the animal studies were conducted in accordance with the standards established in the Guide for the Care and Use of Laboratory Animals, which was published by the Institutional Animal Care and Use Committee (IACUC) of Taipei Medical University (Additional file 1). The animal studies were also performed in accordance with the ARRIVE guideline (Additional file 2). Thirty rats were acclimated for 20 days before dosing, but only 25 of these animals were used the following experiments. All of the rats were kept at 37 °C in groups of five under a 12-h dark/light cycle with ad libitum access to food and water before the surgery. The rats were subjected to MCAO-induced ischemia by the administration of an autologous blood clot, as described in our previous studies [11, 12]. After surgery, the rats were housed individually under similar environmental conditions and were found to be free of apparent infection or inflammation, as well as showing no neurological deficits. In this study, at 24 h after MCA occlusion, the rats were arbitrarily separated into five groups of five rats each, including (group 1) sham-operated; (group 2) orally treated with distilled water for 30 days, followed by thromboembolic occlusion; (groups 3 and 4) treated with aspirin (5 mg/kg) and TRCQT (0.5 g/kg) alone for 30 days, followed by thromboembolic occlusion; and (group 5) treated with TRCQT (0.5 g/kg) combined with aspirin (5 mg/kg), followed by thromboembolic occlusion.

Neurological functional tests
To assess the neurobehavioral scoring of the animals, a sensorimotor integrity was measured for 30 days after MCAO by an investigator with no prior knowledge of the group allocation (Additional file 3) [13]. The neurologic scores were measured by using a 4-point sliding scale. Each rat was examined for resistance to lateral push (score = 4), open field circling (score = 3) and shoulder adduction (score = 2) or contralateral forelimb flexion (score = 1) when held by the tail. Rats extending both forelimbs towards the floor and not showing any other signs of neurologic impairment were scored 0. In this study, all of the rats subjected to MCAO either exhibited a neurologic score of 4 when they were examined 24 h after ischemia or immediately before reperfusion, or were excluded from the study.

Quantification of brain infarct volume
At 24 h after reperfusion, the rats were anesthetized and their brains were removed and cut into 2-mm-thick

slices. The slices were then immersed in a 2% solution of 2,3,5-triphenyltetrazolium chloride (TTC) in phosphate-buffered saline at 37 °C for 30 min and fixed in 4% phosphate buffered formalin. The infarct areas of each slice were determined using a computerized image analyzer (Image-Pro plus). These areas were then summed and multiplied by the slice thickness to give the infarct volumes of each slice, which were calculated according to the method reported by Hsiao's group [11]. None of the animals died during these experiments.

Western blot analysis
After 30 days of TRCQT treatment followed by thrombo-embolic occlusion, the rat brain tissues were collected and homogenized, followed by sonication in a lysis buffer containing 20 mM Tris–HCl (pH 7.5), 1 mM $MgCl_2$, 125 mM NaCl, 1% Triton X-100, 1 mM phenylmethylsulfonyl fluoride, 10 µg/mL leupeptin, 10 µg/mL aprotinin, 25 mM β-glycerophosphate, 50 mM sodium fluoride and 100 µM sodium orthovanadate. The expression levels of TNF-α, phospho-JNK, activated caspase-3 and Bax-2 were analyzed by immunoblotting, as described previously by Rodrigo et al. [14] with minor modifications. A mixture of tris-buffered saline and Tween 20 (TBST) buffer containing 0.1% Tween 20 was used to wash the membranes.

Detection of DNA fragmentation by TUNEL assay
The in situ detection of DNA fragmentation in the brain tissues of the rats was performed 30 days after TRCQT treatment followed by thromboembolic occlusion using a TUNEL detection kit (Millipore, Billerica, Massachusetts, USA). Briefly, brain tissues were fixed in 4% formaldehyde and embedded in paraffin wax. Five micrometer sections of the embedded material were then cut and washed for 30 min in PBS. The sections were then equilibrated in water for 30 min at 37 °C, before being incubated in a mixture of Proteinase K (250 µL) enzyme at 37 °C for 30 min. The proteinase K digestion process was stopped by washing the sections with PBS (four 2-min wash cycles). The sections were then incubated in terminal deoxynucleotidyl transferase (TdT) buffer [2.5 mM Tris–HCl (pH 6.6), 0.2 M potassium cacodylate, 2.5 mM $CoCl_2$, 0.25 mg/mL bovine serum albumin (BSA)] for 10 min, followed by 60 min at 37 °C in a TdT end-labeling cocktail. The TdT end-labeling cocktail was removed and the reaction was stopped, and the resulting sections were washed in PBS. The sections were incubated in Avidin-FITC in the dark for 30 min at 37 °C and then washed in PBS to end the reaction. The sections were then counterstained with PI for 10 min at 37 °C and mounted on a cover slip. Only the green-stained cells were counted as belonging to the apoptotic phenotype and the density of apoptotic cells was detected by immuno-fluorescent

microscopy (TCS SP5, Leica, Mannheim, Germany) by counting the green-stained cells.

Measurements of hydroxyl radical (OH·⁻) formation by electron spin resonance (ESR) spectrometry
ESR experiments were conducted according to the method reported by Chou et al. [15] using a Bruker EMX ESR spectrometer (Billerica, MA, USA). Briefly, a Fenton reaction solution (50 µm $FeSO_4$ + 2 mM H_2O_2) was pretreated with a solvent control (0.1% DMSO) or TRCQT (0.3, 0.7 and 1.3 mg/mL) for 10 min. The rate of hydroxyl radical-scavenging activity was defined by the following equation:

Inhibition rate =
   1 − [signal height (TRCQT)/signal height (control)]

Statistical analysis
The results were expressed as the mean ± SD and were accompanied by the number of observations. The experiments were assessed by analysis of variance (ANOVA), version 9.2 (SAS Inc., Cary, NC, USA), using the Newman–Keuls method. A P value of less than 0.05 was considered statistically significant. Concentration-dependent effects were determined by visual inspection of the results.

Results
Effect of TRCQT, aspirin alone, or in combination on infarct volume
The effects of TRCQT and aspirin alone or in combination on the infarct volumes are shown in Fig. 1A, B. Compared with the group treated with distilled water (group 2), the animals treated with TRCQT alone showed a significant decrease in their infarct volume ($P < 0.001$). In contrast, the group treated with aspirin alone (group 3) did not show any significant effects. A similar effect was also found in rats treated with aspirin combined with TRCQT (group 5) ($P < 0.001$) for 30 days after MCAO compared with the sham-operated (group 1).

Neurobehavioral assessment
Neurological deficit was examined at 24 h after reperfusion and scored on a 4-point scale according to the method described by Bederson's group [13]. The changes observed in the neurological deficit scores of the different groups are shown in Fig. 2. Rats treated with aspirin (group 3) for 30 days after MCAO exhibited a moderate reduction in their neurobehavioral scores compared with the sham-operated group at 24 h after ischemia ($P = 0.0525$). However, rats treated with TRCQT alone (group 4) for 30 days showed a significant reduction in their neurobehavioral deficit score compared with the sham-operated group at 24 h after thromboembolic occlusion ($P = 0.0537$). Notably, rats treated with a

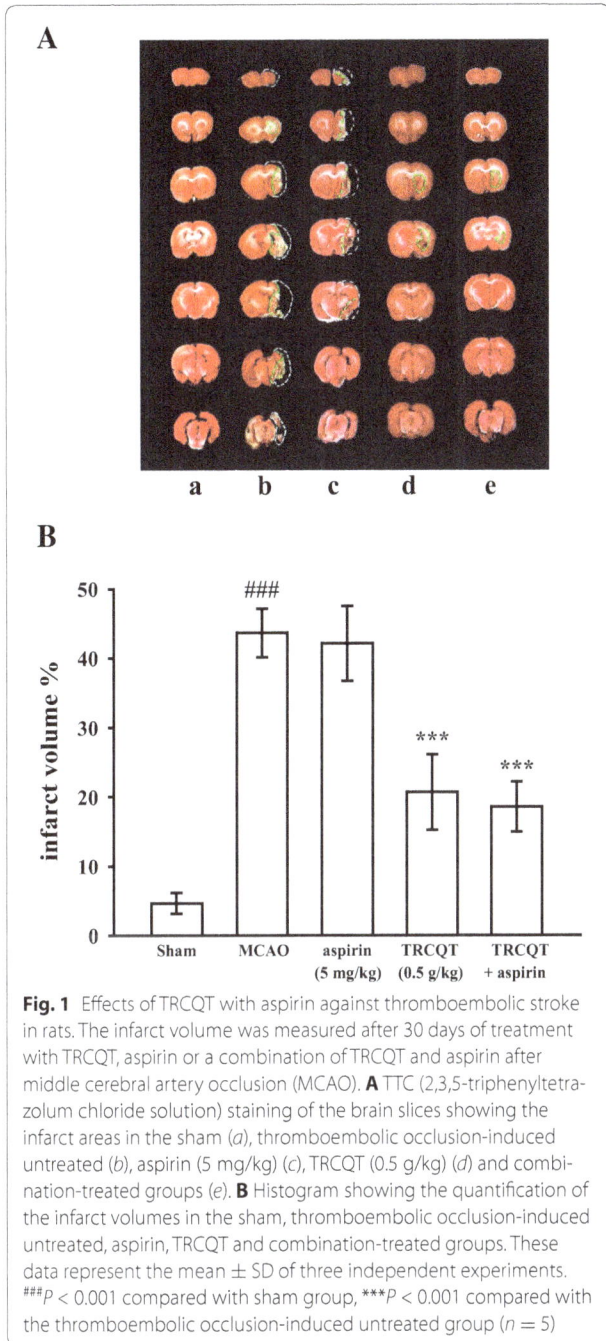

Fig. 1 Effects of TRCQT with aspirin against thromboembolic stroke in rats. The infarct volume was measured after 30 days of treatment with TRCQT, aspirin or a combination of TRCQT and aspirin after middle cerebral artery occlusion (MCAO). **A** TTC (2,3,5-triphenyltetrazolum chloride solution) staining of the brain slices showing the infarct areas in the sham (*a*), thromboembolic occlusion-induced untreated (*b*), aspirin (5 mg/kg) (*c*), TRCQT (0.5 g/kg) (*d*) and combination-treated groups (*e*). **B** Histogram showing the quantification of the infarct volumes in the sham, thromboembolic occlusion-induced untreated, aspirin, TRCQT and combination-treated groups. These data represent the mean ± SD of three independent experiments. ###$P < 0.001$ compared with sham group, ***$P < 0.001$ compared with the thromboembolic occlusion-induced untreated group ($n = 5$)

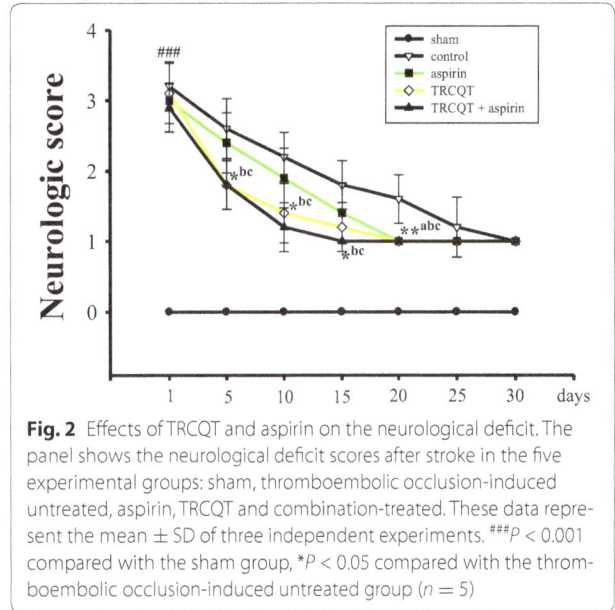

Fig. 2 Effects of TRCQT and aspirin on the neurological deficit. The panel shows the neurological deficit scores after stroke in the five experimental groups: sham, thromboembolic occlusion-induced untreated, aspirin, TRCQT and combination-treated. These data represent the mean ± SD of three independent experiments. ###$P < 0.001$ compared with the sham group, *$P < 0.05$ compared with the thromboembolic occlusion-induced untreated group ($n = 5$)

TRCQT ($P = 0.021$) alone showed significant decreases in the expression of this protein. Moreover, a significant inhibitory effect was observed in the expression of TNF-α in the rats treated with aspirin (0.5 g/kg) combined with TRCQT ($P = 0.02$).

The effects of the TRCQT, aspirin and TRCQT/aspirin combination on the levels of p-JNK are shown in Fig. 3b. Compared with the MCAO-induced group, the rats treated with TRCQT or aspirin alone showed a significant decrease in their p-JNK levels ($P < 0.001$). The rats treated with a combination of aspirin and TRCQT also showed a significant decrease in their expression of p-JNK compared with those from the individual treatment groups ($P < 0.001$).

TRCQT inhibited the apoptosis-related proteins Bax and activated caspase-3 in the ischemic brain tissues

As shown in Fig. 4a, there was a significant increase ($P = 0.015$) in the levels of Bax protein in the MCAO-induced group compared with the sham group. Although the rats treated with aspirin or TRCQT alone showed a significant decrease in the expression of Bax ($P = 0.018$ and 0.013, respectively), this effect was potentiated when these treatments were combined ($P = 0.011$).

The expression of activated caspase-3 did not change in the sham, MCAO-induced or aspirin treated rats (Fig. 4b), but there was significant decrease in the expression levels of this protein in the rats treated with a combination of aspirin and TRCQT ($P = 0.048$). The rats treated with TRCQT alone also showed a considerable decrease in their activated caspase-3 expression, although this effect was not significant.

combination of aspirin and TRCQT showed a better neurobehavioral outcome than those treated those treated with TRCQT or aspirin alone ($P = 0.0119$).

TRCQT enhanced aspirin's inhibitory effect on TNF-α and p-JNK in the ischemic brain

As shown in Fig. 3a, there was a significant increase in the expression levels of TNF-α in the MCAO-induced group, whereas the groups treated with aspirin ($P = 0.043$) or

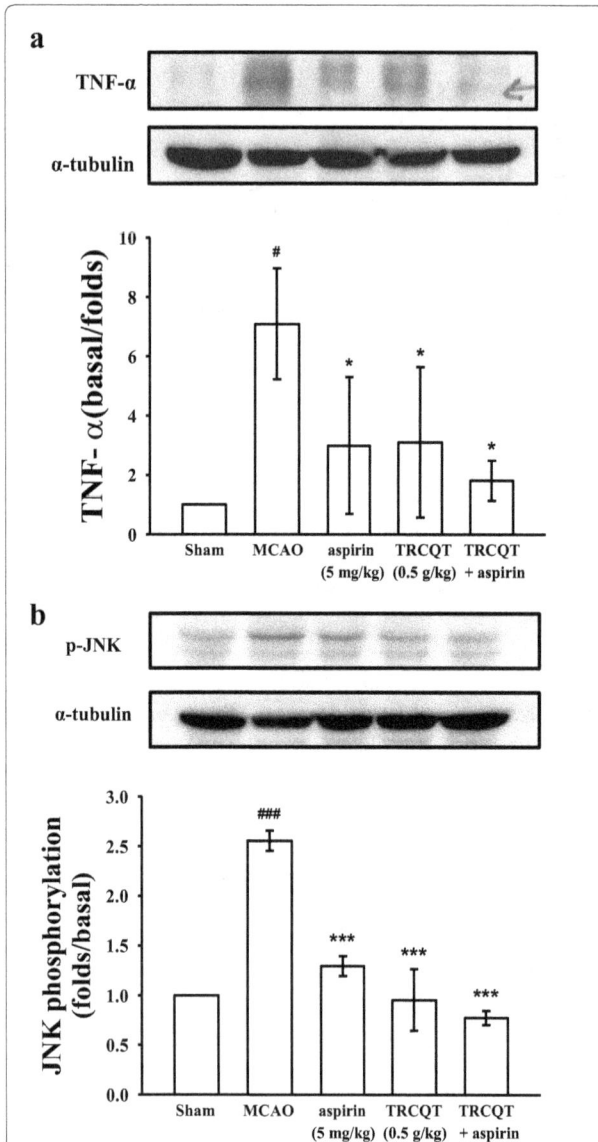

Fig. 3 Effects of TRCQT combined with aspirin on the expressions of TNF-α (**a**) and p-JNK (**b**) in cerebral homogenates 30 days after thromboembolic stroke in rats. The data represent the mean ± SD of three independent experiments. [#] and [###]$P < 0.01$ compared with the sham-operated group, * and ***$P < 0.05$ compared with the thromboembolic occlusion-induced untreated group. Equal loading in each lane was demonstrated by similar intensities of α-tubulin ($n = 5$)

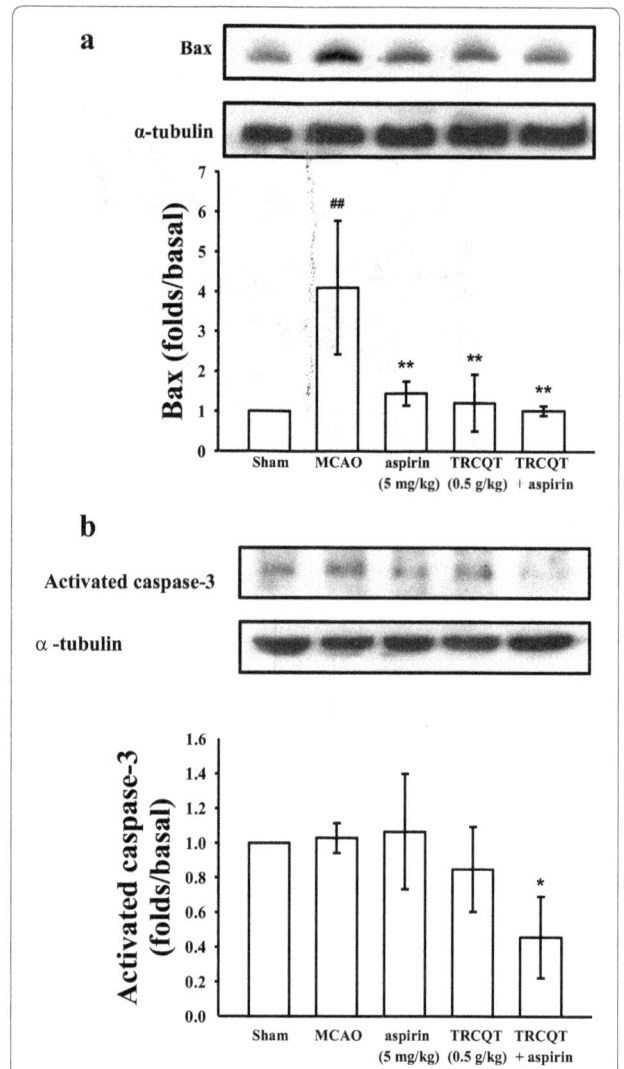

Fig. 4 Effects of TRCQT combined with aspirin on the expression levels of Bax (**a**) and activated caspase-3 (**b**) in cerebral homogenates 30 days after thromboembolic stroke in rats. The data represent the mean ± SD of three independent experiments. [##]Compared with the sham-operated group, **compared with the thromboembolic occlusion-induced untreated group. Equal loading in each lane was demonstrated by similar intensities of α-tubulin ($n = 5$)

Effect of combination of TRCQT and aspirin on DNA fragmentation

Although no TUNEL-positive cells were identified in the sham-operated group (Fig. 5), we did observe a considerable increase in the number of TUNEL-positive cells in the MCAO-induced group. Rats treated with a combination of TRCQT and aspirin showed a noticeable reduction in the number of TUNEL-positive cells, although this effect was not statistically significant.

TRCQT attenuated the in vitro formation of HO· radicals

TRCQT significantly attenuated the Fenton reaction-induced formation of HO· radicals in a concentration-dependent manner (0.3, 0.7 and 1.3 mg/mL) (Fig. 6). Moreover, TRCQT inhibited the formation of HO· radicals to a much greater extent at a concentration of

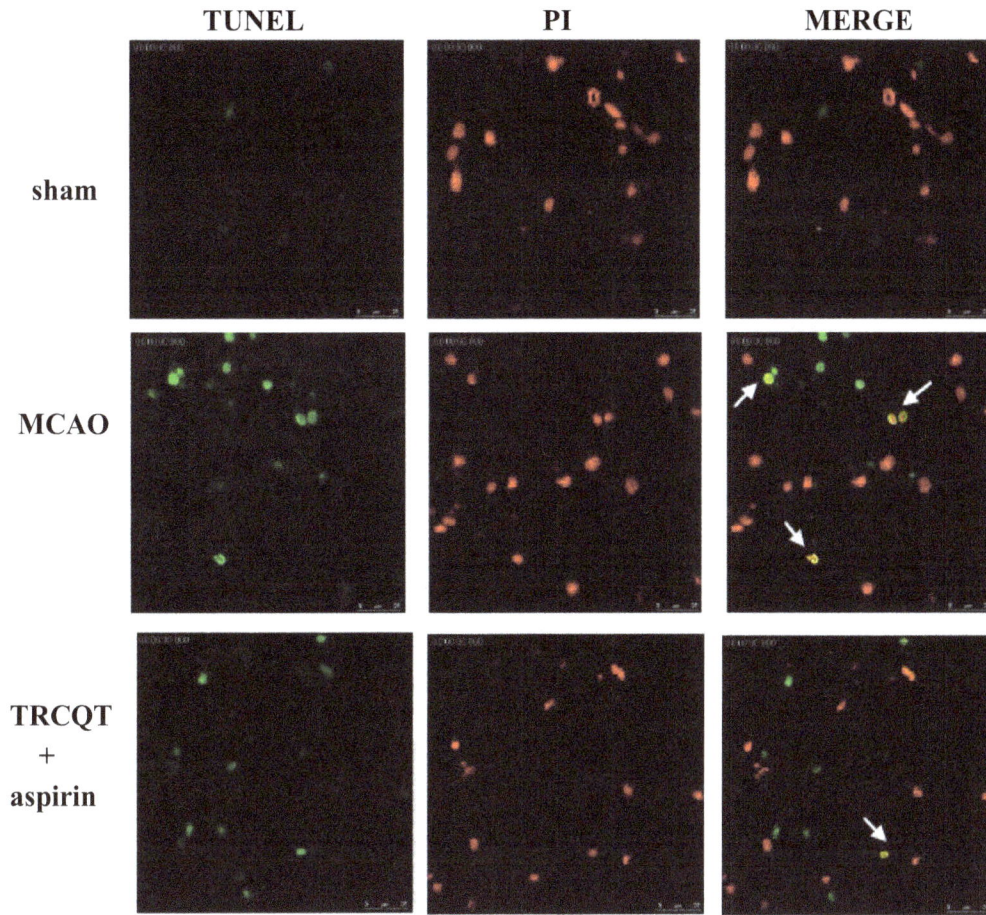

Fig. 5 Effects of a combination of TRCQT and aspirin on DNA fragmentation after MCAO injury in rats. TUNEL staining images of damaged cortex samples collected from each group after TRCQT combined with aspirin administration at high magnification (25 μm). The TUNEL-positive material was localized in the nuclei of the neurons. Numerous TUNEL-positive cells were identified in the thromboembolic occlusion-induced untreated group compared with the sham group and the group treated with a combination of TRCQT and aspirin

1.3 mg/mL compared with a concentration of 0.3 mg/mL ($P < 0.001$).

Discussion

This study demonstrated that the oral treatment with TRCQT or aspirin suppressed thromboembolic stroke in rats and led to an improved neurological outcome by reducing the infarct volume. The treatment of rats with TRCQT or aspirin alone inhibited the expression of TNF-α, p-JNK, activated caspase-3 and Bax, as well as reducing the number of TUNEL positive cells in the ischemic brain regions of these animals. Although the treatment of the rats with TRCQT or aspirin alone resulted in neuroprotective effects, the combination of these two drugs was much more effective. Treatment with TRCQT (0.3, 0.7 and 1.3 mg/mL) led to a significant reduction in the formation of HO· radicals.

Vascular inflammation is mediated by pro-inflammatory cytokines, such as TNF-α [16, 17]. The administration of TNF-α leads to an increase in tissue damage and neurological deficits, thereby aggravating ischemic brain injury [18]. Anti-TNF neutralizing antibodies [19] and the inhibition of soluble TNF-α receptor type 1 [20] have been reported to reduce ischemic damage and improve functional outcome after stroke [21]. The results of our previous study demonstrated that the oral administration of *Tao-Hong-Si-Wu Tang* (THSWT) attenuated the effects of embolic stroke by inhibiting the expression of TNF-α [22]. In this study, the treatment of MCAO-induced rats with TRCQT or aspirin alone led to a reduction in the TNF-α levels. Cerebral ischemia results in an increase in the levels of mitogen activated protein kinases (MAPKs) [23, 24]. Inhibition of the JNK MAPK pathways could therefore improved outcomes in ischemic

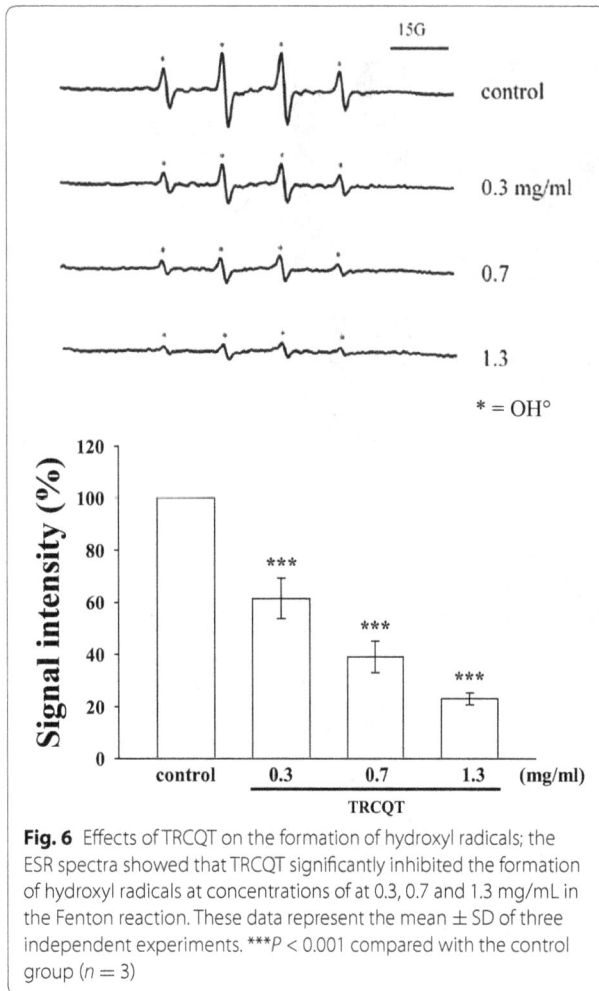

Fig. 6 Effects of TRCQT on the formation of hydroxyl radicals; the ESR spectra showed that TRCQT significantly inhibited the formation of hydroxyl radicals at concentrations of at 0.3, 0.7 and 1.3 mg/mL in the Fenton reaction. These data represent the mean ± SD of three independent experiments. ***$P < 0.001$ compared with the control group ($n = 3$)

The production of reactive oxygen species (ROS) is a significant factor in the neuropathology of stroke [30]. During acute ischemic stroke, ROS can be generated through multiple injury mechanisms, including mitochondrial inhibition, Ca^{2+} overload and reperfusion injury [31]. H_2O_2 is the source of HO· radicals, which can contribute to neuronal injury after cerebral ischemic reperfusion, resulting in neuronal death [32, 33]. The hydroxyl radical-scavenging activity of TRCQT was directly evaluated using an ESR method, and the results revealed that TRCQT scavenged HO· radicals in a concentration-dependent manner.

The screening of traditional Chinese medicines to identify potential neuroprotective agents by evaluating their neuroprotective effects using in vivo and in vitro experimental models of stroke is highly desired. A large amount of clinical information has been gathered over the years pertaining to the use of Chinese medicines treat stroke using indigenous herbal materials [34]. The results of this study should provide researchers with a better understanding of the mechanisms underlying the therapeutic value of using a combination of TRCQT and aspirin to treat thromboembolic stroke.

Conclusions
TRCQT reduced brain infarct volume and improved neurological outcomes by reducing apoptosis, attenuating the expression of TNF-α and p-JNK, and reducing the formation of HO· radicals in MCAO-induced embolic stroke of rats.

brain injury by suppressing the production of inflammatory cytokines [25, 26]. The phosphorylation of JNK can promote stress-induced cell death and regulate the downstream signaling events associated with apoptosis during ischemic injury [27]. In this study, we observed increases in the activation of TNF-α and p-JNK in rats with MCAO-induced brain injury. Notably, the treatment of these rats with TRCQT or aspirin alone led a significant decrease in the activation of these proteins.

Activated caspase-3 occurs following apoptosis in the hippocampus after transient cerebral ischemia-mediated neuronal death [28, 29]. The levels of activated caspase-3 and Bax observed at 30 days after ischemia were higher than those found in the sham rats. Furthermore, the number of TUNEL-positive cells found in the ischemic region increased after MCAO ischemia. The oral administration of TRCQT in combination with aspirin led to significant decreases in the expression levels of Bax and activated caspase-3, as well as a reduction in the number of TUNEL-positive cells.

Abbreviations
CCA: common carotid artery; ESR: electron spin resonance spectrometry; ICA: internal carotid artery; JNK: c-Jun N-terminal kinases; MCAO: middle cerebral artery occlusion; MTT: 2,5-diphenyl tetrazolium bromide; OH⁻: hydroxyl radical; PA: pterygopalatine artery; ROS: reactive oxygen species; TdT: terminal deoxynucleotidyl transferase; TNF-α: tumor necrosis factor-α; TRCQT: Tao-Ren-Cheng-Qi Tang; TTC: 2,3,5-triphenyltetrazolium chloride; TUNEL: terminal deoxynucleotidyl transferase dUTP nick end labeling.

Authors' contributions
LWH and WCS perceived the study. MCY and TLY designed the study. LWH performed ESR study and WCS performed TUNEL assay. NCC performed the Western blot analysis. MCY, TLY, TJ and PAT performed the statistical analysis. TJ and JRS wrote the manuscript. All authors read and approved the final manuscript.

Author details
¹ Graduate Institute of Medical Sciences, College of Medicine, Taipei Medical University, Taipei, Taiwan. ² Department of Internal Medicine, Yuan's General

Hospital, Kaohsiung, Taiwan. [3] Department of Internal Medicine, School of Medicine, Taipei Medical University, Taipei, Taiwan. [4] Department of Microbiology, Institute of Ophthalmology, Joseph Eye Hospital, Tiruchirappalli, Tamil Nadu 620 001, India. [5] Department of Pharmacology, School of Medicine, Taipei Medical University, Taipei, Taiwan.

Acknowledgements
This work was supported by Grants (MOST104-2622-B-038-003 and MOST 104-2320-B-038-045-MY2) from the Ministry of Science and Technology of Taiwan and Yuan's General Hospital-Taipei Medical University (103-YGH-TMU-04).

Competing interests
The authors declare that they have no competing interests.

References

1. Feigin VL, Lawes CMM, Bennett DA, Barker-Collo SL, Parag V. Worldwide stroke incidence and early case fatality reported in 56 population based studies: a systematic review. Lancet Neurol. 2009;8:355–69.
2. Lo EH, Moskowitz MA, Jacobs TP. How brain cells die after stroke. Stroke. 2005;36:189–92.
3. Jiang B, Wang WZ, Chen H, Hong Z, Yang QD, Wu SP, Du XL, Bao QJ. Incidence and trends of stroke and its subtypes in China. Stroke. 2006;37:63–8.
4. Fisher M. Characterizing the target of acute stroke therapy. Stroke. 1997;28:866–72.
5. Zhu XH, Li SJ, Hu HH, Sun LR, Das M, Gao TM. Neuroprotective effects of Xiao-Xu-Ming decoction against ischemic neuronal injury in vivo and in vitro. J Ethnopharmacol. 2010;127:38–46.
6. Li XM, Bai XC, Huang H, Xiao ZJ, Gao TM. Neuroprotective effects of Buyang Huanwu decoction on neuronal injury in hippocampus after transient forebrain ischemia in rats. Neurosci Lett. 2003;346:29–32.
7. Wang L, Zhou GB, Liu P, Song JH, Liang Y, Yan XJ, Xu F, Wang BS, Mao JH, Shen ZX, Chen SJ, Chen Z. Dissection of mechanisms of Chinese medicinal formula Realgar-Indigo naturalis as an effective treatment for promyelocytic leukemia. Proc Natl Acad Sci USA. 2008;105:4826–31.
8. Gong X, Sucher NJ. Stroke therapy in traditional Chinese medicine (TCM): prospects for drug discovery and development. Phytomed. 2002;9:478–84.
9. Shi H, Shi L. The clinical effect of modified Taohongsiwu decoction on diabetes peripheral neuropathy. J Henan Univ Chin Med. 2006;21:38–9.
10. Yang JM. Therapeutic effect observation of 154 cases of coronary artery disease angina using Taohongsiwutang (THSW). China J Mol Med. 2007;17:2268–75.
11. Hsiao G, Lin KH, Chang Y, Chen TL, Tzu NH, Chou DS, Sheu JR. Protective mechanisms of inosine in platelet activation and cerebral ischemic damage. Arterioscler Thromb Vasc Biol. 2005;25:1998–2004.
12. Lee YM, Chang CY, Yen TL, Geraldine P, Lan CC, Sheu JR, Lee JJ. Extract of Antrodia camphorata exerts neuroprotection against embolic stroke in rats without causing the risk of hemorrhagic incidence. Sci World J. 2014;2014:1–8.
13. Bederson JB, Pitts LH, Germano SM, Nishimura MC, Davis RL, Bartkowski HM. Evaluation of 2,3,5-triphenyltetrazolium chloride as a stain for detection and quantification of experimental cerebral infarction in rats. Stroke. 1986;17(6):1304–8.
14. Rodrigo J, Alonso D, Fernandez AP, Serrano J, Richart A, López JC, Santacana M, Martínez-Murillo R, Bentura ML, Ghiglione M, Uttenthal LO. Neuronal and inducible nitric oxide synthase expression and protein nitration in rat cerebellum after oxygen and glucose deprivation. Brain Res. 2001;909:20–45.

15. Chou DS, Hsiao G, Shen MY, Tsai YJ, Chen TF, Sheu JR. ESR spin trapping of a carbon-centered free radical from agonist-stimulated human platelets. Free Rad Biol Med. 2005;39:237–48.
16. Chamorro A, Hallenbeck J. The harms and benefits of inflammatory and immune responses in vascular disease. Stroke. 2006;37:291–3.
17. Barone FC, Feuerstein GZ. Inflammatory mediators and stroke: new opportunities for novel therapeutics. J Cereb Blood Flow Metab. 1999;19:819–34.
18. Barone FC, Arvin B, White RF, Miller A, Webb CL, Willette RN, Lysko PG, Feuerstein GZ. Tumor necrosis factor-alpha. A mediator of focal ischemic brain injury. Stroke. 1997;28:1233–44.
19. Hosomi N, Ban CR, Naya T, Takahashi T, Guo P, Song XY, Kohno M. Tumor necrosis factor-alpha neutralization reduced cerebral edema through inhibition of matrix metalloproteinase production after transient focal cerebral ischemia. J Cereb Blood Flow Metab. 2005;25:959–67.
20. Nawashiro H, Martin D, Hallenbeck JM. Inhibition of tumor necrosis factor and amelioration of brain infarction in mice. J Cereb Blood Flow Metab. 1997;17:229–32.
21. Wang X, Feuerstein GZ, Xu L, Wang H, Schumacher WA, Ogletree ML, Taube R, Duan JJ, Decicco CP, Liu RQ. Inhibition of tumor necrosis factor-alpha-converting enzyme by a selective antagonist protects brain from focal ischemic injury in rats. Mol Pharmacol. 2004;65:890–6.
22. Wu CJ, Chen JT, Yen TL, Jayakumar T, Chou DS, Hsiao G, Sheu JR. Neuroprotection by the traditional Chinese medicine, Tao-Hong-Si-Wu-Tang, against middle cerebral artery occlusion-induced cerebral ischemia in rats. Evid Based Complement Altern Med. 2011;2011:1–9.
23. Irving EA, Barone FC, Reith AD, Hadingham SJ, Parsons AA. Differential activation of MAPK/ERK and p38/SAPK in neurones and glia following focal cerebral ischaemia in the rat. Brain Res Mol Brain Res. 2000;77:65–75.
24. Hayashi T, Sakai K, Sasaki C, Zhang WR, Warita H, Abe K. c-Jun N-terminal kinase (JNK) and JNK interacting protein response in rat brain after transient middle cerebral artery occlusion. Neurosci Lett. 2000;284:195–9.
25. Okami N, Narasimhan P, Yoshioka H, Sakata H, Kim GS, Jung JE, Maier CM, Chan PH. Prevention of JNK phosphorylation as a mechanism for rosiglitazone in neuroprotection after transient cerebral ischemia: activation of dual specificity phosphatase. J Cereb Blood Flow Metab. 2012;33:106–14.
26. Wallace BK, Jelks KA, O'Donnell ME. Ischemia-induced stimulation of cerebral microvascular endothelial cell Na-K-Cl cotransport involves p38 and JNK MAP kinases. Am J Physiol Cell Physiol. 2012;302:505–17.
27. Tournier C, Hess P, Yang DD, Xu J, Turner TK, Nimnual A, Bar-Sagi D, Jones SN, Flavell RA, Davis RJ. Requirement of JNK for stress-induced activation of the cytochrome c-mediated death pathway. Science. 2000;288:870–4.
28. Chen J, Nagayama T, Jin K, Steler RA, Zhu RL, Graham SH, Simon RP. Induction of caspase-3-like protease may mediate delayed neuronal death in the hippocampus after transient cerebral ischemia. J Neurosci. 1998;18:4914–28.
29. Iijima T, Mishima T, Akagawa K, Iwao Y. Mitochondrial hyperpolarization after transient oxygen-glucose deprivation and subsequent apoptosis in cultured rat hippocampal neurons. Brain Res. 2003;993:140–5.
30. Coyle JT, Puttfarcken P. Oxidative stress, glutamate, and neurodegenerative disorders. Science. 1993;262:689–95.
31. Cuzzocrea S, Riley DP, Caputi AP, Salvemini D. Antioxidant therapy: a new pharmacological approach in shock, inflammation, and ischemia/reperfusion injury. Pharmacol Rev. 2001;53:135–59.
32. Zhu DY, Deng Q, Yao HH, Wang DC, Deng Y, Liu GQ. Inducible nitric oxide synthase expression in the ischemic core and penumbra after transient focal cerebra lischemia in mice. Life Sci. 2002;71:1985–96.
33. Ikonomidou C, Kaindl AM. Neuronal death and oxidative stress in the developing brain. Antioxid Redox Signal. 2011;14:1535–50.
34. Gong X, Sucher NJ. Stroke therapy in traditional Chinese medicine (TCM): prospects for drug discovery and development. Phytomedicine. 2002;9:478–84.

12

Gut microbiota was modulated by moxibustion stimulation in rats with irritable bowel syndrome

Xiaomei Wang[1,2*†], Qin Qi[3†], Yuanyuan Wang[3†], Huangan Wu[1,2*], Xiaoming Jin[4], Huan Yao[5], Duiyin Jin[3], Yanan Liu[3] and Cun Wang[3]

Abstract

Background: The pathogenesis of irritable bowel syndrome (IBS) is closely related to intestinal dysbacteriosis and can be controlled by moxibustion treatment. However, the mechanism underlying the therapeutic value of moxibustion in IBS treatment remains unknown.

Methods: An IBS rat model was established by colorectal distention (CRD) stimulus and mustard oil clyster. Sixty-five male rats were randomly divided into six groups: normal, IBS model, moxibustion, electroacupuncture (EA), Bifid-triple Viable Capsule (BTVC) and Pinaverium Bromide (PB) groups. The moxibustion group was treated with mild moxibustion at the bilateral Tianshu (ST25) and Shangjuxu (ST37) for 10 min/day for 7 days, the EA group was given EA at ST25 and ST37 once daily for 7 days, while the BTVC group and PB groups received Bifid-triple Viable Capsule and Pinaverium Bromide solution (at the proportion of 1:0.018) respectively by gavage once daily for 7 days. After the treatment, abdominal withdrawal reflex (AWR) scores were determined based on CRD stimulus, gut microbiota profiling was conducted by 16S rRNA high-throughput sequencing.

Results: Irritable bowel syndrome model rats had significantly increased AWR scores at all intensities (20, 40, 60 and 80 mmHg) compared with the normal group. Moxibustion treatment significantly reduced AWR scores compared with the IBS model group at all intensities. Across all groups the most abundant phyla were *Bacteroidetes* and *Firmicutes* followed by *Proteobacteria* and *Candidatus Saccharibacteria*. At genus level IBS model rats had a higher abundance of *Prevotella*, *Bacteroides* and *Clostridium XI* and a lower abundance of *Lactobacillus* and *Clostridium XIVa* compared with normal rats. These changes in microbiota profiles could however be reversed by moxibustion treatment. Alpha diversity was decreased in IBS model rats compared with normal rats, yet significantly increased in moxibustion- and PB-treated rats compared with IBS rats.

Conclusion: Our findings suggest that moxibustion treats IBS by modulating the gut microbiota.

Keywords: Irritable bowel syndrome, Moxibustion, Gut microbiota, 16S rRNA

*Correspondence: wxm123@vip.sina.com; wuhuangan@126.com
†Xiaomei Wang, Qin Qi and Yuanyuan Wang contributed equally to this work
[1] Shanghai Research Institute of Acupuncture and Meridian, Shanghai University of Traditional Chinese Medicine, 650 South Wanping Road, Xuhui District, Shanghai 200030, China
Full list of author information is available at the end of the article

Background

Irritable bowel syndrome (IBS) is one of the most common gastrointestinal disorders, affecting 10–20% of the population worldwide [1, 2]. IBS is characterized by chronic (continuous or intermittent) abdominal pain, bloating, changes in bowel habit and/or stool property. IBS has a multifactorial etiology that may include colonic dysmotility [3], visceral hypersensitivity [4], brain–gut interactions [5], genetic factors [6], post-infectious low-grade inflammation [7] and altered gut microbiota [8].

Along with the development of microecology theories, the role of the gut microbiota in IBS has been paid increasing attention in recent years. There are trillions of bacteria in the human gut that have co-evolved with us [9]. The predominant phyla in the human gut are *Firmicutes* and *Bacteroidetes*, followed by *Proteobacteria*, *Actinobacteria*, *Fusobacteria* and *Verrucomicrobia* [10]. The human gut is home to a rich variety of microbes. Accordingly, the human intestinal track, particularly the colon, is equipped with sophisticated regulatory mechanisms that facilitate intestinal balance despite complex interaction with the gut microbiota. However, once intestinal balance is disturbed chronic diseases including inflammatory bowel disease [11], allergic diseases [12], obesity [13], colorectal cancer [14] among others [15] may ensue. IBS is closely linked to alterations in gut microbiota composition [16], which can lead to increased permeability of the intestinal mucosal barrier and modulation of cytokine secretion, thus playing a significant role in the pathophysiology of IBS.

Patients with IBS generally have a reduced quality of life [17], underscoring the importance of addressing these symptoms. The treatment of IBS ranges from pharmaceutical to psychological intervention [18]. However, long-term use of currently prescribed therapeutics, such as 5-hydroxytryptamine receptor (5-HT$_3$) antagonists, although partly effective, does have several side effects. Psychological treatment does not have any side effects but it is difficult to apply effectively long-term. Moxibustion is a traditional Chinese therapy used to improve general health and treat chronic conditions by stimulating specific points with heat generated by burning herbal preparations containing dried mugwort leaves [19]. Both temperature-related mechanisms and nontemperature-related mechanisms likely underlie the effects of moxibustion. The latter includes smoke, herbs, and far infrared effects [20]. Growing evidence supports moxibustion as a safe and effective treatment for IBS [21]. Interestingly, moxibustion has been shown to regulate intestinal microbiota [22]. However, few studies have explored the effect of moxibustion on the intestinal microbiota. We therefore used high-throughput sequencing to determine changes in intestinal microbial community structure in an IBS rat model with or without moxibustion treatment. Our results provide new leads regarding the pathogenesis and treatment of IBS.

Materials and methods

The Minimum Standards of Reporting Checklist (Additional file 1) contains details of the experimental design, and statistics, and resources used in this study.

Experimental animals

A total of 65 specific-pathogen free 8-day-old male Sprague–Dawley rats were provided by the Department of Laboratory Animal Science of Shanghai University of Traditional Chinese Medicine. The animals were raised under standard conditions at 25 ± 1 °C with a relative humidity of 50–70% and 12 h light/dark cycle. The rats did not separate from their mother until they were 4 weeks old. All rats were randomly divided into six groups: normal (n = 11), model (n = 11), moxibustion (n = 11), electroacupuncture (EA, n = 10), Bifid-triple Viable Capsule (BTVC, n = 11) and Pinaverium Bromide (PB, n = 11). All animal work was performed according to the protocols approved by the University Animal Care and Use Committee of Shanghai University of Traditional Chinese Medicine [IACUC protocol number: SYXK (Shanghai) 2009-0082] to reduce pain and to avoid damage. All efforts were made to minimize animal suffering. During establishing IBS model rats, operations should be slow and soft to avoid causing pain and distress. After the procedure, the animals were monitored until fully free to move and eat. For animal therapy, be gentle when catching animals, and take appropriate treatment after the animals calm down. At the end of the experiment, animals received a lethal dose of pentobarbital sodium to minimize animal suffering.

Establishment of the IBS rat model

The IBS rat model was established by colorectal distention (CRD) through mechanical and chemical stimulus as previously described [23]. An inflatable balloon (Shanghai Dinghuang Industrial Co., Ltd. China) was slowly inserted rectally about 2 cm into the descending colon of rats. The balloon was distended with 0.5 ml of air, for 1 min and then repeated after 30 min. The same distention was performed for 14 consecutive days between the age of 8 and 21 days. After 4 weeks rest, mustard oil (0.2 ml, 4%, Shanghai Zhixin Chemical Co., Ltd. China.) was injected into the descending colon from the anus once a day for 14 days.

Treatment groups

After successful establishment of the model, rats in the moxibustion group, EA group, BTVC and PB group received their relevant treatments. For the moxibustion group, the ignited moxa stick (0.5 cm in diameter) (Nanyang Hanyi Moxa Co., Ltd. China) was placed 2 cm above the bilateral Tianshu (ST25) and Shangjuxu (ST37) acupoints for 10 min/day for 7 days. ST25 is located bilaterally 5 mm lateral to the intersection between the upper 2/3 and the lower 1/3, in the line between the xiphoid process and the pubic symphysis upper border and ST37 is 5 mm lateral to the anterior tubercle of the tibia and 15 mm below the knee joint [24].

The EA group was given EA at the bilateral Tianshu and Shangjuxu acupoints with Han's Acupoint Nerve Stimulator (Beijing Huawei Industrial Development Corporation. China. LH402A) for sparse–dense waves (frequency of sparse wave: 2 Hz, frequency of dense wave: 10 Hz, intensity: 4 mA) for 20 min, once daily for 7 days. The BTVC and PB groups received Bifid-triple Viable Capsule (Inner Mongolia Shuangqi Pharmaceutical Co., Ltd. China. Lot number: S19980004) and Pinaverium Bromide (Abbott Healthcare SAS. France. Lot number: H20120127), respectively by gavage, once daily for 7 days. The BTVC and PB solutions were prepared as specified for a weight ratio of 1:0.018 for an adult (70 kg) and a rat (200 g). Prepare the required dose of suspension with drinking water. The BTVC solution concentration was 2 mg/ml with a daily dose of 20 mg/kg. The PB solution concentration was 5 mg/ml with a daily dose of 50 mg/kg. The normal and model groups did not receive any treatment. Two rats were died in BTVC group during the treatment by gavage.

Abdominal withdrawal reflex (AWR) scores

Abdominal withdrawal reflex scores were calculated to assess colon sensitivity to CRD after treatments according to Al-Chaer et al. [23]. Distention was produced by inflating a balloon inside the descending colon through the anus; the inflation balloon had four pressure grades: 20, 40, 60 and 80 mmHg. Each CRD lasted about 20 s and was repeated three times. AWR scores were produced blindly with no subjective judgment. The mean score for each rat was used for downstream analysis. The detailed grading rules on AWR scores are as follows: (0) no behavioral response to CRD; (1) occasional head movement at the onset of the stimulus; (2) mild abdominal muscle contraction but no lifting; (3) strong abdominal muscle contraction and the abdomen but not pelvic structure being lifted off the platform; (4) body arching and lifting of pelvic structures off the platform.

Preparation of fecal and colon tissue samples

After calculating the AWR scores, rats were weighed and injected with 2% pentobarbital sodium (Sigma. USA. P3761). The colon samples (5 cm above the anus, 3 cm in length) were rapidly collected from the descending colon, 5 g fecal matter was collected and stored at − 80 °C for 16S rRNA sequencing. Then, colon samples were fixed in 10% paraformaldehyde for hematoxylin–eosin staining for histopathological observation.

Fecal DNA extraction

Bacterial genomic DNA was extracted from all fecal samples using the QIAamp DNAMini Kit (QIAGEN, Germany) according to the manufacturer's instructions. First, 100 mg fecal sample and 1.4 ml buffer ASL were added to a 2 ml tube. Next, 20 µl proteinase K was added to the tube and mixed well before incubation at 56 °C until the sample was fully dissolved. Next 200 µl buffer AL was added to the tube, mixed thoroughly, followed by incubation at 70 °C for 10 min. Subsequently, 200 µl ethanol (96%) was added to the mixture, which was then loaded onto the QIAamp Mini spin column and centrifuged at 8000 rpm for 1 min. The column material was washed with 500 µl buffer AW1 and centrifuged at 8000 rpm for 1 min, then with 500 µl buffer AW2 and centrifuged at 14,000 rpm for 3 min. Finally, the DNA was eluted in 100 µl of AE elution buffer. DNA integrity and fragment size range was assessed by agarose gel electrophoresis, and DNA concentrations were measured using a NanoDrop ND-2000 spectrophotometer (Thermo Fisher Scientific, USA).

Illumina MiSeq sequencing

The V3–V4 region of the bacterial 16S rRNA gene was amplified by polymerase chain reaction (PCR) using universal bacterial primers 341F and 806R [25]. Pooled amplicons were sequenced on a 300 PE Illumina MiSeq. Demultiplexed reads were quality filtered based on sequence length and quality as previously described [26]. Operational taxonomic units (OTUs) were clustered at 97% similarity, and chimeric sequences were removed using UCHIME [27]. Finally, taxonomic assignment of representative sequences was preformed using the Ribosomal Database Project (RDP) MultiClassifier tool [28].

Statistical analyses

AWR scores was analysed using SPSS21.0 software, and data were expressed as mean ± SD (Standard ± Deviation) for normally distributed data and as M (Q_{25}–Q_{75}) for non-normally distributed data. One-way analysis of variance (ANOVA) was performed for normally distributed data and a non-parametric test (Kruskal–Wallis H test.) was used for non-normally distributed data.

Bioinformatic analyses were performed using R 3.2.3 (http://cran.r-project.org). Differences in relative abundance between groups were assessed using the Kruskal–Wallis test. Alpha diversity was calculated using

Simpson's diversity index. Beta diversity was determined by analysis of similarities (ANOSIM) using unweighted UniFrac as distance metric. In addition, OTUs that are differentially abundant were determined using Linear discriminant analysis effect size (LefSE). Results were deemed significant if $P < 0.05$.

Results

Abdominal withdrawal reflex (AWR) scores

As shown in Fig. 1, AWR scores were significantly increased in IBS model rats compared with normal rats at all four CRD pressures ($P < 0.01$). AWR scores were however significantly reduced in IBS model rats following treatment with moxibustion at 20 ($P < 0.05$), 40, 60 and 80 mmHg ($P < 0.01$). AWR scores of the EA, BTVC and PB groups also were significantly lower than in IBS model group (EA group: 20 mmHg $P < 0.05$, 40, 60 and 80 mmHg, $P < 0.01$; BTVC group: 40 mmHg, $P < 0.01$; PB group: 20, 40 and 60 mmHg, $P < 0.05$, 80 mmHg, $P < 0.01$). These results suggest that moxibustion treatment could effectively decrease visceral hypersensitivity as EA, BTVC and PB.

Histological analysis

As shown in Fig. 2, there were no significant differences in histological features between groups. The colonic tissue structure was normal in all groups, and the colonic mucosa epithelium was complete and had regularly arranged glands. There was no congestion, edema, ulcers, inflammatory cell infiltration or other pathological changes in any of the groups.

Gut microbial composition

A total of 3,759,276 high quality raw sequences were obtained using the MiSeq platform (Illumina, San Diego, CA, USA), and 2,802,729 filtered reads were retained after

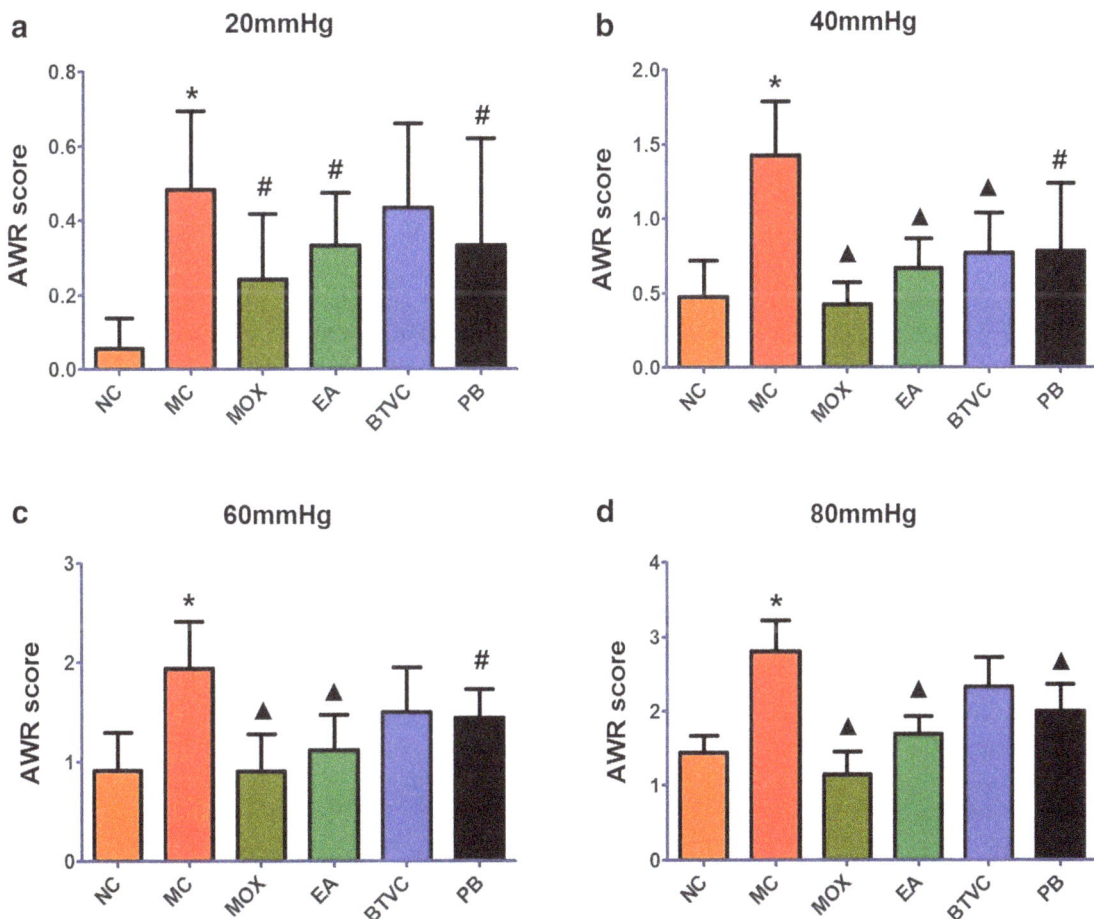

Fig. 1 Abdominal withdrawal reflex (AWR) scores under different distention pressure (**a** 20 mmHg, **b** 40 mmHg, **c** 60 mmHg, **d** 80 mmHg) in different groups. NC: normal group; MC: IBS model group; MOX: moxibustion group; EA: electroacupuncture group; BTVC: Bifid-triple Viable Capsule group; PB: Pinaverium Bromide group. Data are presented as Median, $Q_{25}-Q_{75}$ (n = 7 per group). *$P < 0.01$, versus normal group; #$P < 0.05$, ▲$P < 0.01$, versus model group

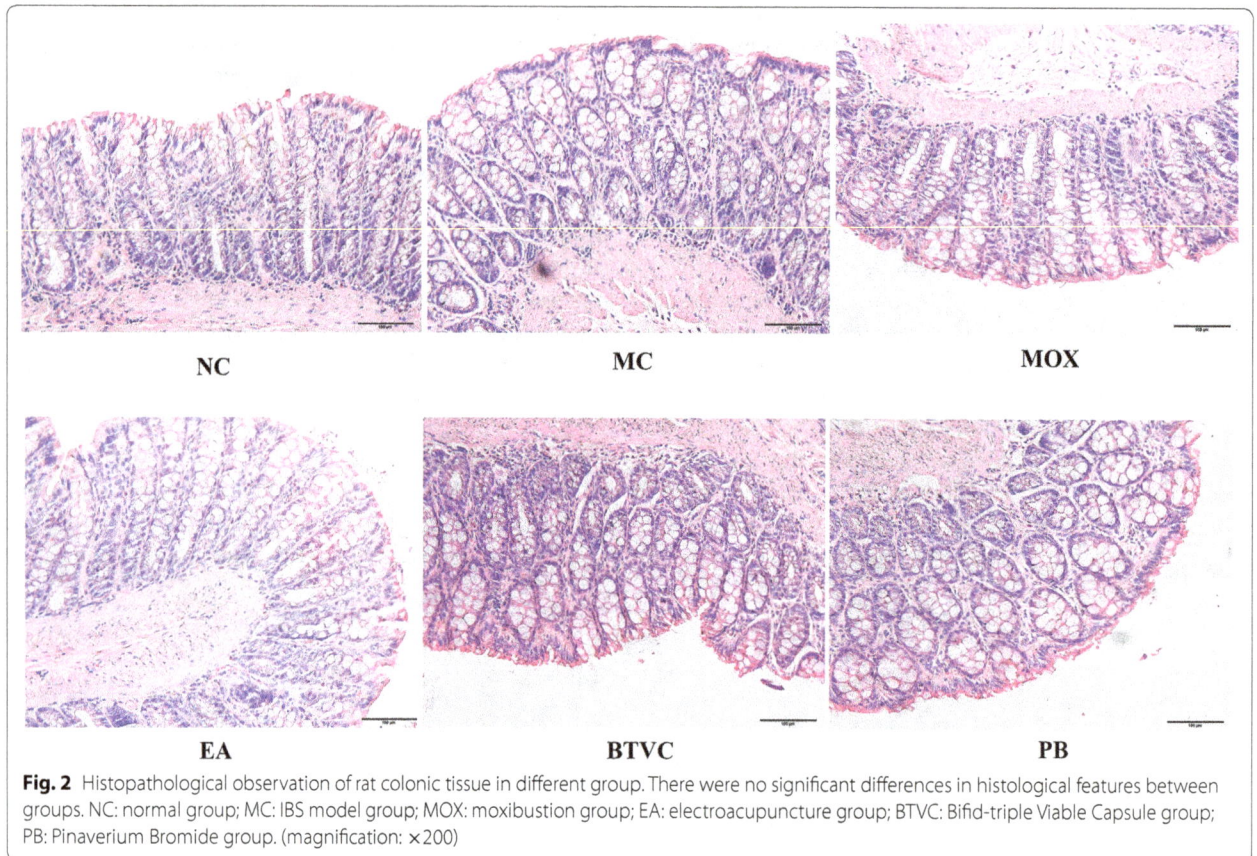

Fig. 2 Histopathological observation of rat colonic tissue in different group. There were no significant differences in histological features between groups. NC: normal group; MC: IBS model group; MOX: moxibustion group; EA: electroacupuncture group; BTVC: Bifid-triple Viable Capsule group; PB: Pinaverium Bromide group. (magnification: ×200)

splicing and quality control with an average of 44,487 reads per sample (ranging from 37,081 to 54,506 reads). Reads were then clustered into OTUs at 97% similarity resulting in 1361 OTUs, which were used for further taxa diversity analysis. In terms of microbial composition, the major phyla present across all groups were *Bacteroidetes* and *Firmicutes*, followed by *Proteobacteria* and *Candidatus Saccharibacteria* (Fig. 3a). At class level, *Bacteroidia* and *Clostridia* were the dominant taxa across all groups, followed by *Bacilli* and *Alphaproteobacteria* (Fig. 3b).

Comparison of gut microbial composition between normal and IBS model rats
At phylum level, both normal and IBS model rats had fecal samples dominated by the phyla *Bacteroidetes* and *Firmicutes*. However, the relative abundance of *Bacteroidetes* and *Firmicutes* varied significantly between groups.

Compared with the normal group the model group had a higher relative abundance of *Bacteroidetes* and a lower relative abundance of *Firmicutes* (Fig. 4a). At genus level, the IBS model group had a higher relative abundance of the genera *Prevotella*, *Bacteroides*, *Barnesiella*, *Paraprevotella*, *Clostridium XI* and *Sphingomonas* compared with normal samples, and a lower relative abundance of *Lactobacillus*, *Clostridium XIVa* and *Oscillibacter* (Fig. 4b).

Comparison of gut microbial composition between IBS model rats with and without moxibustion treatment
Treatment of IBS model rats with moxibustion led to a fecal microbial profile closer to that of normal rats, with decreased levels of *Bacteroidetes* and increased levels of *Firmicutes* following treatment (Fig. 4a). At genus level *Prevotella*, *Bacteroides* and *Clostridium XI* were

(See figure on next page.)
Fig. 3 Comparison of overall community structure at phylum and class level by treatment group. **a** At phylum level, *Bacteroidetes* and *Firmicutes* were the dominant taxa across all groups, followed by *Proteobacteria* and *Candidatus Saccharibacteria*; **b** at class level, *Bacteroidia* and *Clostridia* were the dominant taxa across all groups, followed by *Bacilli* and *Alphaproteobacteria*. NC: normal group; MC: IBS model group; MOX: moxibustion group; EA: electroacupuncture group; BTVC: Bifid-triple Viable Capsule group; PB: Pinaverium Bromide group

a

Phylum Level Barplot

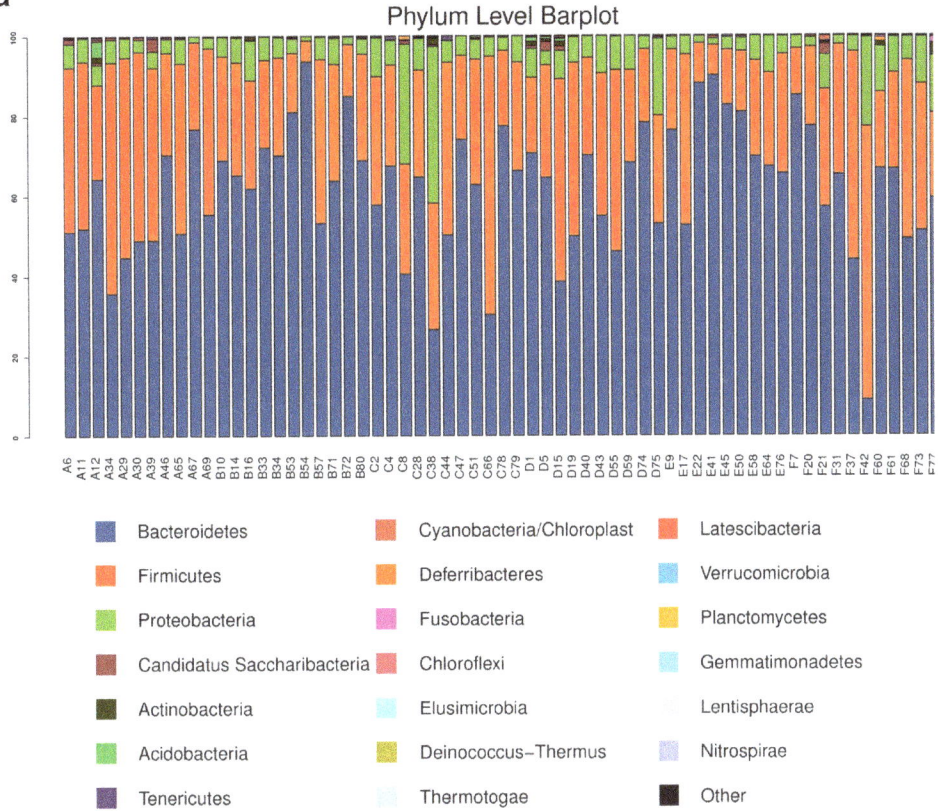

Legend:
- Bacteroidetes
- Firmicutes
- Proteobacteria
- Candidatus Saccharibacteria
- Actinobacteria
- Acidobacteria
- Tenericutes
- Cyanobacteria/Chloroplast
- Deferribacteres
- Fusobacteria
- Chloroflexi
- Elusimicrobia
- Deinococcus–Thermus
- Thermotogae
- Latescibacteria
- Verrucomicrobia
- Planctomycetes
- Gemmatimonadetes
- Lentisphaerae
- Nitrospirae
- Other

b

Class Level Barplot

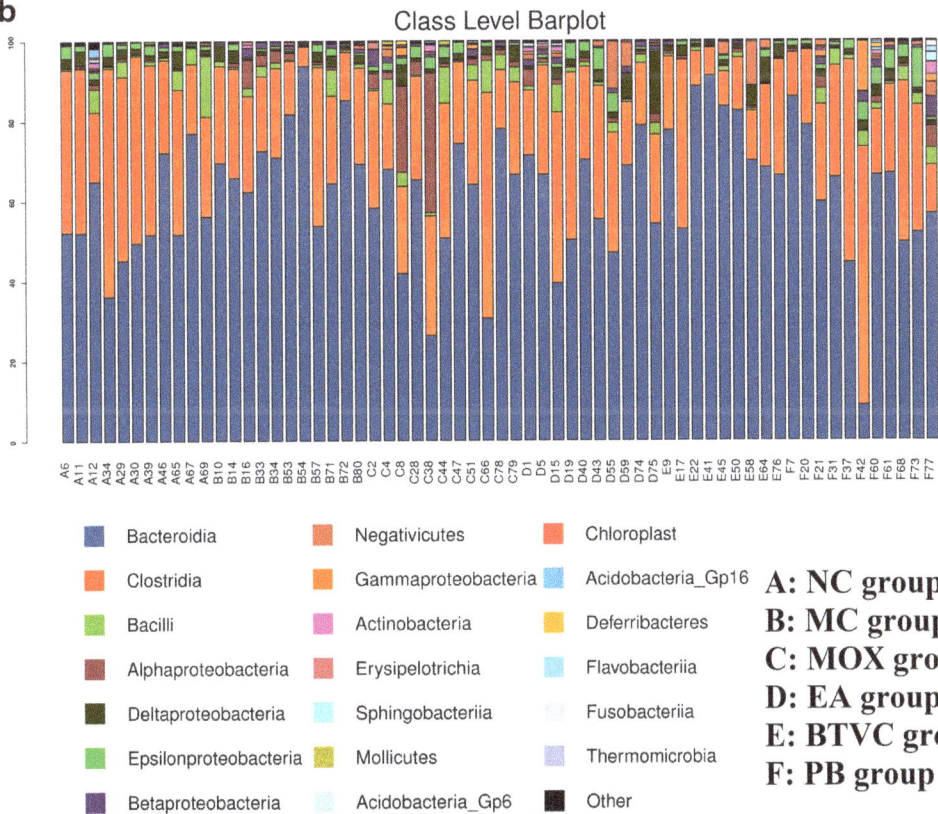

Legend:
- Bacteroidia
- Clostridia
- Bacilli
- Alphaproteobacteria
- Deltaproteobacteria
- Epsilonproteobacteria
- Betaproteobacteria
- Negativicutes
- Gammaproteobacteria
- Actinobacteria
- Erysipelotrichia
- Sphingobacteriia
- Mollicutes
- Acidobacteria_Gp6
- Chloroplast
- Acidobacteria_Gp16
- Deferribacteres
- Flavobacteriia
- Fusobacteriia
- Thermomicrobia
- Other

A: NC group
B: MC group
C: MOX group
D: EA group
E: BTVC group
F: PB group

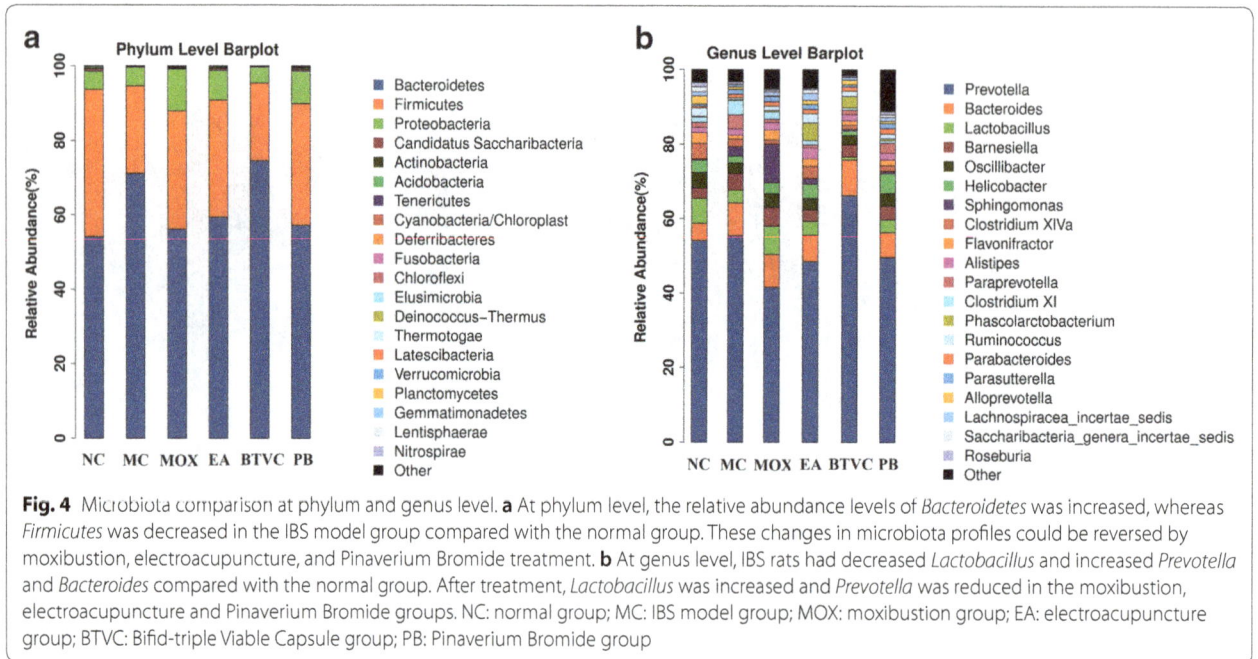

Fig. 4 Microbiota comparison at phylum and genus level. **a** At phylum level, the relative abundance levels of *Bacteroidetes* was increased, whereas *Firmicutes* was decreased in the IBS model group compared with the normal group. These changes in microbiota profiles could be reversed by moxibustion, electroacupuncture, and Pinaverium Bromide treatment. **b** At genus level, IBS rats had decreased *Lactobacillus* and increased *Prevotella* and *Bacteroides* compared with the normal group. After treatment, *Lactobacillus* was increased and *Prevotella* was reduced in the moxibustion, electroacupuncture and Pinaverium Bromide groups. NC: normal group; MC: IBS model group; MOX: moxibustion group; EA: electroacupuncture group; BTVC: Bifid-triple Viable Capsule group; PB: Pinaverium Bromide group

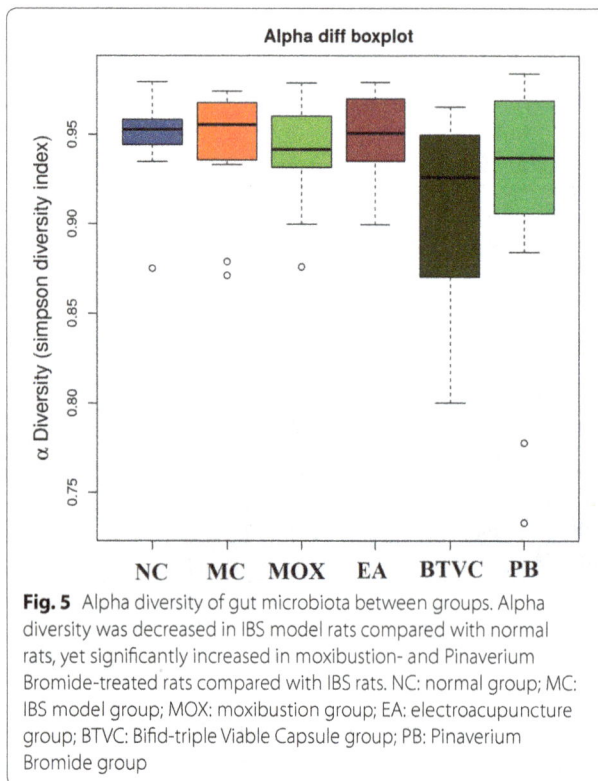

Fig. 5 Alpha diversity of gut microbiota between groups. Alpha diversity was decreased in IBS model rats compared with normal rats, yet significantly increased in moxibustion- and Pinaverium Bromide-treated rats compared with IBS rats. NC: normal group; MC: IBS model group; MOX: moxibustion group; EA: electroacupuncture group; BTVC: Bifid-triple Viable Capsule group; PB: Pinaverium Bromide group

Richness and diversity of gut bacterial communities

Alpha diversity, as measured by Simpson's diversity index (Fig. 5), was significantly decreased in model compared with normal rats ($P = 0.01$). However, alpha diversity was increased following moxibustion treatment ($P = 0.015$). The EA, BTVC and PB groups also had higher alpha diversity than the model group, which suggests that all these treatments increase gut microbial diversity. With respect to beta diversity, principal coordinates analysis (PCoA) demonstrated significant differences between normal and model groups on the second axis (Fig. 6), suggesting that disease may be the factor influencing microbial community composition. However, the first and second principal coordinates only accounted for 15.04% and 8.93% of the total variations respectively, indicating that there are other factors affecting the IBS rats microbial community or more-refined analysis needed. The microbial community composition from EA group was more similar to PB group, and moxibustion was more similar to BTVC on the first axis.

Fecal biomarkers of IBS and different treatments

Linear discriminant analysis effect size (LEfSe), a biomarker discovery tool for high dimensional data, was used to determine which OTUs were differentially abundant between normal and model samples and model and different treatments samples and hence potential biomarkers of IBS and different treatments (Fig. 7a, b). A total of 37 OTUs at different taxonomic levels were differentially abundant ($P < 0.05$) between

decreased in moxibustion-treated IBS rats while *Lactobacillus* and *Clostridium XIVa* were increased in moxibustion-treated IBS rats (Fig. 4b). The relative abundance values were presented in Additional file 2: Table S1.

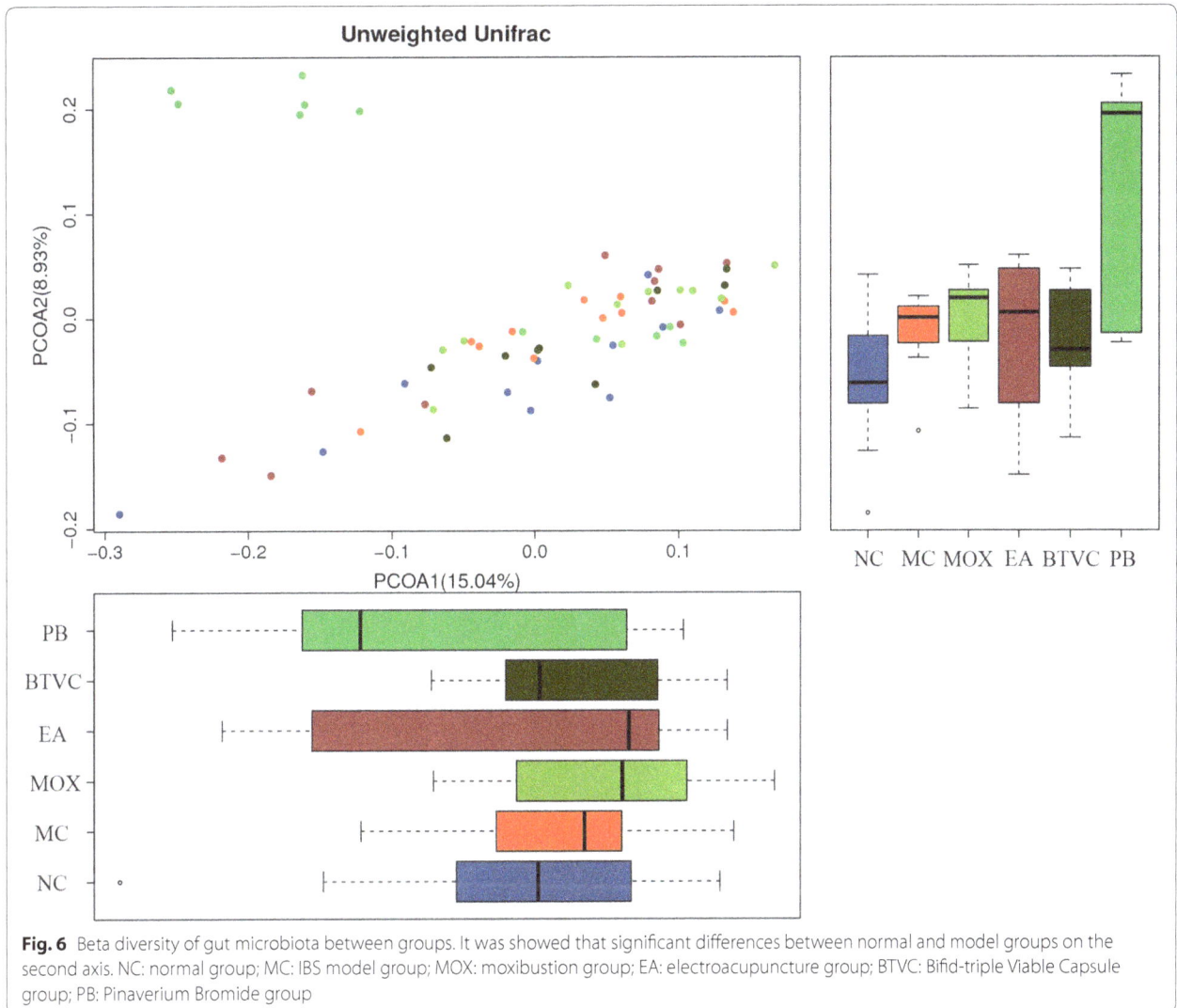

Fig. 6 Beta diversity of gut microbiota between groups. It was showed that significant differences between normal and model groups on the second axis. NC: normal group; MC: IBS model group; MOX: moxibustion group; EA: electroacupuncture group; BTVC: Bifid-triple Viable Capsule group; PB: Pinaverium Bromide group

normal and model samples. At phylum level, the relative abundance of *Bacteroidetes* and *Firmicutes* were increased and decreased in IBS model rats, respectively. At class level *Bacterodia*, *Alphaproteobacteria*, *Betaproteobacteria* and *Erysipelotrichia* were highly enriched in IBS model rats, while *Epsilonproteobacteria* and *Clostridia* were enriched in normal rats. At order level, *Bacteroidales*, *Sphingomonadales*, *Burkholderiales* and *Erysipelotrichales* were significantly enriched in the IBS model rats. At family level *Porphyromonadaceae*, *Peptostreptococcaceae*, *Sphingomonadaceae*, *Sutterellaceae*, *Burkholderiales* and *Erysipelotrichaceae* were enriched in IBS model rats, while *Helicobacteraceae*, *Ruminococcaceae* and *Lachnospiraceae* were enriched in normal rats. Similarly, the genera *Advenella*, *Psychrobacter*, *Clostridium XI*, *Sphingomonas*, *Parasutterella* and *Aquabacterium* were significantly more abundant in IBS model rats, whereas normal rats were enriched

with *Clostridium IV*, *Butyricicoccus*, *Saccharibacteria*, *Helicobacter*, *Ruminococcus*, *Clostridium XIVa*, and *Faecalibacterium*. These results are represented by heatmap analyses on a per-sample basis in Fig. 7c.

A total of 14 OTUs at different taxonomic levels were differentially abundant (P < 0.05) between MC and MOX group. Among them, compared with MC group, the relative abundance of *Ruminococcaceae*, *Enterobacteriaceae*, *Clostridiaceae1*, *Enterobacteriales*, *Escherichia Shigella*, *Clostridiumsensustricto*, *Butyricicoccus* and *Enterorhabdus* were significant abundant in MOX group which may be the potential biomarkers of the moxibustion to treat UC (Fig. 8a, b). A total of 17 OTUs at different taxonomic levels were differentially abundant (P < 0.05) between MC and EA group. Similarly, the relative abundance of *Negativicutes*, *Selenomonadales*, *Gammaproteobacteria*, *Buttiauxella*, *Bacillaceae2*, *Butyricicoccus*, *Enterobacteriales*, *Enterobacteriaceae* and *Virgibacillus* were significant

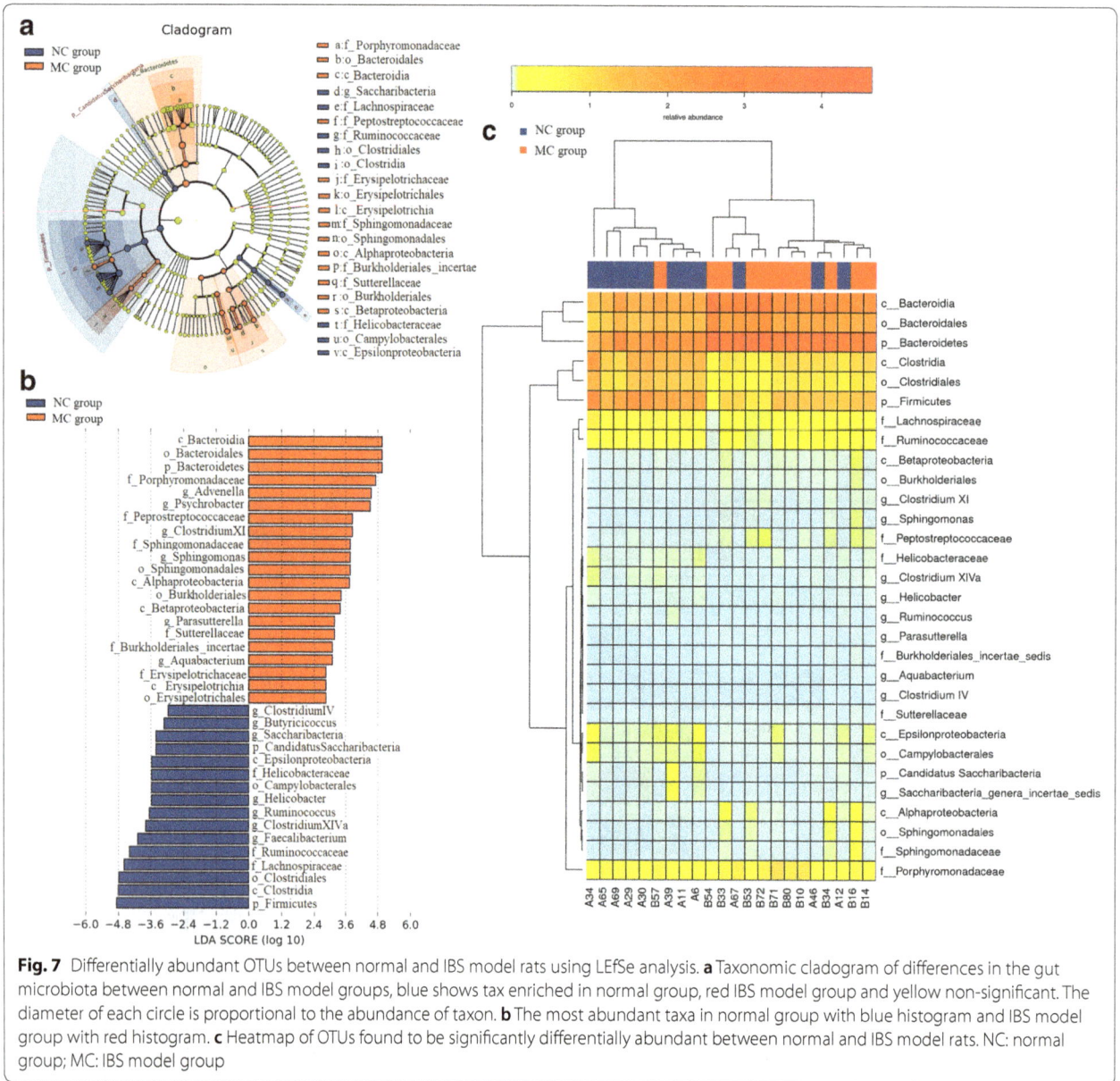

Fig. 7 Differentially abundant OTUs between normal and IBS model rats using LEfSe analysis. **a** Taxonomic cladogram of differences in the gut microbiota between normal and IBS model groups, blue shows tax enriched in normal group, red IBS model group and yellow non-significant. The diameter of each circle is proportional to the abundance of taxon. **b** The most abundant taxa in normal group with blue histogram and IBS model group with red histogram. **c** Heatmap of OTUs found to be significantly differentially abundant between normal and IBS model rats. NC: normal group; MC: IBS model group

abundant in EA group which may be the potential biomarkers of the electroacupuncture to treat UC (Fig. 8c, d). Interestingly, *Butyricicoccus, Enterobacteriales* and *Enterobacteriaceae* were significant abundant both in MOX and EA group then MC group.

A total of 26 OTUs at different taxonomic levels were differentially abundant (P < 0.05) between MC and BTVC group. Among them, *Clostridiales IncertaesedisXI* and *Parvimonas* were significant abundant in BTVC group then MC group (Fig. 9a, b). A total of 81 OTUs at different taxonomic levels were differentially abundant (P < 0.05) between MC and PB group. Compared with MC group, there were 69 taxa significant abundant in

PB group which may be the potential biomarkers of the Pinaverium Bromide to treat UC, such as *Ruminococcus, Butyricicoccus, Fusobacteria, Deinococcales, Thermotogae, Vibrionales, Epsilonproteobacteria* and so on (Fig. 9c, d).

Discussion

IBS is characterized by several symptoms, including abdominal pain, that can seriously affect quality of life. Visceral hypersensitivity (enhanced intestinal perception) plays a significant role in such abdominal pain and discomfort [4]. In this study, we applied AWR scores to assess visceral hypersensitivity in rats. We found

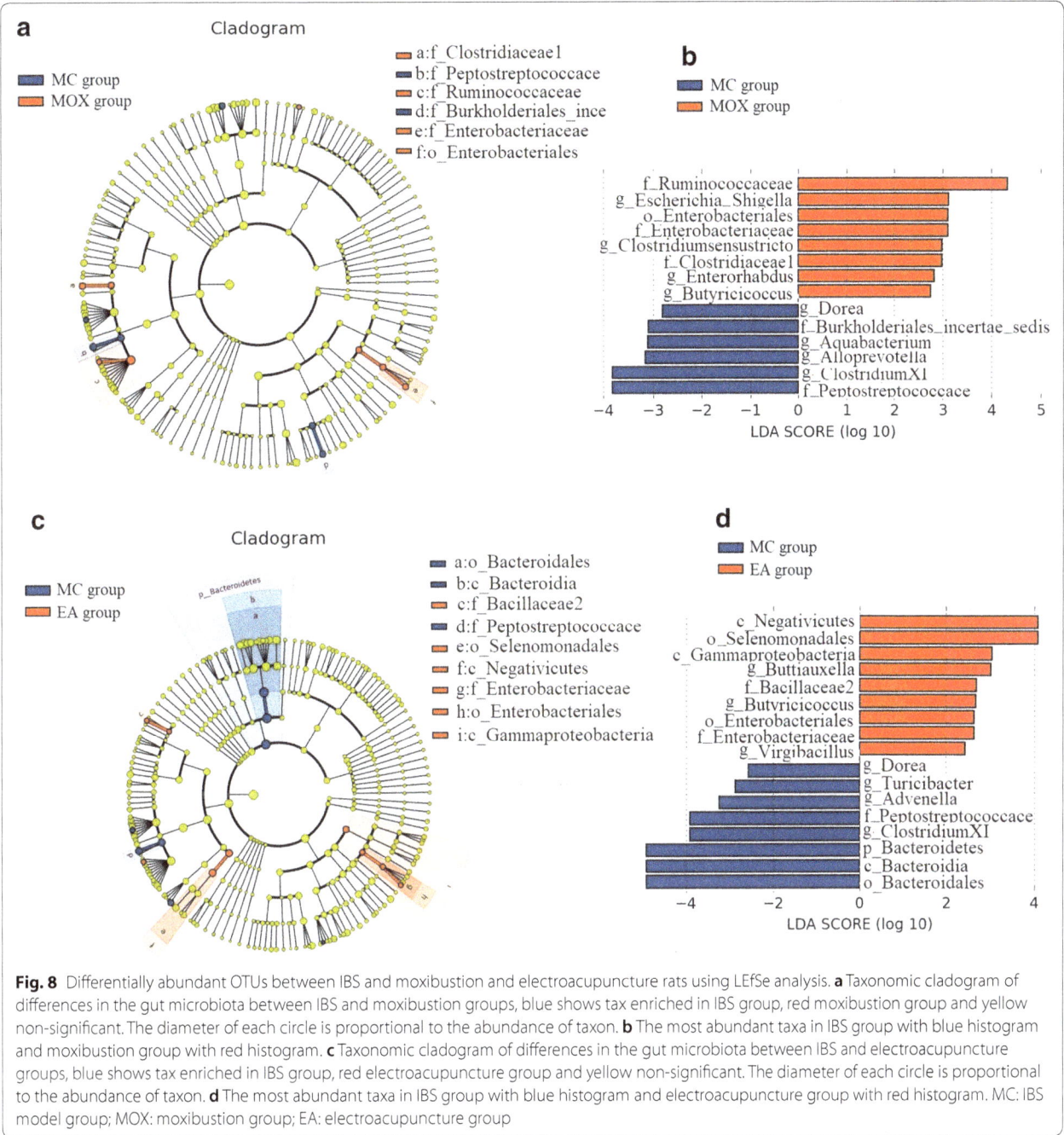

Fig. 8 Differentially abundant OTUs between IBS and moxibustion and electroacupuncture rats using LEfSe analysis. **a** Taxonomic cladogram of differences in the gut microbiota between IBS and moxibustion groups, blue shows tax enriched in IBS group, red moxibustion group and yellow non-significant. The diameter of each circle is proportional to the abundance of taxon. **b** The most abundant taxa in IBS group with blue histogram and moxibustion group with red histogram. **c** Taxonomic cladogram of differences in the gut microbiota between IBS and electroacupuncture groups, blue shows tax enriched in IBS group, red electroacupuncture group and yellow non-significant. The diameter of each circle is proportional to the abundance of taxon. **d** The most abundant taxa in IBS group with blue histogram and electroacupuncture group with red histogram. MC: IBS model group; MOX: moxibustion group; EA: electroacupuncture group

(See figure on next page.)

Fig. 9 Differentially abundant OTUs between IBS and Bifid-triple Viable Capsule and Pinaverium Bromide rats using LEfSe analysis. **a** Taxonomic cladogram of differences in the gut microbiota between IBS and Bifid-triple Viable Capsule groups, blue shows tax enriched in IBS group, red Bifid-triple Viable Capsule group and yellow non-significant. The diameter of each circle is proportional to the abundance of taxon. **b** The most abundant taxa in IBS group with blue histogram and Bifid-triple Viable Capsule group with red histogram. **c** Taxonomic cladogram of differences in the gut microbiota between IBS and Pinaverium Bromide groups, blue shows tax enriched in IBS group, red Pinaverium Bromide group and yellow non-significant. The diameter of each circle is proportional to the abundance of taxon. **d** The most abundant taxa in IBS group with blue histogram and Pinaverium Bromide group with red histogram. MC: IBS model group; BTVC: Bifid-triple Viable Capsule group; PB: Pinaverium Bromide group

a

Cladogram

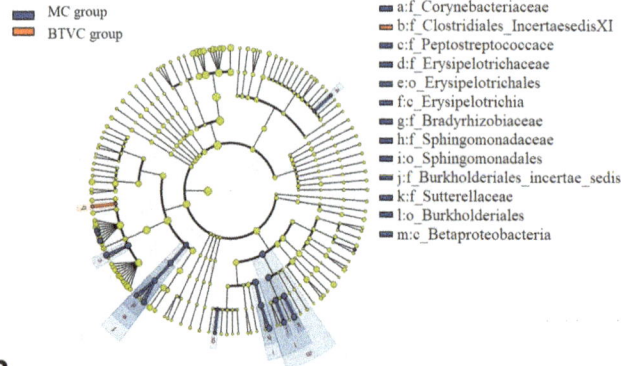

b

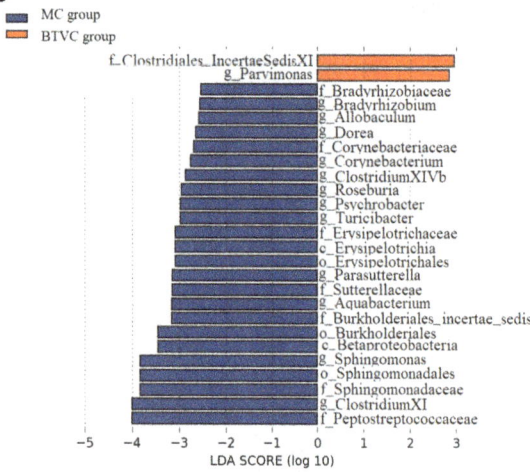

c

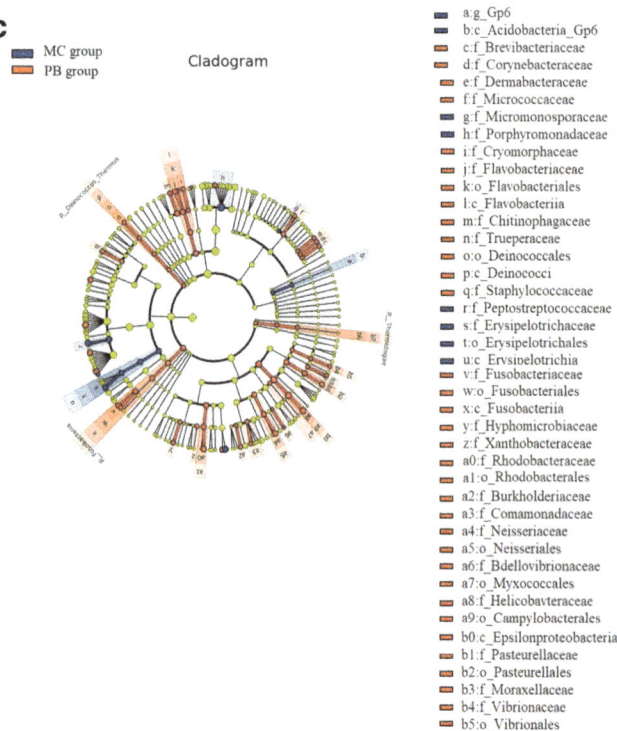

d

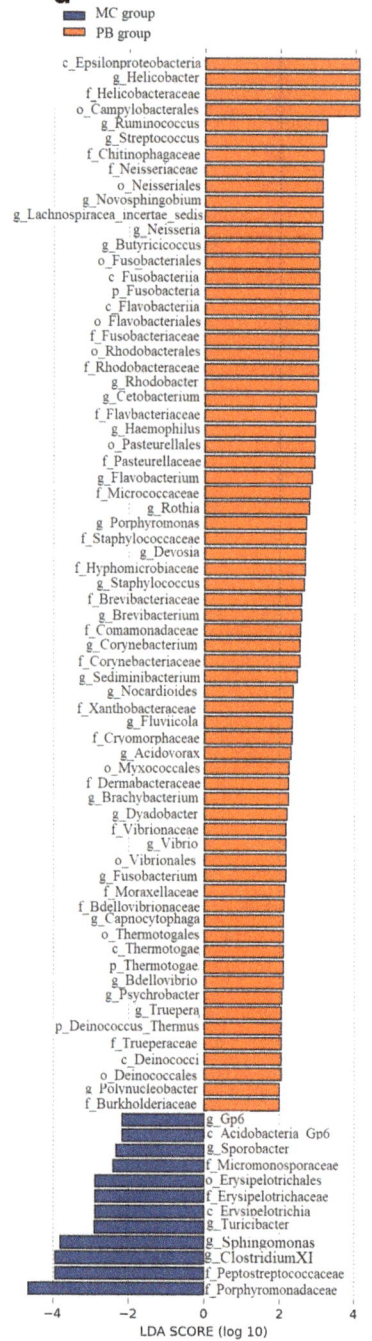

that AWR scores of IBS model rats were significantly increased compared with normal rats. Certain studies have shown that patients with IBS have a higher pain sensitivity and lower pain threshold than normal subjects [29]—our results support these findings. More importantly, AWR scores of IBS rats were significantly decreased in moxibustion, EA, BTVC and PB groups, which demonstrates that moxibustion and EA can effectively alleviated abdominal pain by increasing pain threshold and decreasing visceral hypersensitivity in IBS rats as Pinaverium Bromide and Bifid-triple Viable Capsule. Several studies have reported that electroacupuncture [30], probiotic [31] and Pinaverium Bromide [32] have therapeutic effect for IBS. Our findings indicate that moxibustion may potentially be used as an alternative treatment to Bifid-triple Viable Capsule and Pinaverium Bromide.

The intestinal microbiota profoundly affects human health through various means. Commensal bacteria promote proper functioning of the physical and biochemical barrier against pathogens as well as immune system development [33]. Intestinal bacteria and their metabolic products interact with the host gut mucosal surface thereby shaping the host immune system. Under healthy conditions the host's response to these bacterial signals will result in immune tolerance. Normal intestinal microbiota play a critical role in promoting immune system development, sustaining normal immune function, and preventing infection by pathogens [34]. However, when dysbacteriosis occurs the balance between tolerance towards commensals and immune activation in response to pathogens may be lost, which may lead to a range of diseases.

Tianshu and Shangjuxu acupoints are ancient and classical acupoint combination for intestinal diseases such as diarrhea and abdominal pain [35]. Numerous studies suggest that dysbacteriosis is closely related to the pathophysiology of IBS [36]. Moxibustion has proven benefits in treating IBS [37]. However, ours is the first study to examine the effect of moxibustion on the gut microbiota in IBS. We analyzed changes in gut microbiota between IBS and normal rats and the effect of moxibustion therapy on the gut microbiota.

We found that the intestinal microbial composition of IBS rats differed from that of normal rats. IBS rats had significantly decreased alpha diversity and increased relative abundance of *Bacteroidetes*, which is consistent with previous reports [38]. Several studies have now reported that IBS patients and IBS model rats have significantly reduced levels of *Lactobacillus* [39, 40]. *Lactobacillus* is a major component of the commensal bacterial flora of the human intestinal tract, and is fre-

quently used as a probiotic as it induces the production of large quantities of anti-inflammatory interleukins that improve intestinal barrier function, thus preventing the development of colitis [41]. Several studies have shown that *Lactobacillus GG*—a specific probiotic strain of *Lactobacillus* (ATCC 53103)—effectively treats IBS in humans and rats [42–44]. Indeed, in our study, *Lactobacillus* was decreased in IBS rats, as were *Clostridium XIVa* and *Oscillibacter*. Further, *Prevotella*, *Bacteroides* and *Clostridium XI* were increased in IBS model rats. Interestingly however, these IBS-related changes in gut microbiota could be normalized by moxibustion treatment, after which the relative abundance of *Lactobacillus* and *Clostridium XIVa* increased, while *Prevotella*, *Bacteroides* and *Clostridium XI* decreased. In addition, moxibustion treatment led to increased gut microbiota diversity, as did the other treatments considered in this study (EA, BTVC, and PB) to varying degrees.

We conducted LEfSe to discover distinctive features at all levels which may be the potential biomarkers of the IBS. Twenty-one features were discovered by LEfSe, and the relative abundance of *Bacteroidia*, *Bacteroidales* and *Bacteroidetes*, which exhibited the top three highest LDA score suggesting that these features may be closely related to IBS. We have also identified some potential markers that may play a therapeutic role in different treatments. It was an interesting finding that *Butyricicoccus*, *Enterobacteriales* and *Enterobacteriaceae* were significant abundant both in MOX and EA group compared to MC group. This suggests that moxibustion and electroacupuncture may have some similar therapeutic targets. Although we have found some potential biomarkers, how to regulate these markers by moxibustion and electroacupuncture still requires further research.

Conclusions

Our findings suggest that moxibustion treats IBS by modulating the gut microbiota. We demonstrate that moxibustion could potentially be used to regulate gut microbiota imbalances and therefore to treat patients with IBS.

Abbreviations

IBS: irritable bowel syndrome; CRD: colorectal distention; EA: electroacupuncture; BTVC: Bifid-triple Viable Capsule; PB: Pinaverium Bromide; AWR: abdominal withdrawal reflex; 5-HT$_3$: 5-hydroxytryptamine receptor; PCR: polymerase chain reaction; OTUs: operational taxonomic units; RDP: Ribosomal Database Project; PCoA: principal coordinates analysis; ANOVA: one-way analysis of variance; ANOSIM: analysis of similarities; LEfSe: Linear discriminant analysis effect size.

Authors' contributions

WX and WH conceived and designed the study. WX and QQ wrote the main manuscript text. WY, LY and JD performed animal experiments and collected data. JX and YH analyzed data. WC prepared figures and tables. All authors reviewed the manuscript. All authors read and approved the final manuscript.

Author details

[1] Shanghai Research Institute of Acupuncture and Meridian, Shanghai University of Traditional Chinese Medicine, 650 South Wanping Road, Xuhui District, Shanghai 200030, China. [2] Key Laboratory of Acupuncture and Immunological Effects, Shanghai University of Traditional Chinese Medicine, Shanghai 200030, China. [3] Yueyang Clinical Medical College, Shanghai University of Traditional Chinese Medicine, Shanghai 200437, China. [4] Stark Neurosciences Research Institute & Department of Anatomy and Cell Biology, Indiana University School of Medicine, Indianapolis, IN 46202, USA. [5] Department of Radiation Oncology, Indiana University School of Medicine, Indianapolis, IN 46202, USA.

Acknowledgements

Sequencing data analysis was supported by Realbio Genomics Institute.

Competing interests

The authors declare that they have no competing interests.

Consent for publication

Not applicable.

Funding

This work was supported by the Natural Science Foundation of Shanghai (Grant Number 14ZR1438700), the National Basic Research Programme of China (973 programme, Grant Number 2015CB554501) and National Natural Science Foundation of China (Grant Number 81473758).

References

1. Canavan C, West J, Card T. The epidemiology of irritable bowel syndrome. Clin Epidemiol. 2014;6:71–80.
2. Zeber-Lubecka N, Kulecka M, Ambrozkiewicz F, Paziewska A, Goryca K, Karczmarski J, et al. Limited prolonged effects of rifaximin treatment on irritable bowel syndrome-related differences in the fecal microbiome and metabolome. Gut Microbes. 2016;7:397–413.
3. Lee OY. Asian motility studies in irritable bowel syndrome. J Neurogastroenterol Motil. 2010;16:120–30.
4. Barshop K, Staller K. New pathways, new targets: visceral hypersensitivity pathogenesis in irritable bowel syndrome. Clin Transl Gastroenterol. 2016;7:e146.
5. Lee YJ, Paek KS. Irritable bowel syndrome: emerging paradigm in pathophysiology. World J Gastroenterol. 2014;20:2456–69.
6. Ratanasirintrawoot S, Israsena N. Stem cells in the intestine: possible roles in pathogenesis of irritable bowel syndrome. J Neurogastroenterol Motil. 2016;22:267–382.
7. Ringel Y, Maharshak N. Intestinal microbiota and immune function in the pathogenesis of irritable bowel syndrome. Am J Physiol Gastrointest Liver Physiol. 2013;305:529–41.
8. Bennet S, Öhman L, Simrén M. Gut microbiota as potential orchestrators of irritable bowel syndrome. Gut Liver. 2015;9:318–31.
9. Qin J, Li R, Raes J, Arumugam M, Burgdorf KS, Manichanh C, et al. A human gut microbial gene catalog established by metagenomic sequencing. Nature. 2010;464:59–65.
10. Khan I, Yasir M, Azhar EI, Kumosani T, Barbour EK, Bibi F, et al. Implication of gut microbiota in human health. CNS Neurol Disord Drug Targets. 2014;13:1325–33.
11. Ubeda C, Pamer EG. Antibiotics, microbiota, and immune defense. Trends Immunol. 2012;33:459–66.
12. Huang Y, Chen Z. Inflammatory bowel disease related innate immunity and adaptive immunity. Am J Transl Res. 2016;8:2490–7.
13. Penders J, Gerhold K, Thijs C, Zimmermann K, Wahn U, Lau S, et al. New insights into the hygiene hypothesis in allergic diseases: mediation of sibling and birth mode effects by the gut microbiota. Gut Microbes. 2014;5:239–44.
14. Pickett-Blakely O. Obesity and irritable bowel syndrome: a comprehensive review. Gastroenterol Hepatol. 2014;10:411–6.
15. Marchesi JR, Dutilh BE, Hall N, Peters WH, Roelofs R, Boleij A, et al. Towards the human colorectal cancer microbiome. PLoS ONE. 2011;6:e20447.
16. Lopetuso LR, Scaldaferri F, Bruno G, Petito V, Franceschi F, Gasbarrini A. The therapeutic management of gut barrier leaking: the emerging role for mucosal barrier protectors. Eur Rev Med Pharmacol Sci. 2015;19:1068–76.
17. Zhu LM, Huang D, Shi LL, Liang LX, Xu T, Chang M, et al. Intestinal symptoms and psychological factors jointly affect quality of life of patients with irritable bowel syndrome with diarrhea. Health Qual Life Outcomes. 2015;13:49.
18. Shi Y, Chen YH, Yin XJ, Wang AQ, Chen XK, Lu JH, et al. Electroacupuncture versus moxibustion for irritable bowel syndrome: a randomized, parallel-controlled trial. Evid Based Complement Altern Med. 2015;2015:361786.
19. Yoon SL, Grundmann O, Koepp L, Farrell L. Management of irritable bowel syndrome (IBS) In adults: conventional and complementary/alternative approaches. Altern Med Rev. 2011;16:134–51.
20. Chiu JH. How does moxibustion possibly work? Evid Based Complement Altern Med. 2013;2013:198584.
21. Huang RJ, Zhao JM, Wu LY, Dou CZ, Liu HR, Weng ZJ, et al. Mechanisms underlying the analgesic effect of moxibustion on visceral pain in irritable bowel syndrome: a review. Evid Based Complement Altern Med. 2014;2014:895914.
22. Wang XM, Lu Y, Wu LY, Yu SG, Zhao BX, Hu HY, et al. Moxibustion inhibits interleukin-12 and tumor necrosis factor alpha and modulates intestinal flora in rat with ulcerative colitis. World J Gastroenterol. 2012;18:6819–28.
23. Al-Chaer ED, Kawasaki M, Pasricha PJ. A new model of chronic visceral hypersensitivity in adult rats induced by colon irritation during postnatal development. Gastroenterology. 2000;119:1276–85.
24. Weng ZJ, Wu LY, Zhou CL, Dou CZ, Shi Y, Liu HR, et al. Effect of electroacupuncture on P2X3 receptor regulation in the peripheral and central nervous systems of rats with visceral pain caused by irritable bowel syndrome. Purinergic Signal. 2015;11(3):321–9.
25. Takahashi S, Tomita J, Nishioka K, Hisada T, Nishijima M. Development of a prokaryotic universal primer for simultaneous analysis of Bacteria and Archae using next-generation sequencing. PLoS ONE. 2014;9:e105592.
26. Vicente CS, Ozawa S, Hasegawa K. Composition of the cockroach gut microbiome in the presence of parasitic nematodes. Microbes Environ. 2016;31:314–20.
27. Xu J, Chen X, Yu S, Su Y, Zhu W. Effects of early intervention with sodium butyrate on gut microbiota and the expression of inflammatory cytokines in neonatal piglets. PLoS ONE. 2016;11:e0162461.
28. Wang Q, Garrity GM, Tiedje JM, Cole JR. Naive Bayesian classifier for rapid assignment of rRNA sequences into the new bacterial taxonomy. Appl Environ Microbiol. 2007;73:5261–7.
29. Keszthelyi D, Troost FJ, Masclee AA. Irritable bowel syndrome: methods, mechanisms, and pathophysiology. Methods to assess visceral hypersensitivity in irritable bowel syndrome. Am J Physiol Gastrointest Liver Physiol. 2012;303:141–54.
30. Zhao JM, Chen L, Zhou CL, Shi Y, Li YW, Shang HX, et al. Comparison of electroacupuncture and moxibustion for relieving visceral hypersensitivity in rats with constipation-predominant irritable bowel syndrome. Evid Based Complement Altern Med. 2016;2016:9410505.
31. Cui S, Hu Y. Multistrain probiotic preparation significantly reduces symptoms of irritable bowel syndrome in a double-blind placebo-controlled study. Int J Clin Exp Med. 2012;5(3):238–44.
32. Hou X, Chen S, Zhang Y, Sha W, Yu X, Elsawah H, et al. Quality of life in patients with irritable bowel syndrome (IBS), assessed using the IBS–quality of life (IBS-QOL) measure after 4 and 8 weeks of treatment with mebeverine hydrochloride or pinaverium bromide: results of an international prospective observational cohort study in Poland, Egypt, Mexico and China. Clin Drug Invest. 2014;34(11):783–93.
33. Zeng MY, Cisalpino D, Varadarajan S, Hellman J, Warren HS, Cascalho M, et al. Gut microbiota-induced immunoglobulin G controls systemic infection by symbiotic bacteria and pathogens. Immunity. 2016;44:647–58.

34. Furusawa Y, Obata Y, Fukuda S, Endo TA, Nakato G, Takahashi D, et al. Commensal microbe-derived butyrate induces the differentiation of colonic regulatory T cells. Nature. 2013;504:446–50.
35. Zhang HS, Wang FC. Application of combination of he-mu points and combination of shu-yuan in syndrome differentiation of zang- and fu-organs. Zhongguo Zhen Jiu. 2006;26(5):378–80.
36. Öhman L, Törnblom H, Simrén M. Crosstalk at the mucosal border: importance of the gut microenvironment in IBS. Nat Rev Gastroenterol Hepatol. 2015;12:36–49.
37. Kondo T, Kawamoto M. Acupuncture and moxibustion for stress-related disorders. Biopsychosoc Med. 2014;8:7.
38. Ponnusamy K, Choi JN, Kim J, Lee SY, Lee CH. Microbial community and metabolomic comparison of irritable bowel syndrome faeces. J Med Microbiol. 2011;60:817–27.
39. Goepp J, Fowler E, McBride T, Landis D. Frequency of abnormal fecal bio-markers in irritable bowel syndrome. Glob Adv Health Med. 2014;3:9–15.
40. Sheikh Sajjadieh MR, Kuznetsova LV, Bojenko VB. Dysbiosis in ukrainian children with irritable bowel syndrome affected by natural radiation. Iran J Pediatr. 2012;22:364–8.
41. Patel R, DuPont HL. New approaches for bacteriotherapy: prebiotics, new-generation probiotics, and synbiotics. Clin Infect Dis. 2015;60:108–21.
42. Kianifar H, Jafari SA, Kiani M, Ahanchian H, Ghasemi SV, Grover Z, et al. Probiotic for irritable bowel syndrome in pediatric patients: a randomized controlled clinical trial. Electron Physician. 2015;7:1255–60.
43. Shavakhi A, Minakari M, Farzamnia S, Peykar MS, Taghipour G, Tayebi A, et al. The effects of multi-strain probiotic compound on symptoms and quality-of-life in patients with irritablebowel syndrome: a randomized placebo-controlled trial. Adv Biomed Res. 2014;3:140.
44. Tiequn B, Guanqun C, Shuo Z. Therapeutic effects of *Lactobacillus* in treating irritable bowel syndrome: a meta-analysis. Intern Med. 2015;54:243–9.

13

Techniques for extraction and isolation of natural products

Qing-Wen Zhang[1]* 🆔, Li-Gen Lin[1] and Wen-Cai Ye[2]*

Abstract

Natural medicines were the only option for the prevention and treatment of human diseases for thousands of years. Natural products are important sources for drug development. The amounts of bioactive natural products in natural medicines are always fairly low. Today, it is very crucial to develop effective and selective methods for the extraction and isolation of those bioactive natural products. This paper intends to provide a comprehensive view of a variety of methods used in the extraction and isolation of natural products. This paper also presents the advantage, disadvantage and practical examples of conventional and modern techniques involved in natural products research.

Keywords: Natural products, Extraction, Isolation, Natural medicine, Chromatography, Phytochemical investigation

Background

Natural medicines, such as traditional Chinese medicine (TCM) and Ayurveda, were formed and developed in the daily life of ancient people and in the process of their fight against diseases over thousands of years, and they have produced a positive impact on the progress of human civilization. Today, natural medicines not only provide the primary health-care needs for the majority of the population in developing countries but have attracted more and more attention in developed countries due to soaring health-care costs and universal financial austerity. In the USA, approximately 49% of the population has tried natural medicines for the prevention and treatment of diseases [1]. Chemicals known to have medicinal benefits are considered to be "active ingredients" or "active principles" of natural medicines. Natural products have provided the primary sources for new drug development. From the 1940s to the end of 2014, nearly half of the FDA approved chemical drugs for the treatment of human diseases were derived from or inspired by natural products [2, 3]. Natural products offer more drug-like features to molecules from combinatorial chemistry in terms of functional groups, chirality, and structural complexity [4, 5].

The amounts of active ingredients in natural medicines are always fairly low. The lab-intensive and time-consuming extraction and isolation process has been the bottle neck of the application of natural products in drug development. There is an urgent need to develop effective and selective methods for the extraction and isolation of bioactive natural products. This review intends to provide a comprehensive view of a variety of methods used in the extraction and isolation of natural products.

Extraction

Extraction is the first step to separate the desired natural products from the raw materials. Extraction methods include solvent extraction, distillation method, pressing and sublimation according to the extraction principle. Solvent extraction is the most widely used method. The extraction of natural products progresses through the following stages: (1) the solvent penetrates into the solid matrix; (2) the solute dissolves in the solvents; (3) the solute is diffused out of the solid matrix; (4) the extracted solutes are collected. Any factor enhancing the diffusivity and solubility in the above steps will facilitate the extraction. The properties of the extraction solvent, the particle size of the raw materials, the solvent-to-solid ration, the

*Correspondence: qwzhang@umac.mo; chywc@aliyun.com
[1] State Key Laboratory of Quality Research in Chinese Medicine, Institute of Chinese Medical Sciences, University of Macau, Macao, People's Republic of China
[2] Institute of Traditional Chinese Medicine & Natural Products, and Guangdong Provincial Engineering Research Center for Modernization of TCM, College of Pharmacy, Jinan University, Guangzhou 510632, People's Republic of China

extraction temperature and the extraction duration will affect the extraction efficiency [6–10].

The selection of the solvent is crucial for solvent extraction. Selectivity, solubility, cost and safety should be considered in selection of solvents. Based on the law of similarity and intermiscibility (like dissolves like), solvents with a polarity value near to the polarity of the solute are likely to perform better and vice versa. Alcohols (EtOH and MeOH) are universal solvents in solvent extraction for phytochemical investigation.

Generally, the finer the particle size is, the better result the extraction achieves. The extraction efficiency will be enhanced by the small particle size due to the enhanced penetration of solvents and diffusion of solutes. Too fine particle size, however, will cost the excessive absorption of solute in solid and difficulty in subsequent filtration.

High temperatures increase the solubility and diffusion. Temperatures that too high, however, may cause solvents to be lost, leading to extracts of undesirable impurities and the decomposition of thermolabile components.

The extraction efficiency increases with the increase in extraction duration in a certain time range. Increasing time will not affect the extraction after the equilibrium of the solute is reached inside and outside the solid material.

The greater the solvent-to-solid ratio is, the higher the extraction yield is; however, a solvent-to-solid ratio that is too high will cause excessive extraction solvent and requires a long time for concentration.

The conventional extraction methods, including maceration, percolation and reflux extraction, usually use organic solvents and require a large volume of solvents and long extraction time. Some modern or greener extraction methods such as super critical fluid extraction (SFC), pressurized liquid extraction (PLE) and microwave assisted extraction (MAE), have also been applied in natural products extraction, and they offer some advantages such as lower organic solvent consumption, shorter extraction time and higher selectivity. Some extraction methods, however, such as sublimation, expeller pressing and enfleurage are rarely used in current phytochemical investigation and will not discussed in this review. A brief summary of the various extraction methods used for natural products is shown in Table 1.

Maceration

This is a very simple extraction method with the disadvantage of long extraction time and low extraction efficiency. It could be used for the extraction of thermolabile components.

Ćujić et al. achieved high yields of total phenols and total anthocyanins from chokeberry fruit at an optimized condition with 50% ethanol, a solid–solvent ratio of 1:20 and particle size of 0.75 mm, which suggested that maceration was a simple and effective method for the extraction of phenolic compounds from chokeberry fruit [11]. A study on the extraction of catechin (**1**, Fig. 1) from *Arbutus unedo* L. fruits using maceration, microwave-assisted and ultrasound extraction techniques showed that microwave-assisted extraction (MAE) was the most effective, but a lower temperature was applied in maceration with nearly identical extraction yields, which can be translated into economic benefits [12]. Jovanović et al. evaluated the extraction efficiency of polyphenols from *Serpylli herba* using various extraction techniques (maceration, heat assisted extraction and ultrasonic-assisted extraction). Based on the content of total polyphenols, ultrasonic-assisted extraction produced the highest total flavonoids yield and no statistically significant difference were found between maceration and heat assisted extraction [13]. *Cajanus cajan* leaves are used in Chinese folk medicine for the treatment of hepatitis, chickenpox and diabetes. Flavonoids are the bioactive compounds. Jin et al. compared extraction rates of orientoside (**2**), luteolin (**3**), and total flavonoids from *C. cajan* leaves by microwave-assisted method, reflux extraction, ultrasound-assisted extraction, and maceration extraction. The extraction efficiency of orientoside, luteolin, and total flavonoids was found to be the lowest in the extract from maceration method [14].

Percolation

Percolation is more efficient than maceration because it is a continuous process in which the saturated solvent is constantly being replaced by fresh solvent.

Zhang et al. compared the percolation and refluxing extraction methods to extract *Undaria pinnatifida*. They found that the contents of the major component, fucoxanthin (**4**, Fig. 2), from the percolation extraction method was higher than that from the refluxing method while there was no significant difference in extract yield between the two methods [15]. Goupi patch is a compound Chinese medicine preparation consisting of 29 Chinese medicines. Fu et al. used the whole alkaloids content determined by acid–base titration as the index and optimized the ethanol percolation method as soaking the medicine with 55% alcohol for 24 h and then percolating with 12 times the amount of 55% alcohol [16]. When using the extracting rate of sinomenine (**5**) and

Table 1 A brief summary of various extraction methods for natural products

Method	Solvent	Temperature	Pressure	Time	Volume of organic solvent consumed	Polarity of natural products extracted
Maceration	Water, aqueous and non-aqueous solvents	Room temperature	Atmospheric	Long	Large	Dependent on extracting solvent
Percolation	Water, aqueous and non-aqueous solvents	Room temperature, occasionally under heat	Atmospheric	Long	Large	Dependent on extracting solvent
Decoction	Water	Under heat	Atmospheric	Moderate	None	Polar compounds
Reflux extraction	Aqueous and non-aqueous solvents	Under heat	Atmospheric	Moderate	Moderate	Dependent on extracting solvent
Soxhlet extraction	Organic solvents	Under heat	Atmospheric	Long	Moderate	Dependent on extracting solvent
Pressurized liquid extraction	Water, aqueous and non-aqueous solvents	Under heat	High	Short	Small	Dependent on extracting solvent
Supercritical fluid extraction	Supercritical fluid (usually S-CO_2), sometimes with modifier	Near room temperature	High	Short	None or small	Nonpolar to moderate polar compounds
Ultrasound assisted extraction	Water, aqueous and non-aqueous solvents	Room temperature, or under heat	Atmospheric	Short	Moderate	Dependent on extracting solvent
Microwave assisted extraction	Water, aqueous and non-aqueous solvents	Room temperature	Atmospheric	Short	None or moderate	Dependent on extracting solvent
Pulsed electric field extraction	Water, aqueous and non-aqueous solvents	Room temperature, or under heat	Atmospheric	Short	Moderate	Dependent on extracting solvent
Enzyme assisted extraction	Water, aqueous and non-aqueous solvents	Room temperature, or heated after enzyme treatment	Atmospheric	Moderate	Moderate	Dependent on extracting solvent
Hydro distillation and steam distillation	Water	Under heat	Atmospheric	Long	None	Essential oil (usually non-polar)

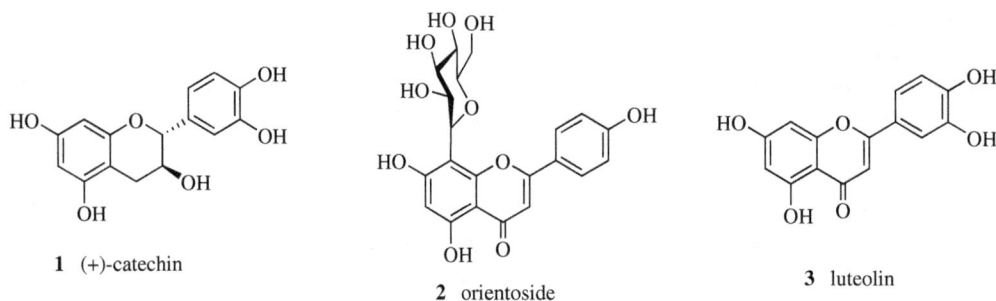

Fig. 1 Structures of compounds **1–3**

1 (+)-catechin

2 orientoside

3 luteolin

ephedrine hydrochloride (**6**) as the index, Gao developed another optimized percolation method: soaking the medicine with 70% ethanol for 24 h and then percolating with 20 times the amount of 70% ethanol. The transfer rates of sinomenine and ephedrine hydrochloride were 78.23 and 76.92%, respectively [17].

Decoction

The extract from decoction contains a large amount of water-soluble impurities. Decoction cannot be used for the extraction of thermolabile or volatile components.

The ginsenosides (**7–31**) in ginseng encounter hydrolysis, dehydration, decarboxylation and addition reactions

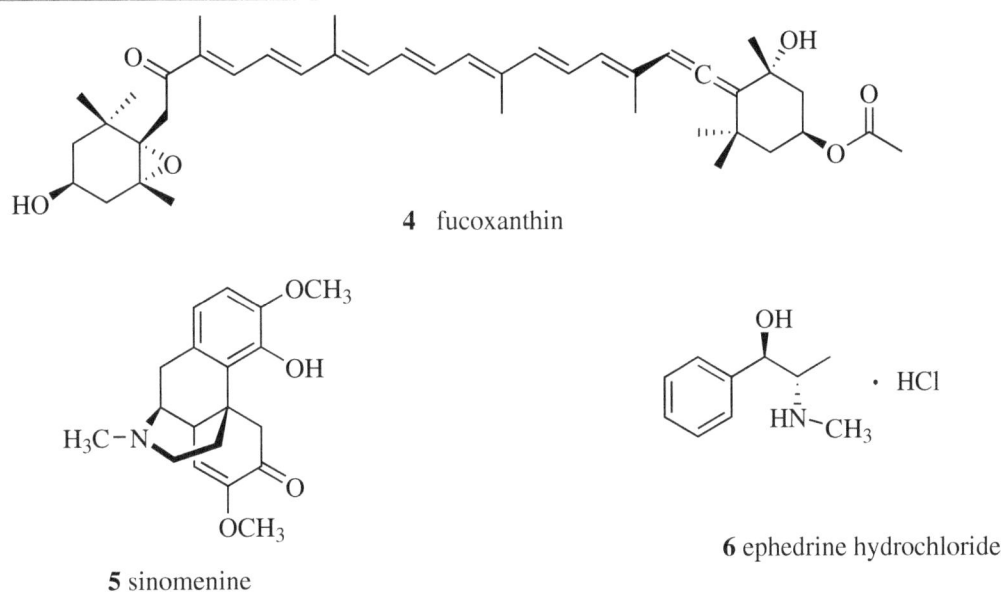

Fig. 2 Structures of compounds **4–6**

during decocting (Fig. 3) [18]. Zhang et al. investigated the chemical transformation of a famous TCM preparation, Danggui Buxue Tang, an herbal decoction containing Astragali Radix and Angelicae Sinensis Radix. They found that two flavonoid glycosides, calycosin-7-O-β-D-glucoside (**32**, Fig. 4) and ononin (**33**), in Astragali Radix, could be hydrolyzed to form calycosin (**34**) and formononetin (**35**), respectively, during decocting. The hydrolysis efficiency was strongly affected by pH, temperature, and the amount of herbs [19]. Two compounds of TCM, Sanhuang Xiexin Tang (SXT) and Fuzi Xiexin Tang (FXT), have been used in China for the treatment of diseases such as diabetes for thousands of years. SXT is composed of Rhei Radix et Rhizoma, Scutellariae Radix and Coptidis Rhizoma while FXT is produced by adding another TCM, Aconiti Lateralis Radix Preparata, in SXT. Zhang et al. applied an UPLC-ESI/MS method to monitor 17 active constituents in SXT and FXT decoctions and macerations. The decoction process might enhance the dissolution of some bioactive compounds compared with the maceration process. The contents of 11 constituents [benzoylaconine (**36**), benzoylhypaconine (**37**), benzoylmesaconine (**38**), berberine (**39**), coptisine (**40**), palmatine (**41**), jatrorrhizine (**42**), aloe-emodin (**43**) and emodin (**44**), baicalin (**45**), wogonoside (**46**)] in decoctions of SXT and FXT were significantly higher than those in macerations of SXT and FXT. The β-glucuronidase in herbs could catalyze the hydrolysis of the glucuronic acid group from glycosides (baicalin and wogonoside) to transfer into aglycones [baicalein (**47**) and wogonin (**48**)]. The high temperature in the decoction process

deactivated the activity of the β-glucuronidase and prevented the transformation of glycosides to their aglycones, which led to the discovery of the higher contents of baicalin and wogonoside in decoctions as well as the higher contents of baicalein and wogonin in macerations. The interaction between chemicals from different herbs was also observed. The diester-diterpenoid alkaloids were not detected in the decoction and maceration of FXT, but diester-diterpenoid alkaloid hypaconitine (**49**) was found in the decoction of the single herb Aconiti Lateralis Radix Preparata. The constituents of the other three herbs in FXT might promote the transformation from diester-diterpenoid alkaloids in Aconiti Lateralis Radix Preparata to other less toxic monoester-diterpenoid alkaloids, which might explain the mechanism of toxicity reduction and efficacy enhancement of TCM by formulation [20].

Reflux extraction

Reflux extraction is more efficient than percolation or maceration and requires less extraction time and solvent. It cannot be used for the extraction of thermolabile natural products.

Refluxing with 70% ethanol provided the highest yield of the natural bio-insecticidal, didehydrostemofoline (**50**, Fig. 5) (0.515% w/w of the extract), from *Stemona collinsiae* root among the extracts prepared by different extraction methods (sonication, reflux, Soxhlet, maceration and percolation) [21]. Zhang compared the extraction efficiency of active ingredients (baicalin (**45**, Fig. 4) and puerarin (**51**) from a TCM compound composing seven herbs with two different methods, decoction and

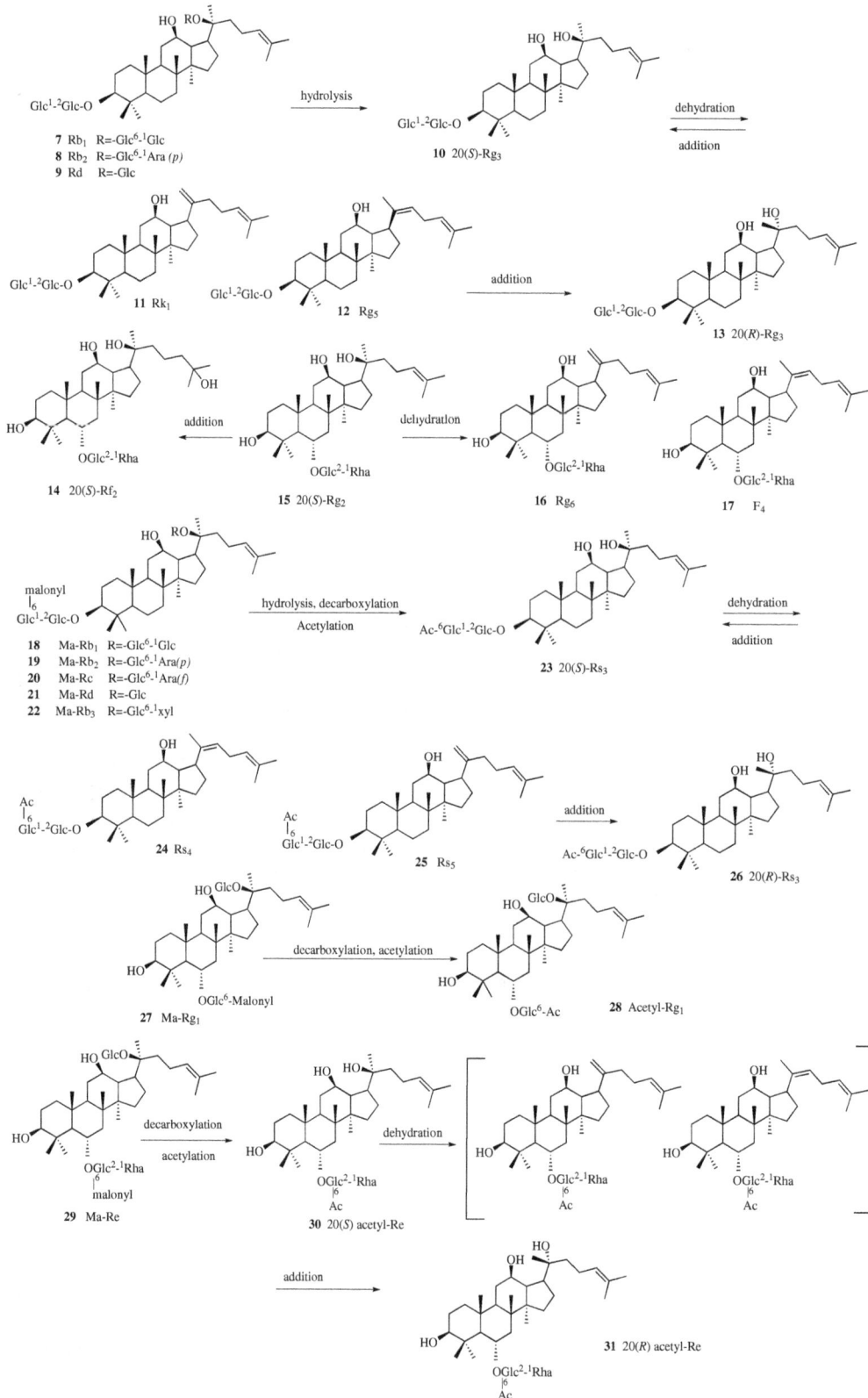

Fig. 3 Possible mechanisms of the chemical conversion of ginsenosides (**7–31**) in decoction

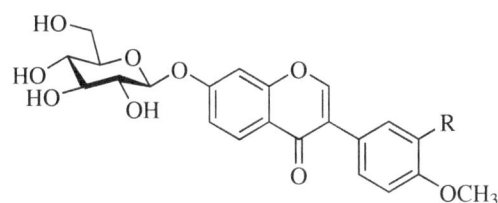

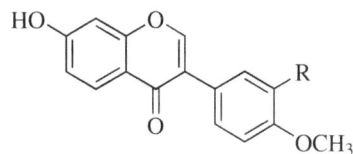

32 calycosin-7-*O*-*β*-D-glucoside   R= OH
33 ononin   R=H

34 calycosin   R= OH
35 formononetin   R= H

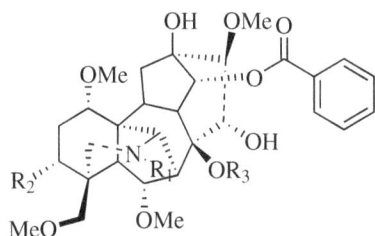

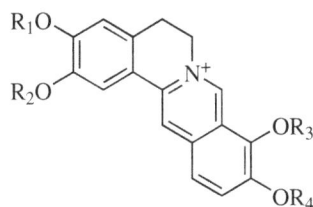

36 benzoylaconine R_1=C_2H_5 R_2=OH R3=H
37 benzoylhypaconine R_1=CH_3 R_2=H R3=H
38 benzoylmesaconine R_1=CH_3 R_2=OH R3=H
49 hypaconitine R_1=CH_3 R_2=H R3=$COCH_3$

	R_1	R_2	R_3	R_4
39 berberine		CH_2		CH_3 CH_3
40 coptisine		CH_2		CH_2
41 palmatine	CH_3	CH_3	CH_3	CH_3
42 jatrorrhizine	H	CH_3	CH_3	CH_3
78 columbamine	CH_3	H	CH_3	CH_3
79 groenlandicine	H	CH_3		CH_2

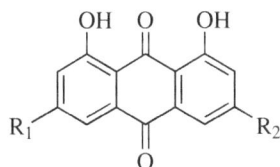

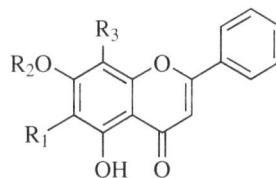

43 aloe-emodin R_1=H R_2=CH_2OH
44 emodin R_1=CH_3 R_2=OH

45 baicalin R_1=OH R_2=GluA R_3=H
46 wogonoside R_1=H R_2=GluA R_3=OCH_3
47 baicalein R_1=OH R_2=H R_3=H
48 wogonin R_1=H R_2=H R_3=OCH_3

Fig. 4 Structures of compounds **32–48** and **78–79**

reflux. The reflux method was found to be better than the decoction method and the highest yields of baicalin and puerarin were obtained from the reflux method with 60% ethanol as the extraction solvent [22].

Soxhlet extraction

The Soxhlet extraction method integrates the advantages of the reflux extraction and percolation, which utilizes the principle of reflux and siphoning to continuously extract the herb with fresh solvent. The Soxhlet extraction is an automatic continuous extraction method with high extraction efficiency that requires less time and solvent consumption than maceration or percolation. The

high temperature and long extraction time in the Soxhlet extraction will increase the possibilities of thermal degradation.

Wei et al. obtained ursolic acid (**52**, Fig. 6) from the TCM Cynomorium (Cynomorii Herba) with a yield of 38.21 mg/g by Soxhlet extraction [23]. The degradation of catechins in tea was also observed in Soxhlet extraction due to the high extraction temperature applied. The concentrations of both total polyphenols and total alkaloids from the Soxhlet extraction method at 70 °C decreased compared to those from the maceration method applied under 40 °C [24, 27].

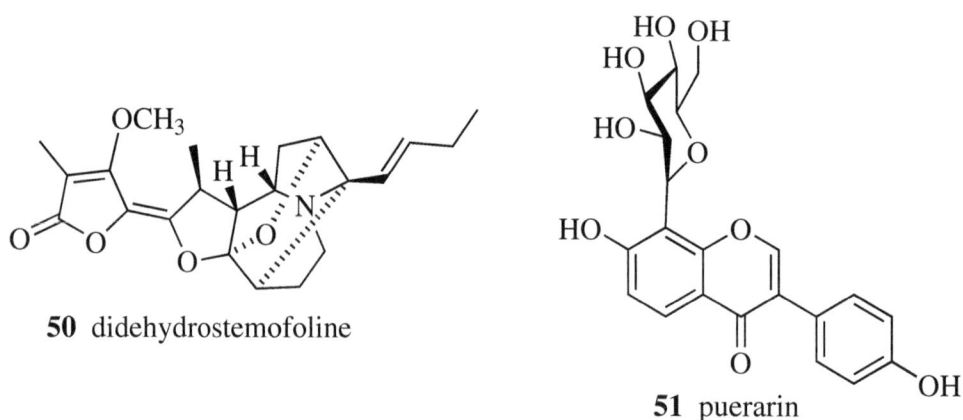

50 didehydrostemofoline

51 puerarin

Fig. 5 Structures of compounds **50–51**

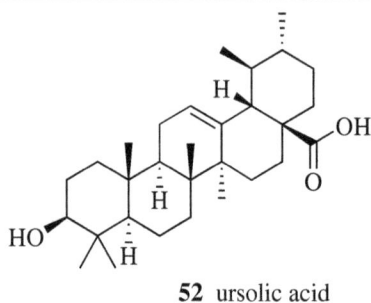

52 ursolic acid

Fig. 6 Structure of compounds **52**

Pressurized liquid extraction (PLE)

Pressurized liquid extraction (PLE) has also been described as accelerated solvent extraction, enhanced solvent extraction, pressurized fluid extraction, accelerated fluid extraction, and high pressure solvent extraction by different research groups. PLE applies high pressure in extraction. High pressure keeps solvents in a liquid state above their boiling point resulting in a high solubility and high diffusion rate of lipid solutes in the solvent, and a high penetration of the solvent in the matrix. PLE dramatically decreased the consumption of extraction time and solvent and had better repeatability compared to other methods.

Pressurized liquid extraction has been successfully applied by the researchers at the University of Macau and other institutes in extracting many types of natural products including saponins, flavonoids and essential oil from TCM [8, 25–27]. Some researchers believed PLE could not be used to extract thermolabile compounds due to the high extraction temperature, while others believed it could be used for the extraction of thermolabile compounds because of the shorter extraction time used in

PLE. Maillard reactions occurred when PLE was used at 200 °C to extract antioxidants from grape pomace [28]. Anthocyanins are thermolabile. Gizir et al. successfully applied PLE to obtain an anthocyanin-rich extract from black carrots because the degradation rate of anthocyanins is time-dependent, and the high-temperature-short-duration PLE extraction conditions could overcome the disadvantage of high temperature employed in the extraction [29].

Supercritical fluid extraction (SFE)

Supercritical fluid extraction (SFE) uses supercritical fluid (SF) as the extraction solvent. SF has similar solubility to liquid and similar diffusivity to gas, and can dissolve a wide variety of natural products. Their solvating properties dramatically changed near their critical points due to small pressure and temperature changes. Supercritical carbon dioxide (S-CO_2) was widely used in SFE because of its attractive merits such as low critical temperature (31 °C), selectivity, inertness, low cost, non-toxicity, and capability to extract thermally labile compounds. The low polarity of S-CO_2 makes it ideal for the extraction of non-polar natural products such as lipid and volatile oil. A modifier may be added to S-CO_2 to enhance its solvating properties significantly.

Conde-Hernández extracted the essential oil of rosemary (*Rosmarinus officinalis*) by S-CO_2 extraction, hydro distillation and steam distillation. He found that both yields of essential oil and antioxidant activity of SFC extract were higher than those from other two methods [30]. S-CO_2 modified with 2% ethanol at 300 bar and 40 °C gave higher extracting selectivity of vinblastine (**53**, Fig. 7) (an antineoplastic drug) from *Catharanthus roseus*, which is 92% more efficient for vinblastine extraction compared to traditional extraction methods [31].

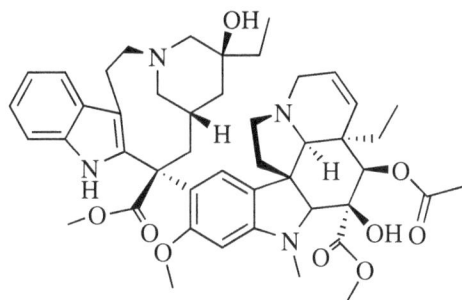

53 vinblastine

Fig. 7 Structure of compounds **53**

Ultrasound assisted extraction (UAE)

Ultrasonic-assisted extraction (UAE), also called ultrasonic extraction or sonication, uses ultrasonic wave energy in the extraction. Ultrasound in the solvent producing cavitation accelerates the dissolution and diffusion of the solute as well as the heat transfer, which improves the extraction efficiency. The other advantage of UAE includes low solvent and energy consumption, and the reduction of extraction temperature and time. UAE is applicable for the extraction of thermolabile and unstable compounds. UAE is commonly employed in the extraction of many types of natural products [32, 33].

Jovanović et al. achieved a higher yield of polyphenols from *Thymus serpyllum* L. by UAE at an optimized condition (50% ethanol as solvent; 1:30 solid-to-solvent ratio; 0.3 mm particle size and 15 min time) than maceration and heat-assisted extraction methods [13]. Wu et al. found that there was no statistically significant difference for extracting ginsenosides, including ginsenosides Rg1 (**54**, Fig. 8) and Rb1 (**7**, Fig. 3), chikusetsusaponins V (**55**), IV (**56**) and IVa (**57**), and pseudoginsenoside RT1 (**58**), from the TCM Panacis Japonici Rhizoma between UAE and reflux using 70% aqueous methanol to extract for 30 min [34]. Guo et al. found both the reflux method and UAE had the advantages of time-saving, convenient operation and high extract yield and that UAE is relatively better than reflux methods for TCM Dichroae Radix using the extract yield and content of febrifugine (**59**) as the indexes [35].

Microwave assisted extraction (MAE)

Microwaves generate heat by interacting with polar compounds such as water and some organic components in the plant matrix following the ionic conduction and dipole rotation mechanisms. The transfers of heat and mass are in the same direction in MAE, which generates a synergistic effect to accelerate extraction and improve extraction yield. The application of MAE provides many advantages, such as increasing the extract yield,

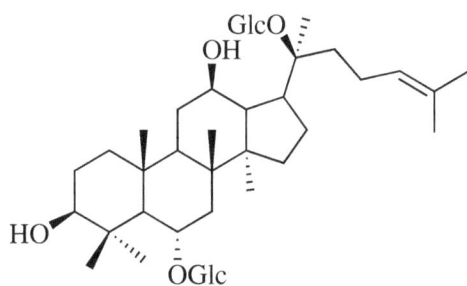

54 ginsenoside Rg1

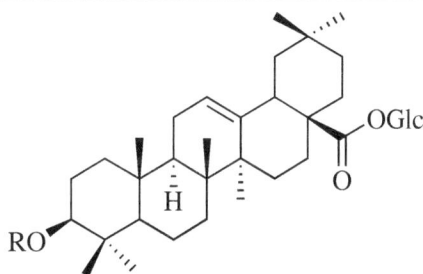

55 chikusetsusaponin V   R=-GluA^2-^{1}Glc
56 chikusetsusaponin IV   R=-GluA^4-^{1}Ara
57 chikusetsusaponin IVa   R=-GluA
58 pseudoginsenoside RT1 R=-GluA^2-^{1}Xyl

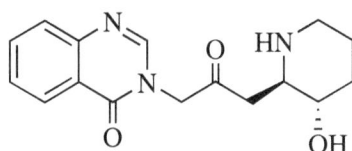

59 febrifugine

Fig. 8 Structures of compounds **54–59**

decreasing the thermal degradation and selective heating of vegetal material. MAE is also regraded as a green technology because it reduces the usage of organic solvent. There are two types of MAE methods: solvent-free extraction (usually for volatile compounds) and solvent extraction (usually for non-volatile compounds) [36, 37].

Chen optimized the conditions for MAE to extract resveratrol (**60**, Fig. 9) from the TCM Polygoni Cuspidati Rhizoma et Radix (the rhizome and radix of *Polygonum cuspidatum*) by orthogonal experiment. An extraction yield of 1.76% of resveratrol was obtained from the optimized conditions as follows: extraction time 7 min, 80% ethanol, ratio of liquid to solid 25:1 (ml:g), microwave power 1.5 kw [38]. Benmoussa et al. employed the enhanced solvent-free MAE method for the extraction of essential oils from *Foeniculum vulgare* Mill. seeds at atmospheric pressure without any addition of solvent or water. The yield and aromatic profile in the enhanced

solvent-free MAE extract was similar to those extracted by hydro distillation and cost only one-sixth of the time of hydro distillation [39]. Xiong et al. developed an MAE to extract five main bioactive alkaloids, liensinine (**61**), neferine (**62**), isoliensinine (**63**), dauricine (**64**), and nuciferin (**65**), from the TCM Nelumbinis Plumula (lotus plumule, the green embryo of *Nelumbo nucifera* seeds) using univariate approach experiments and central composite design. The MAE conditions was optimized as follows: 65% methanol as the extraction solvent, microwave power of 200 W and extraction time of 260 s [40, 44].

Pulsed electric field (PEF) extraction
Pulsed electric field extraction significantly increases the extraction yield and decreased the extraction time because it can increase mass transfer during extraction by destroying membrane structures. The effectiveness of PEF treatment depends on several parameters including

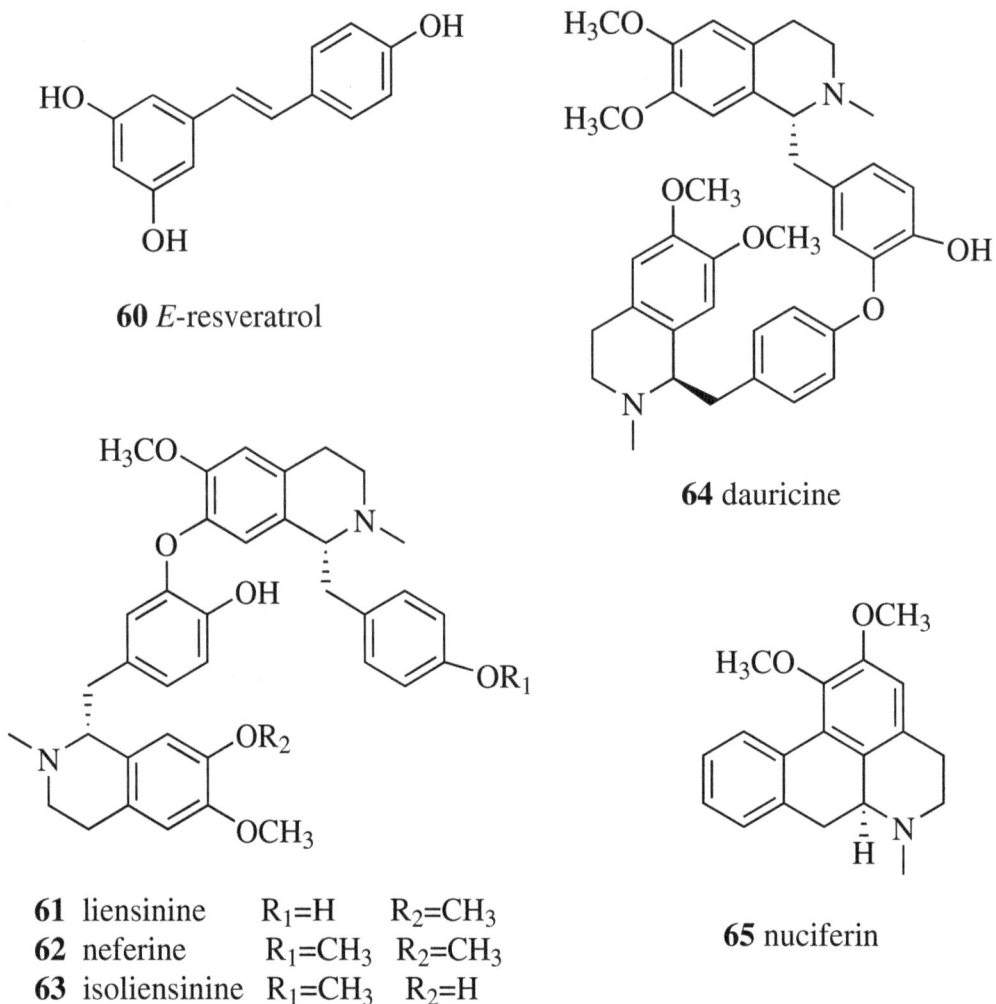

Fig. 9 Structures of compounds **60–65**

field strength, specific energy input, pulse number and treatment temperature. PEF extraction is a non-thermal method and minimizes the degradation of the thermolabile compounds.

Hou et al. obtained the highest yield of the ginsenosides (12.69 mg/g) by PEF using the conditions of 20 kV/cm electric field intensity, 6000 Hz frequency, 70% ethanol–water solution, and 150 l/h velocity. The yield of the ginsenosides of the PEF extraction method is higher than those of MAE, heat reflux extraction, UAE and PLE. The entire PEF extraction process took less than 1 s and much less than the other tested methods [41]. In a study of antioxidants extracted from Norway spruce bark, Bouras found that much higher phenolic content (eight times) and antioxidant activity (30 times) were achieved after the PEF treatment compared to untreated samples [42].

Enzyme assisted extraction (EAE)

The structure of the cell membrane and cell wall, micelles formed by macromolecules such polysaccharides and protein, and the coagulation and denaturation of proteins at high temperatures during extraction are the main barriers to the extraction of natural products. The extraction efficiency will be enhanced by EAE due to the hydrolytic action of the enzymes on the components of the cell wall and membrane and the macromolecules inside the cell which facilitate the release of the natural product. Cellulose, α-amylase and pectinase are generally employed in EAE.

Polysaccharide is one of the bioactive ingredients in the TCM Astragali Radix. Chen et al. studied the EAE of polysaccharide from the radix of *Astragalus membranaceus* using various enzymes and found that glucose oxidase offered better performance in extracting polysaccharide than the other seven enzymes tested (amyloglucosidase,

hemicellulase, bacterial amylase, fungal amylase, pectinase, cellulose and vinozyme). The polysaccharide yield under the optimized EAE condition using glucose oxidase increased more than 250% compared with that from non-enzyme treated method [43]. The extraction yield of chlorogenic acid (**66**, Fig. 10) from *Eucommia ulmoides* leaves was greatly improved when using cellulase and ionic liquids [44]. Strati el al. found that carotenoid and lycopene (**67**) extraction yields from tomato waste were increased by the use of pectinase and cellulase enzymes. Compared to the non-enzyme treated solvent extraction method, sixfold and tenfold higher yields of the two target compounds were obtained in samples treated with cellulase and pectinase, respectively [45].

Hydro distillation and steam distillation

Hydro distillation (HD) and steam distillation (SD) are commonly used methods for the extraction of volatile oil. Some natural compounds encounter decomposition in HD and SD.

The chemical composition and antibacterial activity of the primary essential oil and secondary essential oil from *Mentha citrata* were significantly affected by distillation methods. Both primary essential oil and secondary essential oil yields by HD were higher than those by SD [46, 50]. Yahya and Yunus found that the extraction time did affect the quality of the essential patchouli oil extracted. When the extraction time increased, the contents of some components decreased or increased [47].

Separation methods

The components in the extract from above methods are complex and contain a variety of natural products that require further separation and purification to obtain the active fraction or pure natural products. The separation

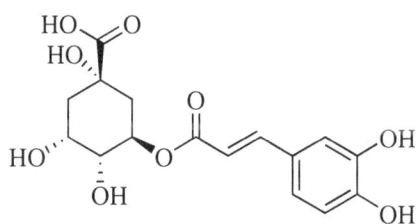

66 chlorogenic acid

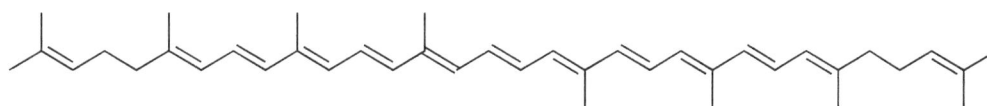

67 lycopene

Fig. 10 Structures of compounds **66–67**

depends on the physical or chemical difference of the individual natural product. Chromatography, especially column chromatography, is the main method used to obtain pure natural products from a complex mixture.

Separation based on adsorption properties

Adsorption column chromatography is widely used for the separation of natural products, especially in the initial separation stage, due to its simplicity, high capacity and low cost of adsorbents such as silica gel and macroporous resins. The separation is based on the differences between the adsorption affinities of the natural products for the surface of the adsorbents. The selection of adsorbents (stationary phase) as well as the mobile phase is crucial to achieve good separation of natural products, maximize the recovery of target compounds and avoid the irreversible adsorption of target compounds onto the adsorbents.

Silica gel is the most widely used adsorbent in phytochemical investigation. It was estimated that nearly 90% of phytochemical separation (preparative scale) was based on silica gel. Silica gel is a polar absorbent with silanol groups. Molecules are retained by the silica gel through hydrogen bonds and dipole–dipole interactions. Thus, polar natural products are retained longer in silica gel columns than nonpolar ones. Sometimes, certain polar natural products might undergo irreversible chemisorption. The deactivation of silica gel by adding water before use or using a water-containing mobile phase will weaken the adsorption. Severe tailing may occur when separating alkaloids on silica gel, and the addition of a small amount of ammonia or organic amines such as triethylamine may reduce the tailing. Twelve alkaloids belonging to the methyl chanofruticosinate group including six new alkaloids, prunifolines A–F (**68–73**, Fig. 11), were obtained from the leaf of *Kopsia arborea* by initial silica gel column chromatography using gradient MeOH–CHCl₃ as the mobile phase followed by centrifugal TLC using ammonia saturated Et₂O–hexane or EtOAc/hexane systems as the eluent [48].

Alumina (aluminum oxide) is a strong polar adsorbent used in the separation of natural products especially in the separation of alkaloids. The strong positive field of Al^{3+} and the basic sites in alumina affecting easily polarized compounds lead to the adsorption on alumina that is different from that on silica gel. The application of alumina in the separation of natural products has decreased significantly in recent years because it can catalyze dehydration, decomposition or isomerization during separation. Zhang and Su reported a chromatographic protocol using basic alumina to separate taxol (**74**, Fig. 11) from the extract of *Taxus cuspidate* callus cultures and found the recovery of taxol was more than 160%. They found

that the increase of taxol came from the isomerization of 7-*epi*-taxol (**75**) catalyzed by alumina. It was also found that a small amount of taxol could be decomposed to baccatin III (**76**) and 10-deacetylbaccatin III (**77**) in the alumina column [49]. Further investigation into the separation of taxol on acidic, neutral and basic alumina indicated that the Lewis souci and the basic activity cores on the surface of alumina induced the isomerization of 7-*epi*-taxol to taxol [50].

The structures of polyamides used in chromatography contain both acryl and amide groups. Hydrophobic and/or hydrogen bond interaction will occur in polyamide column chromatography depending on the composition of the mobile phase. When polar solvents such as aqueous solvents are used as the mobile phase, the polyamides act as the non-polar stationary phase and the chromatography behavior is similar to reversed-phase chromatography. In the contrast, the polyamides act as the polar stationary phase and the chromatography behavior is similar to normal phase chromatography. Polyamide column chromatography is a conventional tool for the separation of natural polyphenols including anthraquinones, phenolic acids and flavonoids, whose mechanisms are ascribed to hydrogen bond formation between polyamide absorbents, mobile phase and target compounds. Gao et al. studied the chromatography behavior of polyphenols including phenolic acids and flavonoids on polyamide column. It was found that the polyamide functioned as a hydrogen bond acceptor, and the numbers of phenolic hydroxyls and their positions in the molecule affected the strength of adsorption [51]. In addition to polyphenols, the separation of other types of natural products by polyamide column chromatography were also reported. The total saponins of Kuqingcha can be enriched by polyamide column chromatography, which significantly reduced the systolic pressure of SHR rat [52]. Using a mixture of dichloromethane and methanol in a gradient as the eluent, the seven major isoquinoline alkaloids in Coptidis Rhizoma including berberine (**39**), coptisine (**40**), palmatine (**41**), jatrorrhizine (**42**), columbamine (**78**), groenlandicine (**79**) (Fig. 4), and magnoflorine (**80**, Fig. 11) were separated in one-step polyamide column chromatography [53].

Adsorptive macroporous resins are polymer adsorbents with macroporous structures but without ion exchange groups that can selectively adsorb almost any type of natural products. They have been widely used either as a standalone system, or as part of a pretreatment process for removing impurities or enriching target compounds due to their advantages, which include high adsorptive capacity, relatively low cost, easy regeneration and easy scale-up. The adsorptive mechanisms of adsorptive macroporous resins include electrostatic forces,

68 prunifoline A

69 prunifoline B R$_1$=OMe, R$_2$=COOMe
70 prunifoline C R$_1$=H,   R$_2$=H

71 prunifoline D R$_1$=H,   R$_2$=H
72 prunifoline E R$_1$ R$_2$=OCH$_2$O
73 prunifoline F R$_1$=H,   R$_2$=OMe

74   taxol   7S
75   7-epi-taxol 7R

76 baccatin III   R=CH$_3$CO
77 10-deacetylbaccatin III R=H

80 magnoflorine

81 PTS R$_1$, R$_2$=H or glycosyl
87 notoginsenoside R1 R$_1$=Glc^2-^{1}Xyl R$_2$=Glc
88 ginsenoside Re   R$_1$=Glc^2-^{1}Rha R$_2$=Glc

82 PDS R$_1$, R$_2$=H or glycosyl

83 brasiliensic acid

84 isobrasiliensic acid

85 xanthochymol R=

86 guttiferone E   R=

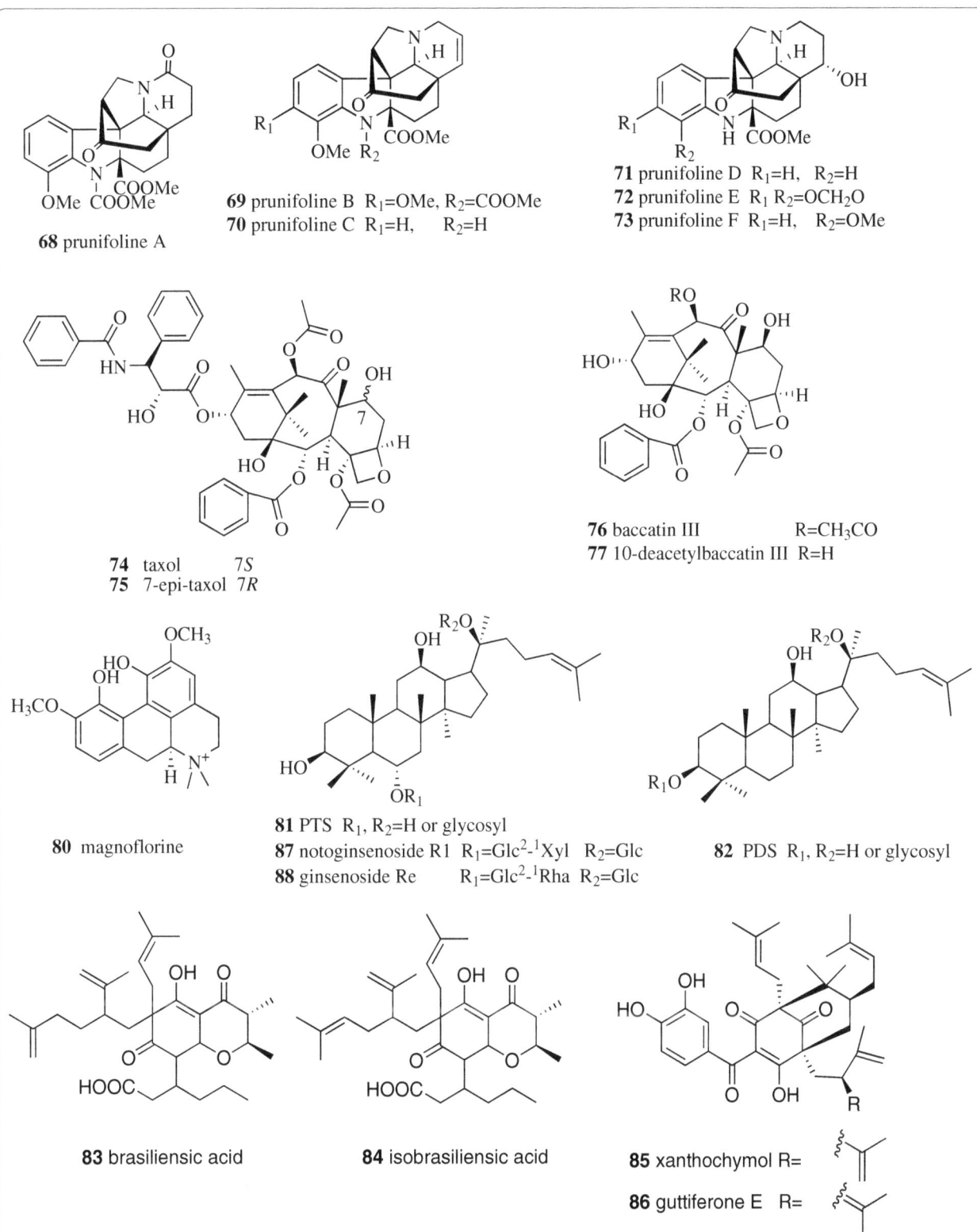

Fig. 11 Structures of compounds **68–88**

hydrogen bonding, complex formation and size-sieving actions between the resins and the natural products in solution. Surface area, pore diameter and polarity are the key factors affecting the capacity of the resins [54]. 20(*S*)-protopanaxatriol saponins (PTS) (**81**) and 20(*S*)-protopanaxadiol saponins (PDS) (**82**, Fig. 11) are known as two major bioactive components in the root of *Panax notoginseng*. PTS and PDS were successfully separated with 30 and 80% (v/v) aqueous ethanol solutions from the D101 macroporous resin column, respectively. The chromatography behaviors of PDS and PTS were close to reversed-phase chromatography when comparing the chromatographic profiles of macroporous resin column chromatography to the HPLC chromatogram on a Zorbax SB-C$_{18}$ column [55]. Recently, Meng et al. obtained the total saponins of Panacis Japonici Rhizoma (PJRS) using D101 macroporous resin. The contents of the four major saponins, chikusetsusaponins V (**55**), IV (**56**) and IVa (**57**), and pseudoginsenoside RT1 (**58**) (Fig. 8), in the obtained PJRS was more than 73%. The PJRS served as the standard reference for quality control of Panacis Japonici Rhizoma [56]. Some researchers assumed that the principal adsorptive mechanism between macroporous resins and polyphenols was associated with the hydrogen bonding formation between the oxygen atom of the ether bond of the resin and the hydrogen atom of phenolic hydroxyl group of the phenol. The hydrogen bonding interaction force was significantly affected by the pH value of the solution [57, 58].

Silver nitrate is another useful solid support in the separation of natural products. Those natural products containing the π electrons reversibly interact with silver ions to form polar complexes. The greater the number of double bonds or aromaticity of the natural product, the stronger the complexation forms. Silver nitrate is typically impregnated on silica gel (SNIS) or alumina for separation. Several research groups reported the separation of fatty acids on SNIS [59–61]. Wang et al. reported the isolation of zingiberene from ginger oleoresin by SNIS column chromatography [62]. A pair of isomers, brasiliensic acid (**83**, Fig. 11) and isobrasiliensic acid (**84**), were separated from *Calophyllum brasiliense* by Lemos et al. on an SNIS column [63, 69]. Some research groups also applied silver nitrate in the two-phase system in high-speed counter-current chromatography (HSCCC) to improve the separation. Xanthochymol (**85**) and guttiferone E (**86**) are a pair of π bond benzophenone isomers from *Garcinia xanthochymus* by AgNO$_3$-HSCCC. The elution order of the π bond isomers in this AgNO$_3$-HSCCC separation is internal π bond (earlier) < terminal, which is identical to that observed from SNIS column chromatography [64].

Separation based on partition coefficient

Partition chromatography (PC) follows the liquid–liquid extraction principle based on the relative solubility in two different immiscible liquids. In the early stage, one liquid phase was coated to a solid matrix (silica gel, carbon, cellulose, etc.) as the stationary phase and another liquid phase was employed as the mobile phase. The disadvantage of an easily removed stationary phase and unrepeatable results has led to this kind of PC being rarely used today. The bonded-phase, in which the liquid stationary phase is chemically bound to the inert support, which is used as the stationary phase overcomes those drawbacks. Commercially available alkyl such as C8 and C18, aryl, cyano and amino substituted silanes are often used as bonded phases, which are widely used to separate a variety of natural products, especially in the final purification step.

Three PTS (notoginsenoside R1 (**87**) (Fig. 11), ginsenosides Rg1 (**55**) (Fig. 8) and Re (**88**) (Fig. 11)) and two PDS [ginsenosides Rb1 (**7**) and Rd (**9**)] (Fig. 3) were well separated in a C18 column using the EtOH–H$_2$O system as the mobile phase [65]. A novel polyacrylamide-based silica stationary phase was synthesized by Cai et al. and was successfully applied in the separation of galactooligosaccharides and saponins of *Paris polyphylla* with EtOH–H$_2$O as the mobile phase [66].

Counter-current chromatography (CCC) is kind of PC that holds the liquid stationary phase by gravity or centrifugal force. CCC has rarely been used in early stages due to its poor stationary retention, long separation time and labor intensive process. CCC was significantly improved in the 1980s, however, when modern CCC, including HSCCC and centrifugal partition chromatography (CPC), were developed. The hydrodynamic CCC systems such as HSCCC have a planetary rotation movement around two rotating axes with no rotating seals, which offers a low pressure drop process. Hydrostatic CCC, e.g., centrifugal partition chromatography, uses only one rotating axis and has a series of interconnecting chambers to trap the stationary phase which offers a higher retention of the stationary phase and a higher system pressure than that of HSCCC. The high system pressure in CPC prevents the improvement of the resolution by increasing the length of the column. High performance CCC (HPCCC) represents a new generation of hydrodynamic CCC and works in the same way as HSCCC, but with a much higher g-level. The HPCCC instruments generate more than 240 g, while early HSCCC equipment gave g-levels of less than 80 g. HPCCC shortens the separation time to less than an hour compared to several hours in previous HSCCC and can achieve at least ten times the throughput of an HSCCC instrument [67]. Compared to the conventional column separation method using a solid stationary phase, both hydrostatic and hydrodynamic CCC systems offer some advantages including the elimination of irreversible adsorption and peak tailing, high loading capacity, high sample recovery, minimal risk of sample denaturation and low solvent consumption. The limitation of CCC is that it only separates the compounds in a relatively narrow polarity window. Over the past 20 years, HSCCC, HPCCC and CPC attracted great attention in separation science and have been widely used in the separation of natural products. Tang et al. developed an HSCCC method using a two-phase solvent system comprising ethyl acetate–*n*-butanol–ethanol–water (4:2:1.5:8.5, v/v/v/v) to separate six flavone *C*-glycosides (**89**–**94**, Fig. 12), including two novel compounds from *Lophatherum gracile* [68]. HSCCC, HPCCC and CPC have also been successfully applied in the separation of volatile oil, which is difficult to separate via conventional column chromatography. Six volatile compounds (curdione (**95**), curcumol (**96**), germacrone (**97**), curzerene (**98**), 1,8-cineole (**99**) and *β*-elemene (**100**)) were isolated by CPC from the essential oil of *Curcuma wenyujin* using a nonaqueous two-phase solvent system consisting of petroleum ether–acetonitrile–acetone (4:3:1 v/v/v) [69]. Four major sesquiterpenoids (ar-turmerone (**101**), *α*-turmerone (**102**), *β*-turmerone (**103**), and *E*-atlantone (**104**)) with similar structures were separated from the essential oil of *Curcuma longa* in a single HSCCC run using a two-phase solvent system composed of *n*-heptane–ethyl acetate–acetonitrile–water (9.5/0.5/9/1, v/v) and each compound achieved over 98% purity [70]. Linalool (**105**), terpinen-4-*ol* (**106**), *α*-terpineol (**107**), *p*-anisaldehyde (**108**), anethole (**109**) and foeniculin (**110**) were successfully isolated from the essential oil of *Pimpinella anisum* by HPCCC using a stepwise gradient elution [71]. Li et al. developed a CPC method for the separation of patchouli alcohol (**111**) with a nonaqueous ether–acetonitrile (1:1, v/v) solvent system. More than 2 g of patchouli alcohol with over 98% purity were isolated from 12.5 g of essential oil over a 240 ml column [72]. The large volume (several liters) column has been adopted in commercial hydrostatic CCC and hydrodynamic CCC equipment for pilot/industrial scale separation. Few reports could be obtained due to commercial confidentiality. It is difficult to judge whether hydrostatic or hydrodynamic CCC is better for industrial applications. Users might select different types of CCC instrument for different purposes. When the stationary phase is poorly retained in hydrodynamic CCC due to high viscosity and small density differences between the mobile and stationary phases, the hydrostatic CCC is more practical than hydrodynamic CCC because the retention of the stationary phase of hydrostatic CCC is less sensitive to the physical properties of liquid systems

and will have a higher retention of the stationary phase. When the stationary phase is well retained in hydrodynamic CCC, higher separation efficiency will be obtained from hydrodynamic CCC than from hydrostatic CCC with the same liquid system and similar column volumes because hydrostatic CCC has relatively low partition efficiency due to a limited degree of mixing, and the hydrodynamic system provides efficient mixing to yield a high partition efficiency.

Separation based on the molecular size
The separation of natural products by membrane filtration (MF) or gel filtration chromatography (GFC) is based on their molecular sizes.

Membrane filtration (MF)
In MF, the semipermeable membrane allows smaller molecules to pass through and retains the larger molecules. MF of natural products could be characterized as microfiltration, ultrafiltration, and nanofiltration based on the pore size of the membrane applied.

Membrane filtration has been a powerful tool for the concentration, clarification and removal of impurities in the lab, as well as in the food and pharmaceutical industries. The contents of total phenols (338%), chlorogenic acid (**66**) (Fig. 10) (483%), theobromine (**112**, Fig. 13) (323%), caffeine (**113**) (251%), condensed tannins (278%) and saponins (211%) in the aqueous extract of *Ilex paraguariensis* were significantly increased by nanofiltration [73, 80]. Coupling membrane filtration is applied when a single membrane filtration step is not satisfactory. A sequence of microfiltration, ultrafiltration and nanofiltration was applied in the isolation of bioactive components from olive leaf extract. Microfiltration followed by ultrafiltration removed the impurities larger than 5 kDa. Nanofiltration recovered the antioxidative and antibacterial polyphenols and flavonoids, and the content of the major component, oleuropein (**114**), in the nanofiltration retentate was concentrated approximately ten times [74].

Gel filtration chromatography (GFC)
Gel filtration chromatography is also known as gel permeation chromatography or size exclusion chromatography. The small molecules have a longer retention time in GFC than large molecules.

Sephadex is formed by cross-linking dextran, and the G-types of Sephadex were used for the separation of hydrophilic compounds such as peptides [75], oligosaccharides and polysaccharides [76].

Sephadex LH20, a hydroxypropylated derivative of Sephadex G25, has both hydrophobic and hydrophilic natures. An adsorption mechanism was also involved in separation using Sephadex LH-20. Sephadex LH-20 can

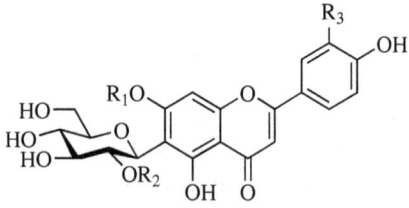

89 luteolin 6-*C*-*β*-D-galactopyranosiduronic acid (1-2)-*β*-D-
glucopyranoside   R₁=H   R₂=GalUA R₃=OH
90 isoorientin   R₁=H   R₂=H   R₃=OH
91 swertiajaponin   R₁=CH₃ R₂=H   R₃=OH
92 apigenin 6-C-*β*-D-galactopyranosiduronic acid (1-2)-*β*-*D*-
glucopyranoside   R₁=H   R₂=GalUA R₃=H

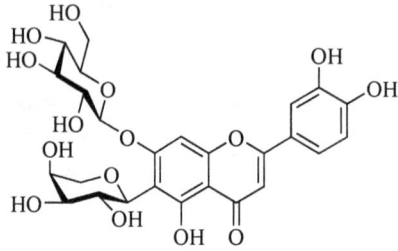

93 luteolin 6-*C*-*α*-L-arabinopyranosyl-7-*O*-*β*-D-glucopyranoside

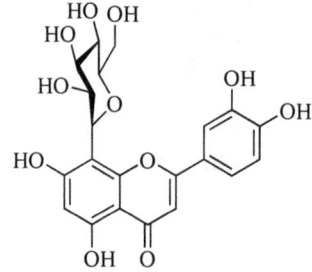

94 orientin

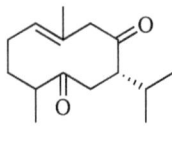

95 curdione

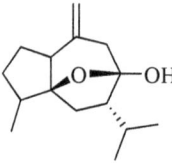

96 curcumol

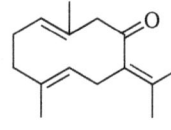

97 germacrone

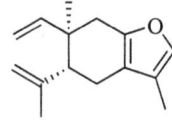

98 curzerene

99 1,8-cineole

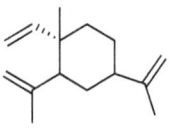

100 *β*-elemene

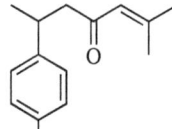

101 ar-turmerone

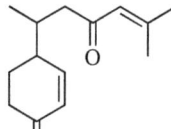

102 *α*-turmerone

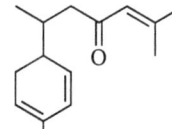

103 *β*-turmerone

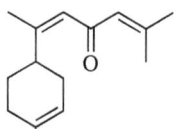

104 *β*-atlantone

105 linalool

106 terpinen-4-ol

107 *α*-terpineol

108 *p*-anisaldehyde

109 anethole

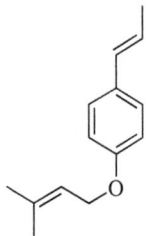

110 foeniculin

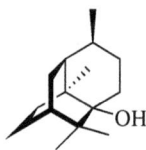

111 patchouli alcohol

Fig. 12 Structures of compounds **89–111**

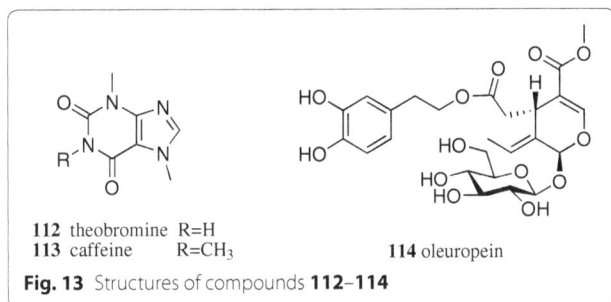

112 theobromine R=H
113 caffeine   R=CH₃

114 oleuropein

Fig. 13 Structures of compounds **112–114**

be used for the separation of a wide variety of natural products in either an aqueous or non-aqueous solvent system. The feruloylated arabinoxylan oligosaccharides of perennial cereal grain intermediate wheat were well separated by Sephadex LH-20 using 100% water as the mobile phase [77]. Three new pyrimidine diterpenes, axistatins 1–3 (**115–117**, Fig. 14) along with three known formamides (**118–120**) were isolated from the anti-cancer active CH_2Cl_2 fraction of *Agelas axifera* over Sephadex LH-20 columns with a series of solvent systems [CH_3OH, CH_3OH–CH_2Cl_2 (3:2), hexane–CH_3OH–2-propanol (8:1:1), hexane–toluene–CH_2Cl_2–EtOH (17:1:1:1) and exane–EtOAc–CH_3OH (4:5:1)], followed by purification using Prep-HPLC [78, 85, 87].

Polyacrylamide (bio-gel P) [79] and cross-linked agarose [80] were also used in the separation of natural products.

Separation based on ionic strength

Ion-exchange chromatography (IEC) separates molecules based on the differences in their net surface charge. Some natural products, such as alkaloids and organic acids possessing a functional group capable of ionization, might be separated by IEC. The charged molecules could be caught and released by ion-exchange resin by changing the ionic strength of the mobile phase (e.g., changing pH or salt concentration). Cation ion-exchange resins were used for the separation of alkaloids, while the anion ion-exchange resins were used for the separation of natural organic acids and phenols.

The positively charged anthocyanins were separated from the neutral polyphenolic compounds in the XAD-7 treated *Actinidia melanandra* fruit (kiwifruit) extract using Dowex 50WX8 cation ion-exchange resin [81]. Feng and Zhao used semi-preparative chromatography to separate (−)epigallocatechin-gallate [**121**, Fig. 15)] and (−)epicatechin-gallate (**122**) in tea crude extract with polysaccharide-based weakly acidic gel CM-Sephadex C-25 [82]. A new alkaloid, fumonisin B₆ (**123**), along with a known alkaloid, fumonisin B₂ (**124**), was isolated by IEC over Strata X-C mixed-mode RP-cation-exchange resin followed by reverse-phase chromatography from the fungus *Aspergillus niger* NRRL 326 cultures extract [83].

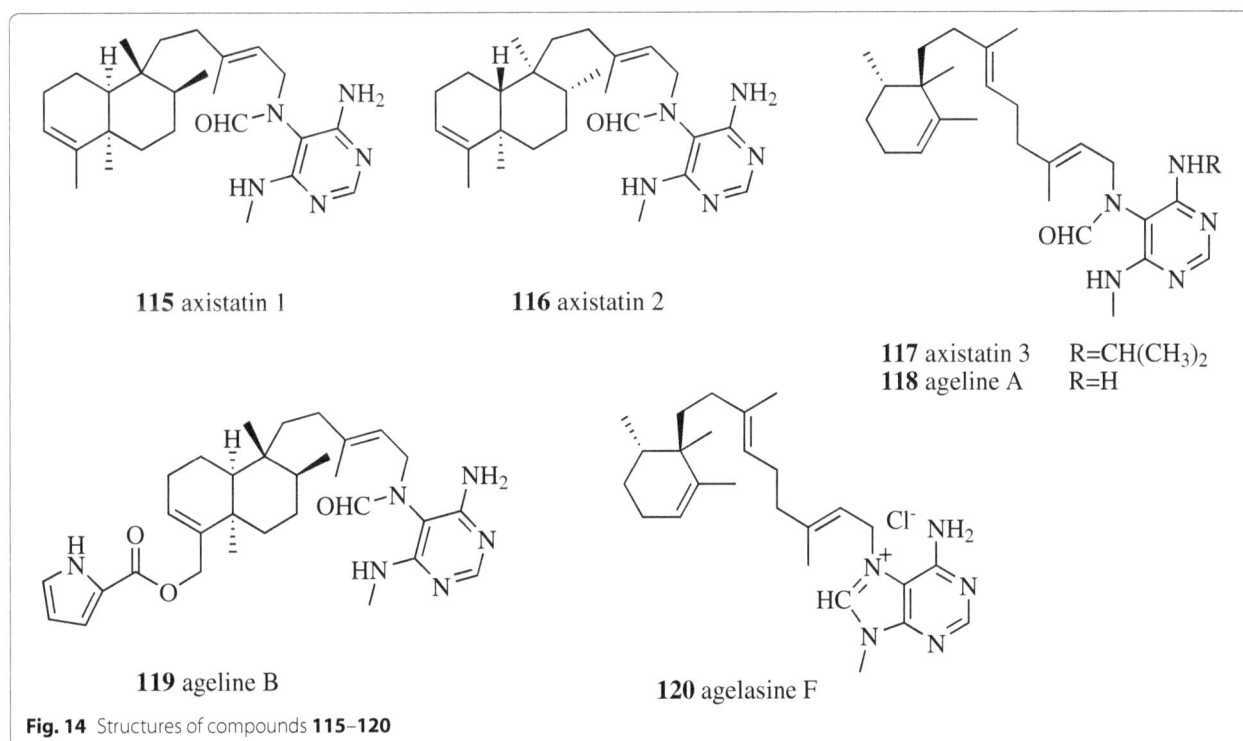

115 axistatin 1

116 axistatin 2

117 axistatin 3   R=CH(CH₃)₂
118 ageline A   R=H

119 ageline B

120 agelasine F

Fig. 14 Structures of compounds **115–120**

Other modern separation techniques
Molecular distillation (MD)
Molecular distillation separates the molecular by distillation under vacuum at a temperature far below its boiling point. It is a suitable distillation method for separating thermosensitive and high-molecular-weight compounds. Borgarello et al. obtained a thymol (**125**, Fig. 16) enrichment fraction from oregano essential oil by molecular distillation modeled by artificial neural networks. The obtained fraction had antioxidant properties and could stabilize the sunflower oil [84]. Three kinds of phthalates were effectively removed from sweet orange oil by molecular distillation under the optimal conditions (evaporation temperature of 50 °C, evaporator pressure of 5 kPa and a feed flow rate of 0.75 ml/min) [85].

Preparative gas chromatography (Prep-GC)
Gas chromatography (GC) with high separation efficiency and fast separation and analysis makes it potentially the ideal preparative method for the separation of volatile compounds. The injection port, column, split device and trap device of GC equipment must be modified for preparative separation due to a lack of commercial Prep-GC [86].

Five volatile compounds, namely, curzerene (**98**) (6.6 mg), β-elemene (**100**, Fig. 12) (5.1 mg), curzerenone (**126**) (41.6 mg), curcumenol (**127**) (46.2 mg), and curcumenone (**128**) (21.2 mg) (Fig. 17), were separated from the methanol extract of Curcuma Rhizome by Prep-GC over a stainless steel column packed with 10% OV-101 (3 m × 6 mm, i.d.) after 83 single injections (20 μl) [87]. Prep-GC was also applied for the separation of natural isomers. A total of 178 mg of *cis*-asarone (**129**) and 82 mg of *trans*-asarone (**130**) were obtained from the essential oil of *Acorus tatarinowii* after 90 single injections (5 μl)

on the same column as above [88]. Prep-GC has become an important separation method for natural volatile compounds; however, a heavier sample load and the large-diameter preparative column employed decreased the efficiency [89]. Meanwhile, the disadvantages of Prep-GC, including the lack of commercial Prep-GC equipment, consumption of a large volume of carrier gas, the decomposition of thermolabile compounds under high operation temperature, the difficulties of fraction collection, and low production, still restrict the usage of Prep-GC.

Supercritical fluid chromatography (SFC)
SFC uses supercritical fluid as the mobile phase. SFC integrates the advantages of both GC and liquid chromatography (LC) as the supercritical fluids possess properties of high dissolving capability, high diffusivity and low viscosity, which allows rapid and efficient separation. Thus, SFC can use a longer column and smaller particles of the stationary phase than HPLC, which provides greater numbers of theoretical plates and better separation. SFC can be used for the separation of non-volatile or thermally labile compounds to which GC is not

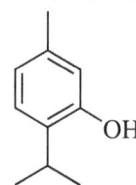
125 thymol
Fig. 16 Structure of compounds **125**

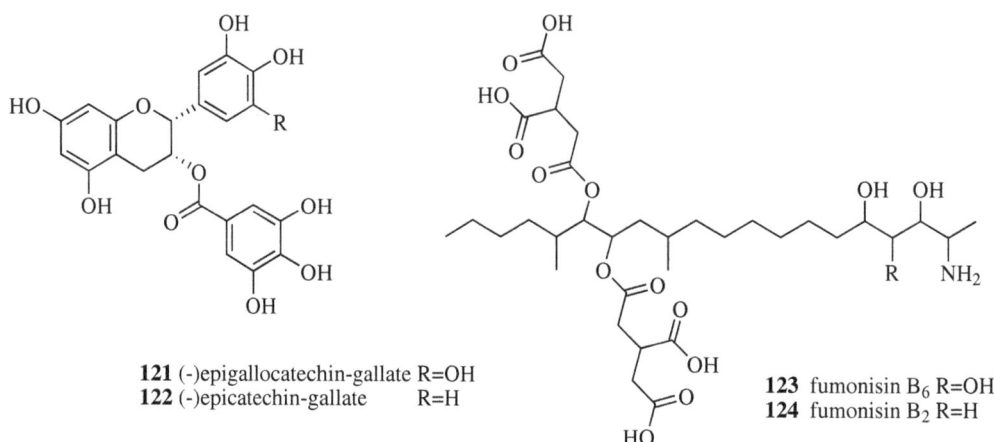
121 (-)epigallocatechin-gallate R=OH
122 (-)epicatechin-gallate R=H
123 fumonisin B₆ R=OH
124 fumonisin B₂ R=H
Fig. 15 Structures of compounds **121**–**124**

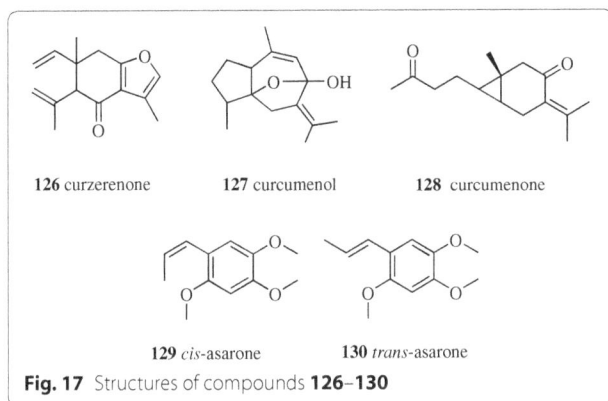

Fig. 17 Structures of compounds **126–130**

126 curzerenone   127 curcumenol   128 curcumenone

129 *cis*-asarone   130 *trans*-asarone

applicable. SFC systems are compatible with a wide range of different detectors including those used in LC and GC systems. The polarity of the widely used mobile phase, S-CO_2, in SFC is close to the polarity of hexane, with the result that SFC was used for the separation of non-polar natural products such as fatty acids, terpenes and essential oils for many years. Eluent modifiers such methanol and acetonitrile enhance the elution strength, which is increasing the interest in separating polar natural products by SFC [90–92].

Zhao et al. successfully separated three pairs of 25 *R/S* diastereomeric spirostanol saponins (**131–136**, Fig. 18) from the TCM Trigonellae Semen (the seed of *Trigonella foenum-graecum*) on two CHIRALPAK IC columns coupled in tandem [93]. Yang et al. applied SFC for the preparative separation of two pairs of 7-epimeric spiro oxindole alkaloids (**137–140**) from stems with hooks of *Uncaria macrophylla* (a herbal source for TCM Uncariae Ramulus Cum Uncis) on a Viridis Prep Silica 2-EP OBD column using acetonitrile containing 0.2% DEA modified S-CO_2. The non-aqueous mobile phase used in SFC prevented the tautomerization of the separated spiro oxindole alkaloids [94]. SFC is also applied in the separation of natural enantiomers. (*R,S*)-goitrin (**141–142**) is the active ingredient of TCM Isatidis Radix. The chiral separation of (*R*) and (*S*) goitrins was successfully achieved by prep-SFC on a Chiralpak IC column using acetonitrile as the organic modifier [95].

Molecular imprinted technology
Molecular imprinted technology has been an attractive separation method in the last decade due to its unique features, which include high selectivity, low cost and easy preparation. Many complementary cavities with the memory of size, shape, and functional groups of the template molecules are generated when the template molecules are removed from the molecular imprinted polymer (MIP). Thus, the template molecule and its analogs will

have the specific recognition and selective adsorption for the MIP. MIPs have been widely used in the separation of natural products or as solid-phase extraction sorbents for sample preparation of herbal materials to enrich the minor compounds.

Ji et al. developed multi-template molecularly imprinted polymers using DL-tyrosine and phenylpyruvic acid as the template molecules to separate dencichine (**143**, Fig. 19) from the water extract of *Panax notoginseng*. Both dencichine and the template molecule of DL-tyrosine (**144**) contain an amino (NH_2) group and a carboxylic acid (COOH) group, and the other template molecule, phenylpyruvic acid (**145**), has an α-keto acid (COCOOH) group that can also be found in the structure of dencichine [96]. Ma et al. developed a preparative separation method to separate solanesol (**146**) from tobacco leaves by flash chromatography based on MIP. The MIP was prepared with methyl methacrylate as the monomer, solanesol as the template molecule and ethylene glycol dimethacrylate as the crosslinker by a suspension polymerization method. A total of 370.8 mg of solanesol with 98.4% purity was separated from the extract of tobacco leaves with a yield of 2.5% of the dry weight of tobacco leaves [97]. You et al. used the thermo-responsive magnetic MIP to separate the three major curcuminoids, curcumin (**147**), demethoxycurcumin (**148**), and bisdemethoxycurcumin (**149**), from the TCM Curcumae Longae Rhizoma (the rhizome of *Curcuma longa*). The designed thermo-responsive magnetic MIP showed good imprinting factor for curcuminoids in a range between 2.4 and 3.1, thermo-responsiveness [lower critical solution temperature at 33.71 °C] and rapid magnetic separation (5 s) [98].

Simulated moving bed chromatography
Simulated moving bed (SMB) chromatography uses multiple columns with stationary phases (bed). The countercurrent movement of the bed is simulated through rotary valves, which periodically switch the inlet (feed and eluent) and outlet (extract and raffinate). The SMB process is a continuous separation method and a powerful tool for the large-scale separation of natural products with the advantage of lower solvent consumption over a shorter period of time.

Two cyclopeptides, cyclolinopeptides C and E (**150–151**, Fig. 20), were obtained from flaxseed oil using a three zone SMBC with eight preparative HPLC normal phase spherical silica gel columns and using absolute ethanol as the desorbent [99]. Kang et al. developed a tandem SMB process consisting of two four-zone SMB units in a series with the same adsorbent particle sizes in Ring I and Ring II to separate paclitaxel (taxol, **74**) (Fig. 11), 13-dehydroxybaccatin III (**152**), and

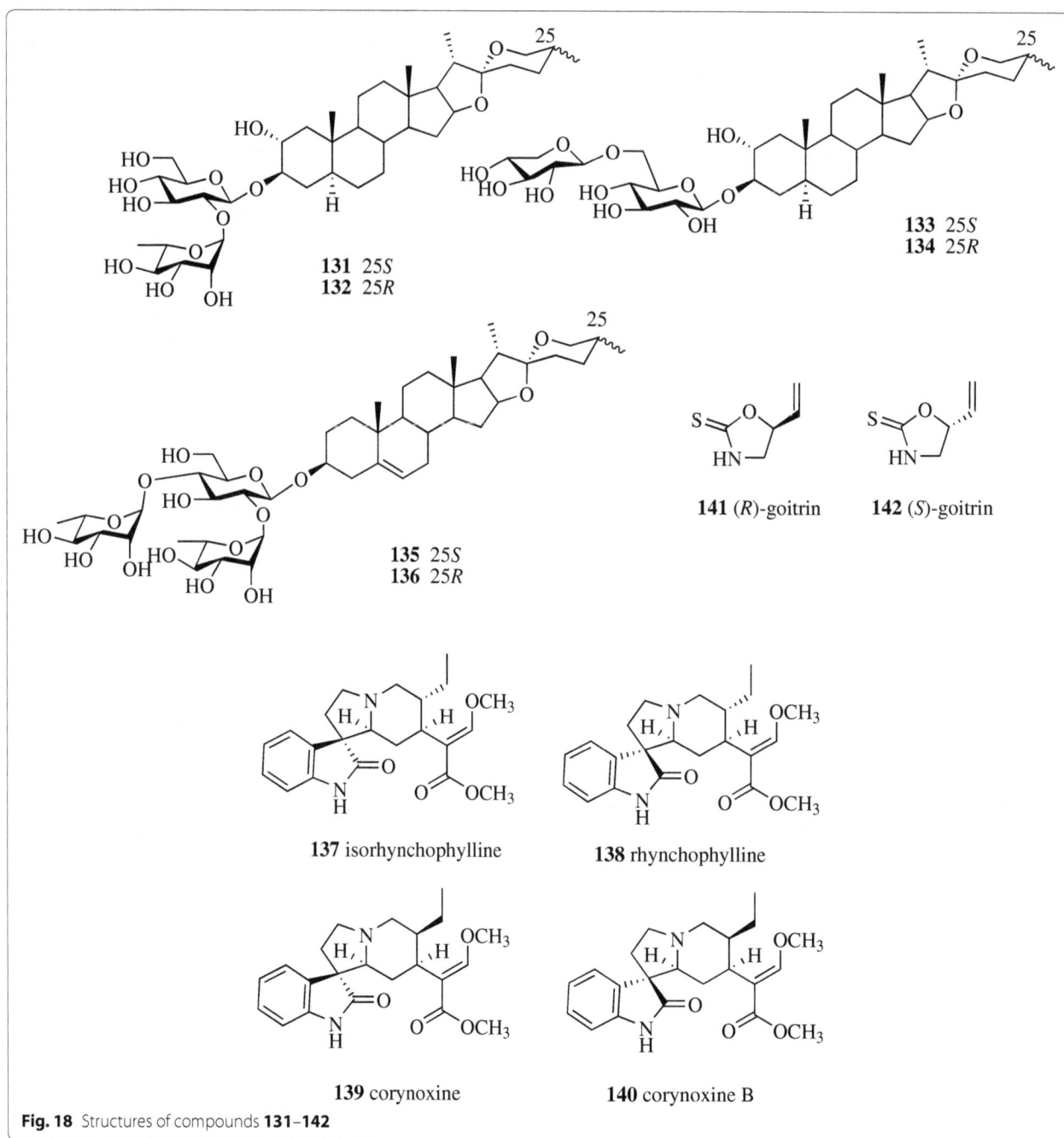

Fig. 18 Structures of compounds **131–142**

10-deacetylpaclitaxel (**153**). Paclitaxel was recovered in the first SMB unit while 13-dehydroxybaccatin III and 10-deacetylpaclitaxel were separated in the second SMB unit [100]. Mun enhanced this SMB chromatography method by using different particle sizes adsorbent in Ring I and Ring II [101]. Supercritical fluids can also be used as the desorbent in SMB chromatography. Liang et al. successfully applied supercritical carbon dioxide with ethanol as the desorbent for a three-zone SMB to

separate resveratrol (**60**) (Fig. 9) and emodin (**44**) (Fig. 4) from a crude extract of the TCM Polygoni Cuspidati Rhizoma et Radix [102].

Multi-dimensional chromatographic separation

The components in the extract subjected to separation were complex, and generally, no pure compound will be separated in one column chromatography. Multi-dimensional separation based on the solid phase extraction

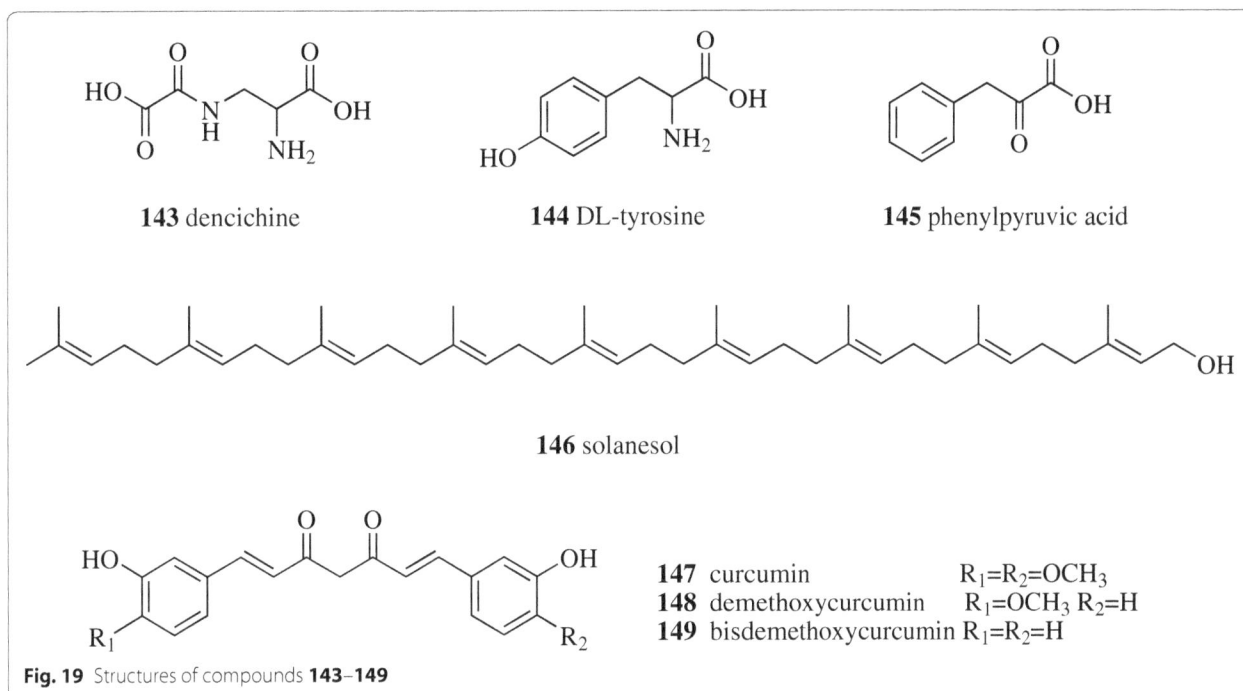

143 dencichine   **144** DL-tyrosine   **145** phenylpyruvic acid

146 solanesol

147 curcumin $R_1=R_2=OCH_3$
148 demethoxycurcumin $R_1=OCH_3$ $R_2=H$
149 bisdemethoxycurcumin $R_1=R_2=H$

Fig. 19 Structures of compounds **143–149**

and coupling of multiple columns with different stationary phases greatly improves the separation efficiency. With more commercial multiple dimensional separation equipment entering the market, the separation of natural products is becoming more rapid, efficient and automated.

Usually, the target compound was enriched by first dimensional separation and purified by last dimensional separation. Multi-dimensional separation can be achieved using the same type separation equipment (LC or GC) or different types of equipment (GC and LC). A novel volatile compound, (2E,6E)-2-methyl-6-(4-methylcyclohex-3-enylidene)hept-2-enal (**154**), was purified by a three-dimensional prep-GC from wampee essential oil [103]. Five antioxidant compounds, including two alkaloids [glusodichotomine AK (**155**) and glusodichotomine B (**156**)] and three flavonoids [tricin (**157**), homoeriodictyol (**158**) (Fig. 21), and luteolin (**3**) (Fig. 1)], were separated using a two-dimensional HPLC (RP/HILIC) method from *Arenaria kansuensis* on a RP-C18HCE and a NP-XAmide preparative columns [104]. Sciarrone et al. exploited the separation of sesquiterpenes in patchouli essential oil by three dimensional Prep-GC. Patchouli alcohol (**111**, Fig. 12) (496 µg) was separated in the first dimension on

a poly(5% diphenyl/95% dimethylsiloxane) column, and 295 µg of α-bulnesene (**159**) was from a second column coated with high molecular weight polyethylene glycol as well as 160 µg α-guaiene (**160**) from the third dimension on an ionic-liquid based column (SLB-IL60) [105]. Pantò et al. applied two three-dimensional approaches (GC–GC–GC and LC–GC–GC) to separate the sesquiterpene alcohols [(Z)-α-santalol (**161**), (Z)-α-*trans* bergamotol (**162**), (Z)-β-santalol (**163**), *epi*-(Z)-β-santalol (**164**), α-bisabolol (**165**), (Z)-lanceol (**166**), and (Z)-nuciferol (**167**)] from the sandalwood essential oil. They found that the first dimensional separation using LC reduced the sample complexity and increased the productivity of low-concentration components [106].

Summary

Natural products have contributed to drug development over the past few decades and continue to do so. The lab-intensive and time-consuming of extraction and isolation processes, however, have hindered the application of natural products in drug development. As technology continues to develop, more and more new automatic and rapid techniques have been created to extract

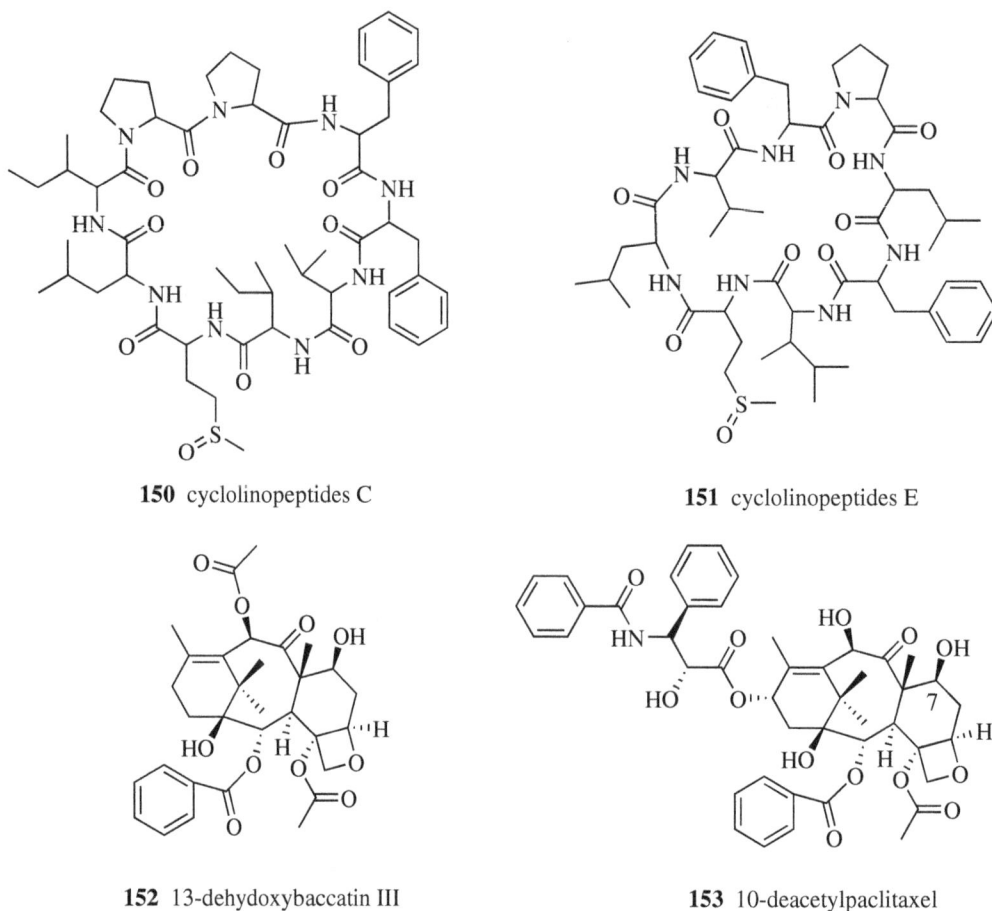

150 cyclolinopeptides C

151 cyclolinopeptides E

152 13-dehydoxybaccatin III

153 10-deacetylpaclitaxel

Fig. 20 Structures of compounds **150–153**

and separate natural products, which might reach the requirement of high-throughput screening.

Regarding extraction, reflux extraction is the most commonly employed technique for preparative separation. The modern extraction methods, also regarded as green extraction methods, including UAE, MAE, SFE and PLE, have also been the subject of increased attention in recent years due to their high extraction yields, selectivity, stability of the target extracts and process safety merits. Some of those green methods have become routine sample preparation methods for analytical purposes.

Regarding isolation, the development of novel packing material could enhance the efficiency of isolation, which

should be researched further. The hyphenation of chromatographic and spectroscopic or spectrometric techniques with the aim of elucidating structures without the need for isolation, such as LC-NMR and LC–MS, is a useful dereplication tool for searching for novel natural products. Although the isolation of pure natural products from complex mixtures remains challenging and we are far from one-step isolation procedures, the application of more selective methods from extraction to fractionation and purification will speed up the time from collecting biological material to isolating the final purified compound.

In conclusion, there is a clear and increasing interest in the extraction and isolation of natural products and their

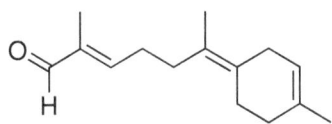

154 (2*E*,6*E*)-2-methyl-6-(4-
methylcyclohex-3-enylidene)hept-2-enal

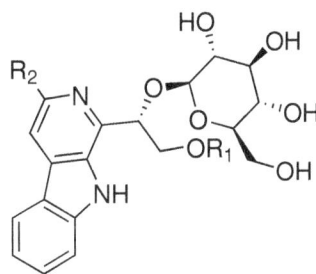

155 glusodichotomine AK R$_1$=CH$_3$ R$_2$=H
156 glusodichotomine B   R$_1$=H   R$_2$=COOH

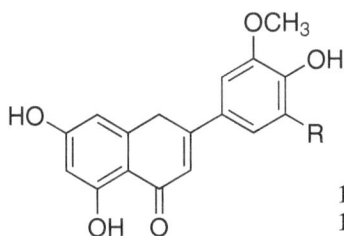

157 tricin   R=OCH$_3$
158 homoeriodictyol R=H

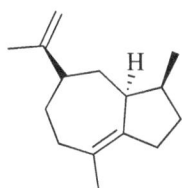

159 α-bulnesene

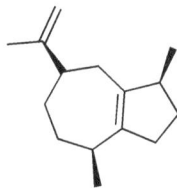

160 α-guaiene

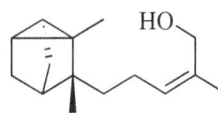

161 (Z)-α-santalol

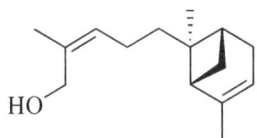

162 (Z)-α-trans bergamotol

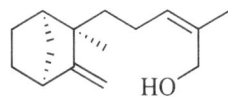

163 (Z)-β-santalol

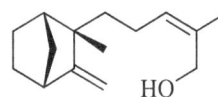

164 epi-(Z)-β-santalol

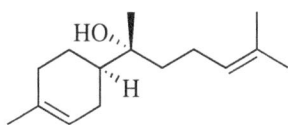

165 α-bisabolol

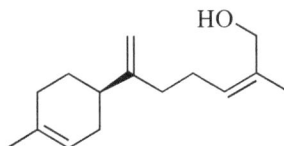

166 (Z)-lanceol

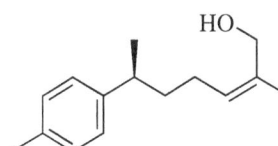

167 (Z)-nuciferol

Fig. 21 Structures of compounds **154–167**

advantageous applications. These specific applications are also conditioning the employed extraction methods and novel stationary phases and mobile phases to be used by these techniques. It is thus expected that these trends will be maintained in the near future as they are mostly motivated by emerging consumer demands and by safety, environmental and regulatory issues.

Abbreviations

CCC: counter-current chromatography; CPC: centrifugal partition chromatography; FXT: Fuzi Xiexin Tang; GC: gas chromatography; GFC: gel filtration chromatography; HD: hydro distillation; HPCCC: high performance counter-current chromatography; HPLC: high-performance liquid chromatography; HSCCC: high-speed counter-current chromatography; IEC: ion-exchange chromatography; LC: liquid chromatography; MAE: microwave assisted extraction; MD: molecular distillation; MF: membrane filtration; MIP: molecular imprinted polymer; PC: partition chromatography; PDS: 20(S)-protopanaxadiol saponins; PEF: pulsed electric field; PLE: pressurized liquid extraction; PJRS: total saponins of Panacis Japonici Rhizoma; Prep-GC: preparative gas chromatography; PTS: 20(S)-protopanaxatriol saponins; S-CO2: supercritical carbon dioxide; SD: steam distillation; SF: supercritical fluid; SFC: supercritical fluid chromatography; SFE: supercritical fluid extraction; SMB: simulated moving bed; SNIS: impregnated on silica gel; SXT: Sanhuang Xiexin Tang; TCM: traditional Chinese medicine; UAE: ultrasonic-assisted extraction.

Authors' contributions

QWZ designed the study, conducted the literature search, extracted and analyzed data, drafted the manuscript, and is the corresponding author. LGL contributed to the critical revisions of the manuscript. WCY co-designed the study and co-developed the full text of the review, and is the co-corresponding author. All authors read and approved the final manuscript.

Acknowledgements

Not applicable.

Competing interests

The authors declare that they have no competing interests.

Consent for publication

Not applicable.

Funding

This work was supported by funding from the Macau Science and Technology Development Fund (FDCT/042/2014/A1), Ministry of Science and Technology of China (No. 2013DFM30080), University of Macau (MYRG2014-00162-ICMS-QRCM and MYRG2016-00046-ICMS-QRCM).

References

1. WHO traditional medicine strategy: 2014–2023; 2013. http://www.who.int/medicines/publications/traditional/trm_strategy14_23/en/. Accessed 29 Dec 2017.
2. Newman DJ, Cragg GM. Natural products as sources of new drugs from 1981 to 2014. J Nat Prod. 2016;79(3):629–61.
3. Newman DJ, Cragg GM. Natural products as sources of new drugs over the 30 years from 1981 to 2010. J Nat Prod. 2012;75(3):311–35.
4. Atanasov AG, Waltenberger B, Pferschy-Wenzig EM, Linder T, Wawrosch C, Uhrin P, Temml V, Wang L, Schwaiger S, Heiss EH, et al. Discovery and resupply of pharmacologically active plant-derived natural products: a review. Biotechnol Adv. 2015;33(8):1582–614.
5. Cragg GM, Newman DJ. Natural products: a continuing source of novel drug leads. Biochim Biophys Acta Gen Subj. 2013;1830(6):3670–95.
6. Li P, Xu G, Li SP, Wang YT, Fan TP, Zhao QS, Zhang QW. Optimizing ultra performance liquid chromatographic analysis of 10 diterpenoid compounds in Salvia miltiorrhiza using central composite design. J Agric Food Chem. 2008;56(4):1164–71.
7. Li P, Yin ZQ, Li SL, Huang XJ, Ye WC, Zhang QW. Simultaneous determination of eight flavonoids and pogostone in Pogostemon cablin by high performance liquid chromatography. J Liq Chromatogr Relat Technol. 2014;37(12):1771–84.
8. Yi Y, Zhang QW, Li SL, Wang Y, Ye WC, Zhao J, Wang YT. Simultaneous quantification of major flavonoids in "Bawanghua", the edible flower of Hylocereus undatus using pressurised liquid extraction and high performance liquid chromatography. Food Chem. 2012;135(2):528–33.
9. Zhou YQ, Zhang QW, Li SL, Yin ZQ, Zhang XQ, Ye WC. Quality evaluation of semen oroxyli through simultaneous quantification of 13 components by high performance liquid chromatography. Curr Pharm Anal. 2012;8(2):206–13.
10. Du G, Zhao HY, Song YL, Zhang QW, Wang YT. Rapid simultaneous determination of isoflavones in Radix puerariae using high-performance liquid chromatography-triple quadrupole mass spectrometry with novel shell-type column. J Sep Sci. 2011;34(19):2576–85.
11. Ćujić N, Šavikin K, Janković T, Pljevljakušić D, Zdunić G, Ibrić S. Optimization of polyphenols extraction from dried chokeberry using maceration as traditional technique. Food Chem. 2016;194:135–42.
12. Albuquerque BR, Prieto MA, Barreiro MF, Rodrigues A, Curran TP, Barros L, Ferreira ICFR. Catechin-based extract optimization obtained from Arbutus unedo L. fruits using maceration/microwave/ultrasound extraction techniques. Ind Crops Prod. 2017;95:404–15.
13. Jovanović AA, Đorđević VB, Zdunić GM, Pljevljakušić DS, Šavikin KP, Godevac DM, Bugarski BM. Optimization of the extraction process of polyphenols from Thymus serpyllum L. herb using maceration, heat- and ultrasound-assisted techniques. Sep Purif Technol. 2017;179:369–80.
14. Jin S, Yang M, Kong Y, Yao X, Wei Z, Zu Y, Fu Y. Microwave-assisted extraction of flavonoids from Cajanus cajan leaves. Zhongcaoyao. 2011;42(11):2235–9.
15. Zhang H, Wang W, Fu ZM, Han CC, Song Y. Study on comparison of extracting fucoxanthin from Undaria pinnatifida with percolation extraction and refluxing methods. Zhongguo Shipin Tianjiaji. 2014;9:91–5.
16. Fu M, Zhang L, Han J, Li J. Optimization of the technology of ethanol extraction for Goupi patch by orthogonal design test. Zhongguo Yaoshi (Wuhan, China). 2008;11(1):75–6.
17. Gao X, Han J, Dai H, Xiang L. Study on optimizing the technological condition of ethanol percolating extraction for Goupi patch. Zhongguo Yaoshi. 2009;12(10):1395–7.
18. Li SL, Lai SF, Song JZ, Qiao CF, Liu X, Zhou Y, Cai H, Cai BC, Xu HX. Decocting-induced chemical transformations and global quality of Du–Shen–Tang, the decoction of ginseng evaluated by UPLC-Q-TOF-MS/MS based chemical profiling approach. J Pharm Biomed Anal. 2010;53(4):946–57.
19. Zhang WL, Chen JP, Lam KYC, Zhan JYX, Yao P, Dong TTX, Tsim KWK. Hydrolysis of glycosidic flavonoids during the preparation of Danggui

Buxue Tang: an outcome of moderate boiling of chinese herbal mixture. Evid Based Complement Altern Med. 2014;2014:608721.

20. Zhang Q, Wang CH, Ma YM, Zhu EY, Wang ZT. UPLC-ESI/MS determination of 17 active constituents in 2 categorized formulas of traditional Chinese medicine, Sanhuang Xiexin Tang and Fuzi Xiexin Tang: application in comparing the differences in decoctions and macerations. Biomed Chromatogr. 2013;27(8):1079–88.

21. Kongkiatpaiboon S, Gritsanapan W. Optimized extraction for high yield of insecticidal didehydrostemofoline alkaloid in *Stemona collinsiae* root extracts. Ind Crops Prod. 2013;41:371–4.

22. Zhang L. Comparison of extraction effect of active ingredients in traditional Chinese medicine compound preparation with two different method. Heilongjiang Xumu Shouyi. 2013;9:132–3.

23. Wei Q, Yang GW, Wang XJ, Hu XX, Chen L. The study on optimization of Soxhlet extraction process for ursolic acid from Cynomorium. Shipin Yanjiu Yu Kaifa. 2013;34(7):85–8.

24. Chin FS, Chong KP, Markus A, Wong NK. Tea polyphenols and alkaloids content using soxhlet and direct extraction methods. World J Agric Sci. 2013;9(3):266–70.

25. Lv GP, Huang WH, Yang FQ, Li J, Li SP. Pressurized liquid extraction and GC–MS analysis for simultaneous determination of seven components in Cinnamomum cassia and the effect of sample preparation. J Sep Sci. 2010;33(15):2341–8.

26. Xu J, Zhao WM, Qian ZM, Guan J, Li SP. Fast determination of five components of coumarin, alkaloids and bibenzyls in Dendrobium spp. using pressurized liquid extraction and ultra-performance liquid chromatography. J Sep Sci. 2010;33(11):1580–6.

27. Xu FX, Yuan C, Wan JB, Yan R, Hu H, Li SP, Zhang QW. A novel strategy for rapid quantification of 20(S)-protopanaxatriol and 20(S)-protopanaxadiol saponins in *Panax notoginseng*, *P. ginseng* and *P. quinquefolium*. Nat Prod Res. 2015;29(1):46–52.

28. Vergara-Salinas JR, Bulnes P, Zuniga MC, Perez-Jimenez J, Torres JL, Mateos-Martin ML, Agosin E, Perez-Correa JR. Effect of pressurized hot water extraction on antioxidants from grape pomace before and after enological fermentation. J Agric Food Chem. 2013;61(28):6929–36.

29. Gizir AM, Turker N, Artuvan E. Pressurized acidified water extraction of black carrot [*Daucus carota* ssp. sativus var. atrorubens Alef.] anthocyanins. Eur Food Res Technol. 2008;226(3):363–70.

30. Conde-Hernández LA, Espinosa-Victoria JR, Trejo A, Guerrero-Beltrán JÁ. CO2-supercritical extraction, hydrodistillation and steam distillation of essential oil of rosemary (Rosmarinus officinalis). J Food Eng. 2017;200:81–6.

31. Falcão MA, Scopel R, Almeida RN, do Espirito Santo AT, Franceschini G, Garcez JJ, Vargas RMF, Cassel E. Supercritical fluid extraction of vinblastine from *Catharanthus roseus*. J Supercrit Fluids. 2017;129:9–15.

32. Barba FJ, Zhu Z, Koubaa M, Sant'Ana AS, Orlien V. Green alternative methods for the extraction of antioxidant bioactive compounds from winery wastes and by-products: a review. Trends Food Sci Technol. 2016;49:96–109.

33. Chemat F, Rombaut N, Sicaire AG, Meullemiestre A, Fabiano-Tixier AS, Abert-Vian M. Ultrasound assisted extraction of food and natural products. Mechanisms, techniques, combinations, protocols and applications. A review. Ultrason Sonochem. 2017;34:540–60.

34. Wu QS, Wang CM, Lu JJ, Lin LG, Chen P, Zhang QW. Simultaneous determination of six saponins in Panacis Japonici Rhizoma using quantitative analysis of multi-components with single-marker method. Curr Pharm Anal. 2017;13(3):289–95.

35. Zt Guo, Xq Luo, Jp Liang, Yang Z, Ai X. Comparative study on extraction of febrifugine from traditional Chinese medicine Dichroa febrifuga by reflux method and ultrasonic method. Shizhen Guoyi Guoyao. 2015;26(6):1532–3.

36. Chemat F, Cravotto G. Microwave-assisted extraction for bioactive compounds. Boston: Springer; 2013.

37. Vinatoru M, Mason TJ, Calinescu I. Ultrasonically assisted extraction (UAE) and microwave assisted extraction (MAE) of functional compounds from plant materials. TrAC Trends Anal Chem. 2017;97:159–78.

38. Chen H. Optimization of microwave-assisted extraction of resveratrol from *Polygonum cuspidatum* sieb et Zucc by orthogonal experiment. Nat Prod Indian J. 2013;9(4):138–42.

39. Benmoussa H, Farhat A, Romdhane M, Bouajila J. Enhanced solvent-free microwave extraction of *Foeniculum vulgare* Mill. essential oil seeds

using double walled reactor. Arabian J Chem 2016. (in press https://doi.org/10.1016/j.arabjc.2016.02.010).

40. Xiong W, Chen X, Lv G, Hu D, Zhao J, Li S. Optimization of microwave-assisted extraction of bioactive alkaloids from lotus plumule using response surface methodology. J Pharm Anal. 2016;6(6):382–8.

41. Hou J, He S, Ling M, Li W, Dong R, Pan Y, Zheng Y. A method of extracting ginsenosides from Panax ginseng by pulsed electric field. J Sep Sci. 2010;33(17–18):2707–13.

42. Bouras M, Grimi N, Bals O, Vorobiev E. Impact of pulsed electric fields on polyphenols extraction from Norway spruce bark. Ind Crops Prod. 2016;80:50–8.

43. Chen H, Zhou X, Zhang J. Optimization of enzyme assisted extraction of polysaccharides from *Astragalus membranaceus*. Carbohydr Polym. 2014;111:567–75.

44. Liu T, Sui X, Li L, Zhang J, Liang X, Li W, Zhang H, Fu S. Application of ionic liquids based enzyme-assisted extraction of chlorogenic acid from *Eucommia ulmoides* leaves. Anal Chim Acta. 2016;903:91–9.

45. Strati IF, Gogou E, Oreopoulou V. Enzyme and high pressure assisted extraction of carotenoids from tomato waste. Food Bioprod Process. 2015;94:668–74.

46. Verma SK, Goswami P, Verma RS, Padalia RC, Chauhan A, Singh VR, Darokar MP. Chemical composition and antimicrobial activity of bergamot-mint (*Mentha citrata* Ehrh.) essential oils isolated from the herbage and aqueous distillate using different methods. Ind Crops Prod. 2016;91:152–60.

47. Yahya A, Yunus RM. Influence of sample preparation and extraction time on chemical composition of steam distillation derived patchouli oil. Proc Eng. 2013;53:1–6.

48. Lim KH, Kam TS. Methyl chanofruticosinate alkaloids from *Kopsia arborea*. Phytochemistry. 2008;69(2):558–61.

49. Zhang Z, Su Z. Recovery of taxol from the extract of *Taxus cuspidata* callus cultures with Al2O3 chromatography. J Liq Chromatogr Relat Technol. 2000;23(17):2683–93.

50. Zhang Z, Su Z. Catalysis mechanism to increase taxol from the extract of *Taxus cuspidate* callus cultures with alumina chromatography. Sep Sci Technol. 2002;37(3):733–43.

51. Gao M, Wang XL, Gu M, Su ZG, Wang Y, Janson JC. Separation of polyphenols using porous polyamide resin and assessment of mechanism of retention. J Sep Sci. 2011;34(15):1853–8.

52. Xs Li, Bq Jiang, Jl Mao. Study on extraction separation and pharmacodynamics of effective components in Kuqingcha. Guangxi Yixue. 2013;35(5):637–8.

53. Yang X, Wang J, Luo J, Kong L. One-step large-scale preparative isolation of isoquinoline alkaloids from rhizoma coptidis chinensis by polyamide column chromatography and their quantitative structure-retention relationship analysis. J Liq Chromatogr Relat Technol. 2012;35(13):1842–52.

54. Li J, Chase HA. Development of adsorptive (non-ionic) macroporous resins and their uses in the purification of pharmacologically-active natural products from plant sources. Nat Prod Rep. 2010;27(10):1493–510.

55. Wan JB, Zhang QW, Ye WC, Wang YT. Quantification and separation of protopanaxatriol and protopanaxadiol type saponins from *Panax notoginseng* with macroporous resins. Sep Purif Technol. 2008;60(2):198–205.

56. Meng FC, Wu QS, Wang R, Li SP, Lin LG, Zhang QW, Chen P. A novel strategy for quantitative analysis of major ginsenosides in Panacis Japonici Rhizoma with a standardized reference fraction. Molecules. 2017;22(12):2067.

57. Wang X, Zhao C, Peng X, Tang K. Adsorption mechanism of methoxy modified macroporous crosslinked resin for phenol. Huaxue Xuebao. 2010;68(5):453–6.

58. Liu W, Zhang S, Zu YG, Fu YJ, Ma W, Zhang DY, Kong Y, Li XJ. Preliminary enrichment and separation of genistein and apigenin from extracts of pigeon pea roots by macroporous resins. Bioresour Technol. 2010;101(12):4667–75.

59. Mander LN, Williams CM. Chromatography with silver nitrate: part 2. Tetrahedron. 2016;72(9):1133–50.

60. Yan Y, Wang X, Liu Y, Xiang J, Wang X, Zhang H, Yao Y, Liu R, Zou X, Huang J, et al. Combined urea-thin layer chromatography and silver nitrate-thin layer chromatography for micro separation and

determination of hard-to-detect branched chain fatty acids in natural lipids. J Chromatogr A. 2015;1425:293–301.

61. Zhang Wm, Zhai Yc, Yang Hj, Zhang Rg, Hao J, Han Jq, Zhang Yl. Silver nitrate-silica gel column chromatography purification linolenic acid in walnut oil. Shipin Gongye Keji. 2015;36(10):229–32.

62. Wang Y, Du Al, Du Aq. Isolation of zingiberene from ginger oleoresin by silver ion coordination column chromatography. Jingxi Huagong. 2012;29(7):672–7.

63. Lemos LMS, Oliveira RB, Sampaio BL, Ccana-Ccapatinta GV, Da Costa FB, Martins DTO. Brasiliensic and isobrasiliensic acids: isolation from Calophyllum brasiliense Cambess. and anti-Helicobacter pylori activity. Nat Prod Res. 2016;30(23):2720–5.

64. Li J, Gao R, Zhao D, Huang X, Chen Y, Gan F, Liu H, Yang G. Separation and preparation of xanthochymol and guttiferone E by high performance liquid chromatography and high speed counter-current chromatography combined with silver nitrate coordination reaction. J Chromatogr A. 2017;1511:143–8.

65. Wan JB, Li P, Yang RL, Zhang QW, Wang YT. Separation and purification of 5 saponins from Panax notoginseng by preparative high-performance liquid chromatography. J Liq Chromatogr Relat Technol. 2013;36(3):406–17.

66. Cai J, Cheng L, Zhao J, Fu Q, Jin Y, Ke Y, Liang X. A novel polyacrylamide-based silica stationary phase for the separation of carbohydrates using alcohols as the weak eluent in hydrophilic interaction liquid chromatography. J Chromatogr A. 2017;1524:153–9.

67. Guzlek H, Wood PL, Janaway L. Performance comparison using the GUESS mixture to evaluate counter-current chromatography instruments. J Chromatogr A. 2009;1216(19):4181–6.

68. Tang Q, Wang Y, Chen M, Zhang Q, Fan C, Huang X, Li Y, Ye W. Application of high-speed counter-current chromatography preparative separation of flavone C-glycosides from Lophatherum gracile. Sep Sci Technol. 2013;48(12):1906–12.

69. Dang YY, Li XC, Zhang QW, Li SP, Wang YT. Preparative isolation and purification of six volatile compounds from essential oil of Curcuma wenyujin using high-performance centrifugal partition chromatography. J Sep Sci. 2010;33(11):1658–64.

70. Zhou YQ, Wang CM, Wang RB, Lin LG, Yin ZQ, Hu H, Yang Q, Zhang QW. Preparative separation of four sesquiterpenoids from Curcuma longa by high-speed counter-current chromatography. Sep Sci Technol. 2017;52(3):497–503.

71. Skalicka-Wozniak K, Walasek M, Ludwiczuk A, Glowniak K. Isolation of terpenoids from Pimpinella anisum essential oil by high-performance counter-current chromatography. J Sep Sci. 2013;36(16):2611–4.

72. Li XC, Zhang QW, Yin ZQ, Zhang XQ, Ye WC. Preparative separation of patchouli alcohol from patchouli oil using high performance centrifugal partition chromatography. J Essent Oil Res. 2011;23(6):19–24.

73. Negrão Murakami AN, de Mello Castanho Amboni RD, Prudêncio ES, Amante ER, de Moraes Zanotta L, Maraschin M, Cunha Petrus JC, Teófilo RF. Concentration of phenolic compounds in aqueous mate (Ilex paraguariensis A. St. Hil) extract through nanofiltration. LWT Food Sci Technol. 2011;44(10):2211–6.

74. Khemakhem I, Gargouri OD, Dhouib A, Ayadi MA, Bouaziz M. Oleuropein rich extract from olive leaves by combining microfiltration, ultrafiltration and nanofiltration. Sep Purif Technol. 2017;172:310–7.

75. Sila A, Bougatef A. Antioxidant peptides from marine by-products: Isolation, identification and application in food systems. A review. J Funct Foods. 2016;21:10–26.

76. Shi L. Bioactivities, isolation and purification methods of polysaccharides from natural products: a review. Int J Biol Macromol. 2016;92:37–48.

77. Schendel RR, Becker A, Tyl CE, Bunzel M. Isolation and characterization of feruloylated arabinoxylan oligosaccharides from the perennial cereal grain intermediate wheat grass (Thinopyrum intermedium). Carbohydr Res. 2015;407:16–25.

78. Pettit GR, Tang YP, Zhang Q, Bourne GT, Arm CA, Leet JE, Knight JC, Pettit RK, Chapuis JC, Doubek DL, et al. Isolation and structures of axistatins 1–3 from the republic of palau marine sponge Agelas axifera hentschel. J Nat Prod. 2013;76(3):420–4.

79. Li J, Cheong K, Zhao J, Hu D, Chen X, Qiao C, Zhang Q, Chen Y, Li S. Preparation of inulin-type fructooligosaccharides using fast protein liquid

80. Tan T, Su ZG, Gu M, Xu J, Janson JC. Cross-linked agarose for separation of low molecular weight natural products in hydrophilic interaction liquid chromatography. Biotechnol J. 2010;5(5):505–10.

81. Comeskey DJ, Montefiori M, Edwards PJB, McGhie TK. Isolation and structural identification of the anthocyanin components of red kiwi-fruit. J Agric Food Chem. 2009;57(5):2035–9.

82. Feng L, Zhao F. Separation of polyphenols in tea on weakly acidic cation-exchange gels. Chromatographia. 2010;71(9):775–82.

83. Månsson M, Klejnstrup ML, Phipps RK, Nielsen KF, Frisvad JC, Gotfredsen CH, Larsen TO. Isolation and NMR characterization of fumonisin B2 and a New fumonisin B6 from Aspergillus niger. J Agric Food Chem. 2010;58(2):949–53.

84. Borgarello AV, Mezza GN, Pramparo MC, Gayol MF. Thymol enrichment from oregano essential oil by molecular distillation. Sep Purif Technol. 2015;153:60–6.

85. Xiong Y, Zhao Z, Zhu L, Chen Y, Ji H, Yang D. Removal of three kinds of phthalates from sweet orange oil by molecular distillation. LWT Food Sci Technol. 2013;53(2):487–91.

86. Wang H, Yang F, Xia Z. Progress in modification of preparative gas chromatography and its applications. Huaxue Tongbao. 2011;74(1):3–9.

87. Yang FQ, Wang HK, Chen H, Chen JD, Xia ZN. Fractionation of volatile constituents from Curcuma rhizome by preparative gas chromatography. J Autom Methods Manage Chem. 2011;2011:6. https://doi.org/10.1155/2011/942467:942467.

88. Zuo HL, Yang FQ, Zhang XM, Xia ZN. Separation of cis- and trans-asarone from Acorus tatarinowii by preparative gas chromatography. J Anal Methods Chem. 2012;2012:5. https://doi.org/10.1155/2012/402081.

89. Ozek T, Demirci F. Isolation of natural products by preparative gas chromatography. Methods Mol Biol. 2012;864:275–300.

90. Speybrouck D, Lipka E. Preparative supercritical fluid chromatography: a powerful tool for chiral separations. J Chromatogr A. 2016;1467:33–55.

91. Hartmann A, Ganzera M. Supercritical fluid chromatography—theoretical background and applications on natural products. Planta Med. 2015;81(17):1570–81.

92. Gibitz Eisath N, Sturm S, Stuppner H. Supercritical fluid chromatography in natural product analysis—an update. Planta Med. 2017; In press.

93. Zhao Y, McCauley J, Pang X, Kang L, Yu H, Zhang J, Xiong C, Chen R, Ma B. Analytical and semipreparative separation of 25 (R/S)-spirostanol saponin diastereomers using supercritical fluid chromatography. J Sep Sci. 2013;36(19):3270–6.

94. Yang W, Zhang Y, Pan H, Yao C, Hou J, Yao S, Cai L, Feng R, Wu W, Guo D. Supercritical fluid chromatography for separation and preparation of tautomeric 7-epimeric spiro oxindole alkaloids from Uncaria macrophylla. J Pharm Biomed Anal. 2017;134:352–60.

95. Nie L, Dai Z, Ma S. Improved chiral separation of (R, S)-goitrin by SFC: an application in traditional Chinese medicine. J Anal Methods Chem. 2016;2016:5. https://doi.org/10.1155/2016/5782942.

96. Ji W, Xie H, Zhou J, Wang X, Ma X, Huang L. Water-compatible molecularly imprinted polymers for selective solid phase extraction of dencichine from the aqueous extract of Panax notoginseng. J Chromatogr B. 2016;1008:225–33.

97. Ma X, Meng Z, Qiu L, Chen J, Guo Y, Yi D, Ji T, Jia H, Xue M. Solanesol extraction from tobacco leaves by Flash chromatography based on molecularly imprinted polymers. J Chromatogr B. 2016;1020:1–5.

98. You Q, Zhang Y, Zhang Q, Guo J, Huang W, Shi S, Chen X. High-capacity thermo-responsive magnetic molecularly imprinted polymers for selective extraction of curcuminoids. J Chromatogr A. 2014;1354:1–8.

99. Okinyo-Owiti DP, Burnett PGG, Reaney MJT. Simulated moving bed purification of flaxseed oil orbitides: unprecedented separation of cyclolinopeptides C and E. J Chromatogr B. 2014;965:231–7.

100. Kang SH, Kim JH, Mun S. Optimal design of a tandem simulated moving bed process for separation of paclitaxel, 13-dehydroxybaccatin III, and 10-deacetylpaclitaxel. Process Biochem. 2010;45(9):1468–76.

101. Mun S. Enhanced performance of a tandem simulated moving bed process for separation of paclitaxel, 13-dehydroxybaccatin III, and 10-deacetylpaclitaxel by making a difference between the adsorbent particle sizes of the two subordinate simulated moving bed units. Process Biochem. 2011;46(6):1329–34.

102. Liang MT, Liang RC, Yu SQ, Yan RA. Separation of resveratrol and emodin by supercritical fluid-simulated moving bed chromatography. J Chromatogr Sep Tech. 2013;4(3):1000175.

103. Sciarrone D, Panto S, Rotondo A, Tedone L, Tranchida PQ, Dugo P, Mondello L. Rapid collection and identification of a novel component from *Clausena lansium* Skeels leaves by means of three-dimensional preparative gas chromatography and nuclear magnetic resonance/infrared/mass spectrometric analysis. Anal Chim Acta. 2013;785:119–25.

104. Cui Y, Shen N, Yuan X, Dang J, Shao Y, Mei L, Tao Y, Wang Q, Liu Z. Two-dimensional chromatography based on on-line HPLC-DPPH bioactivity-guided assay for the preparative isolation of analogue antioxidant compound from *Arenaria kansuensis*. J Chromatogr B. 2017;1046:81–6.

105. Sciarrone D, Panto S, Donato P, Mondello L. Improving the productivity of a multidimensional chromatographic preparative system by collecting pure chemicals after each of three chromatographic dimensions. J Chromatogr A. 2016;1475:80–5.

106. Panto S, Sciarrone D, Maimone M, Ragonese C, Giofre S, Donato P, Farnetti S, Mondello L. Performance evaluation of a versatile multidimensional chromatographic preparative system based on three-dimensional gas chromatography and liquid chromatography-two-dimensional gas chromatography for the collection of volatile constituents. J Chromatogr A. 2015;1417:96–103.

Anti-tumor effects of the American cockroach, *Periplaneta americana*

Yanan Zhao, Ailin Yang, Pengfei Tu* and Zhongdong Hu*

Abstract

Since the incidence of cancer has been on the rise due to increasing exposure to various carcinogenic factors in recent years, cancer has gradually become the first killer to the health of human beings. A growing attention has been paid to anti-cancer effects of traditional Chinese medicine (TCM) with low toxicity and good efficacy. As a kind of TCM, *Periplaneta americana* (*P. americana*) has a good effect on clinical application, and its anti-tumor effects has been increasingly well studied. In this review, the research progress on the anti-tumor effects of *P. americana* was summarized. The main mechanisms of its anti-tumor effects include suppression of tumor cell growth, induction of cell cycle arrest and tumor cell apoptosis, inhibition of angiogenesis, enhancement of immunity, and reversal of tumor drug resistance. This review aims to provide an overview of the research on anti-tumor effects of *P. americana* and aids in its further application as an anti-tumor drug.

Keywords: *Periplaneta americana*, Anti-tumor, Apoptosis, Angiogenesis, Immunity

Background

As one of the leading causes of death in the world, cancer has been the focus of extensive research [1]. According to GLOBOCAN 2012, about 14.1 million new cancer cases and 8.2 million deaths occurred in 2012 worldwide [2]. Meanwhile, there were approximately 3.4 million cancer patients in China in 2012, and the number of cancer deaths was about 2.46 million [3]. Cancer can seriously threaten the patients' quality of life and their survival. Surgery, radiotherapy, and chemotherapy are widely used for the treatment of cancer in the world. However, these methods cannot effectively change the causal interaction of individual factors related to the pathological process. Therefore, it is difficult to completely inhibit tumor recurrence and metastasis. Long-term treatment with these methods may facilitate drug resistance and cause serious side effects in patients [4]. Traditional Chinese medicine (TCM) has a well-established history of high efficiency and low toxicity [5–8]. Tumor treatment with TCM is carried out through the overall regulation of the body [9]. In recent years, cancer therapy using TCM with characteristics of multi-level, multi-link, and multi-target has garnered increasing attention [10–13].

Periplaneta americana, more commonly known as the American cockroach, is the part of Insecta class, Dictyoptera order, and Blattidae family. It is one of the largest, strongest, oldest, and most successful breeding insect groups [14]. The dried worms or fresh adults of *P. americana* are often used as a TCM drug [15]. Its taste is salty and acrid, and its nature is cold. These features can promote blood circulation, remove blood stasis, help digestion, aid in detoxification, and induce diuresis for treating edema. *P. americana* can also be used to treat infantile malnutrition, tonsillitis, body phlegm, carbuncles, sore throat, and insect bites. Modern pharmacological research has revealed that *P. americana* has anti-tumor effects, and is able to enhance immunity, promote tissue repair, stabilize blood pressure, improve microcirculation, protect the liver, and act as an anti-inflammatory, anti-bacterial, and anti-viral agent as well as an analgesic and antioxidant [15, 16].

Clinical application of *P. americana*

Active ingredients isolated from *P. americana* have been developed into clinical drugs in China [17], such as

*Correspondence: pengfeitu@163.com; zdhu@bucm.edu.cn
Modern Research Center for Traditional Chinese Medicine, School of Chinese Materia Medica, Beijing University of Chinese Medicine, No.11 North Third Ring Road, Chaoyang District, Beijing 100029, China

"Xiaozheng Yigan Tablet", "Kangfuxin Liquid", "Ganlong Capsule", and "Xinmailong Injection". "Xiaozheng Yigan Tablet" is an oral tablet with potent anti-tumor effects and anti-bacterial activity. It has been reported to reduce liver inflammation, promote the recovery of liver function, and reduce the degree of liver fibrosis in patients with hepatitis B virus (HBV) infection [18]. Moreover, it has been revealed in a study with 66 cases of primary liver cancer treated with "Xiaozheng Yigan Tablet" that the level of alpha-fetoprotein was reduced and survival time of patients was prolonged [19]. "Kangfuxin Liquid" has been used in clinic for more than 20 years. The main functions of "Kangfuxin Liquid" include eliminating inflammation, reducing swelling, promoting cell proliferation and growth of new granulation tissue, and promoting organism recover. It is mainly applied for stomach and duodenal ulcer, pressure sores, wounds, and burns. Though the curative effect of "Kangfuxin Liquid" is good, its obvious side effects have not been found [20]. "Ganlong Capsule" has a good anti-hepatitis B virus effect and is characteristic of low price, convenient administration, and little side effect [21]. "Xinmailong Injection" has a wide range of therapeutic effects on the cardiovascular system, including improving microcirculation, expanding pulmonary vessels, diuresis, anti-arrhythmic, inhibiting free radical damage, and anti-atherosclerosis. Clinical trials have demonstrated that "Xinmailong Injection" has good therapeutic effect in congestive heart failure and chronic pulmonary heart disease, and the total effective rate is more than 80%. In addition, no obvious untoward reaction was found during treatment [22]. The clinical application of these drugs continue to increase due to limited adverse reactions [16]. Especially, the effect of P. americana on anti-tumor and immune regulation has attracted widespread attention and increasingly become the research focus [23].

Chemical constituents of P. americana

Numerous studies have shown that the main chemical constituents of P. americana include pheromones, proteins, fatty acids and esters, amino acids, alkaloids, alkanes, polysaccharides, isoflavones, cockroach oil, and peptides [16, 24–31]. It was reported that the 50 components of P. americana were separated and identified, most of which were unsaturated fatty acids and esters [26]. Ten cyclic peptides were isolated and purified from P. americana, eight of which were isolated for the first time [27]. Another study identified 23 compounds in P. americana including 16-hydro-7-hexadecenoic acid lactone (35.98%), fatty acids and esters (26.62%), aliphatic aldehyde, stigmast-4-ene-3-one, alkanes, palmitic acid, and linoleic acid [28]. 19 compounds were also separated and identified from P. americana, which mainly included alkanes, octadecadienoic acid, and octadecadienoic

alcohol [29]. P. americana contains more than 16 amino acids, including 7 human essential amino acids and two human semi-essential amino acids [30]. The 70% ethanol extract of P. americana contains amino acid, alkaloid, fatty acids and esters, and pheromones [25]. More than 50 neuropeptides have been identified from P. americana, including allatostatins, pyrokinins, fraps, kinins, and periviscerokinins [31]. In addition, P. americana also contains polysaccharides, cockroach acid, cockroach oil, allergens, chitosan, cytochromes A, B, and C [16, 27].

Pharmacological activity of P. americana

A large number of studies have shown that P. americana has anti-tumor, anti-bacterial, anti-viral, anti-radiation, detumescence, analgesic, and anti-inflammatory effects. In addition, P. americana was shown to protect the liver, promote blood vessel growth, aid in tissue repair, improve microcirculation, and enhance immunity. P. americana also possesses a high antioxidant capacity demonstrated by the clearance of 2,2-diphenylpicrylhydrazyl and OH free radicals [15, 32]. In recent years, the anti-tumor activity of P. americana has become a research focus.

Anti-tumor effects of P. americana

Accumulating evidences have revealed the anti-tumor effects of P. americana on a variety of cancer cells. Herein, we summarized the reported the mechanisms underlying the anti-tumor effects of P. americana.

Inhibition of tumor cell growth

Studies have shown that some TCM drugs can inhibit the growth of tumor cells in vitro and in vivo [12, 33, 34]. These drugs can be used at various stages of tumorigenesis. Mechanistically, these treatments can inhibit the synthesis of DNA, RNA, and proteins, and block the energy metabolism of tumor cells [35]. A previous study has showed that CII-3 from the P. americana caused cytotoxicity in two human lung cancer cell lines [36]. Moreover, P. americana extract inhibited the growth of three human reproductive system cancer cell lines and three human respiratory system tumor cell lines [37, 38]. In addition, P. americana extract suppressed the growth of three human and mouse leukemia cell lines [39]. The 60% ethanol fraction of P. americana organic extracts (PAE60) inhibited tumor growth in S180 tumor-bearing mice by 72.62%. Moreover, PAE60 was determined against 12 human cancer cell lines, and it could effectively inhibited the growth of HL-60, KB, CNE, and BGC823 cells with IC_{50} values <20 μg/mL [23].

Cell cycle arrest

Cell cycle is a complex process involving multiple factors, such as cyclins, cyclin-dependent protein kinases, and cell cycle-dependent protein kinase inhibitors [40,

41]. The abnormal expression of cyclins and cyclin-dependent protein kinases, and loss of cyclin-dependent protein kinase inhibitors can cause uncontrolled cell proliferation and tumor growth [42]. It has been shown that *P. americana* extracts can inhibit the growth of progesterone receptor-negative endometrial cancer cells by blocking the cell cycle via up-regulation of p53 expression and down-regulation of C-erbB-2 expression [43]. *P. americana* extract could arrest the cell cycle of human lung cancer cells H125 in the S phase [44]. Human gastric cancer BGC-823 cells exhibited the cell cycle arrest at G2/M phase in the presence of "Kangfuxin Liquid" that consists of the refined active constituents of *P. americana* [45]. Moreover, *P. americana* extract inhibited the growth of Lewis lung carcinoma (3LL) cells in mice and induced cell cycle arrest in G0/G1 phase [46].

Induction of apoptosis

Apoptosis is a process of programmed cell death, which plays a critical role in cancer development and therapies [47–49]. Multiple genes are involved in apoptosis in cancer cells, such as pro-apoptotic proteins Fas, Bax, p53 and anti-apoptotic proteins Bcl-2, c-myc [50, 51]. Many natural products can induce apoptosis in various human cancer cells, such as gambogic acid, ursolic acid, vinca alkaloids, and camptothecins [8, 52]. *P. americana* extract inhibited the proliferation of human hepatoma cells by inducing apoptosis and reducing the mitochondrial membrane potential, up-regulating Bax, Caspase-9, and Caspase-3 expression, and down-regulating Bcl-2 expression [53]. *P. americana* extracts induced apoptosis in Lewis lung carcinoma (3LL) cells through up-regulation of Fas, Fas receptor (FasR), and p53 gene expression and down-regulation of Bcl-2 expression [54]. In addition, a study revealed that *P. americana* extract induced apoptosis in human hepatocellular carcinoma SMMC-7721 cells via the mitochondrial pathway [55].

Anti-angiogenic effect

Nutrients and oxygen supplied by the vasculature are essential for tumor growth and metastasis. Thus, angiogenesis plays a vital role in tumorigenesis [56, 57]. Vascular endothelial growth factor (VEGF), a major contributor to angiogenesis, promotes the proliferation and migration of endothelial cells, and increases vascular permeability [58, 59]. *P. americana* polypeptides significantly inhibited tumor growth, decreased tumor microvessel density (MVD), and reduced VEGF expression [60]. *P. americana* extract significantly inhibited the tumor growth of H22 tumor-bearing mice and reduced VEGF levels in mice serum [61]. These evidences indicate that the anti-tumor effect of *P. americana* is probably related to angiogenesis inhibition.

Enhancement of immunity

As an important guarantee for the body health, immunity is closely related to the stability of the internal environment. The homeostasis of the organism is destroyed when the immunity of the organism declines, which contributes to occurrence and spread of tumors [62, 63]. Thus, improving body immunity can achieve anti-tumor effect [64]. Tumor necrosis factor alpha (TNF-α) is a multifunctional cytokine with a crucial role in apoptosis, cell survival, and immunity [65, 66]. TNF-α is mainly secreted by monocytes and macrophages and exerts its biological functions through binding to specific receptors on the cell surface and activating intracellular distinct signaling pathways [67]. *P. americana* polypeptide extracts had a strong inhibitory effect on S180 and H22 tumor-bearing mice. The extracts increased the spleen index and thymus gland index of tumor-bearing mice, promoted the proliferation of T lymphocytes, enhanced the phagocytotic function of macrophages, and up-regulated the levels of IL-2, IL-6, IL-12, and TNF-α [68]. Moreover, *P. americana* extracts markedly inhibited tumor growth without causing toxicity of immune organs in S180 tumor-bearing mice, which may be related to an increase in TNF-α in the serum of tumor-bearing mice [69]. *P. americana* could increase the CD4/CD8 ratio of peripheral blood in mice with low immunity [70]. Therefore, *P. americana* extract showed significant anti-tumor activity that might be related to an enhanced immune function in vivo.

Reversal of drug resistance

Chemotherapy is one of the most common and effective methods in cancer treatment. The advancement of molecular biology, biochemistry, and genetic engineering techniques have led to remarkable achievements in the research and development of anti-tumor drugs. However, drug resistance has become a major obstacle for treatment of cancer [71, 72]. Drug resistance is a complex process involving multiple factors in cancer therapy. Thus, it is urgent and important to improve drug resistance in cancer treatment. There is evidence that *P. americana* extract effectively reversed the drug resistance of human hepatoma cells by targeting the multidrug resistance protein (MRP), breast cancer resistance protein (BCRP), and P-glycoprotein (P-gp) [73]. Additionally, human hepatoma HepG2/ADM cell line has biological characteristics of multi-drug resistance, and *P. americana* extract could inhibit the growth of HepG2/ADM cells along with reversal of drug resistance [74].

Conclusion

Periplaneta americana extract has been widely applied in China as an alternative medicine against diseases. The above studies have shown that the anti-tumor effects of

P. americana are attracting more and more attention. This review aimed to provide a clear picture regarding the anti-tumor effects and the underlying mechanisms of *P. americana*. The reported mechanisms of anti-tumor effects of *P. americana* mainly involve inhibition of tumor cell growth, induction of cell cycle arrest and apoptosis, suppression of angiogenesis, enhancement of immunity, and reversal of drug resistance (Fig. 1). However, the specific active constituents and precise mechanisms underlying the anti-cancer activities of *P. americana* remain uncertain. Thus, it is an important research topic to optimize the extraction process and search for the best technological conditions for further

isolation and purification of the anti-tumor constituents of *P. americana*. Additionally, the mechanisms of anti-tumor effects of *P. americana* remain to be further identified. More exploration remain to be performed, such as effects of *P. americana* on cancer metastasis or autophagy. It may be promising to conduct further investigation of PAE60 on the identification of active chemical constituents and relevant pharmacological mechanisms. To be sure, further exploration of anti-cancer drug from *P. americana* will provide potent scientific basis for clinical use of *P. americana* and contribute to the development of novel anti-cancer drugs with high efficiency and low toxicity.

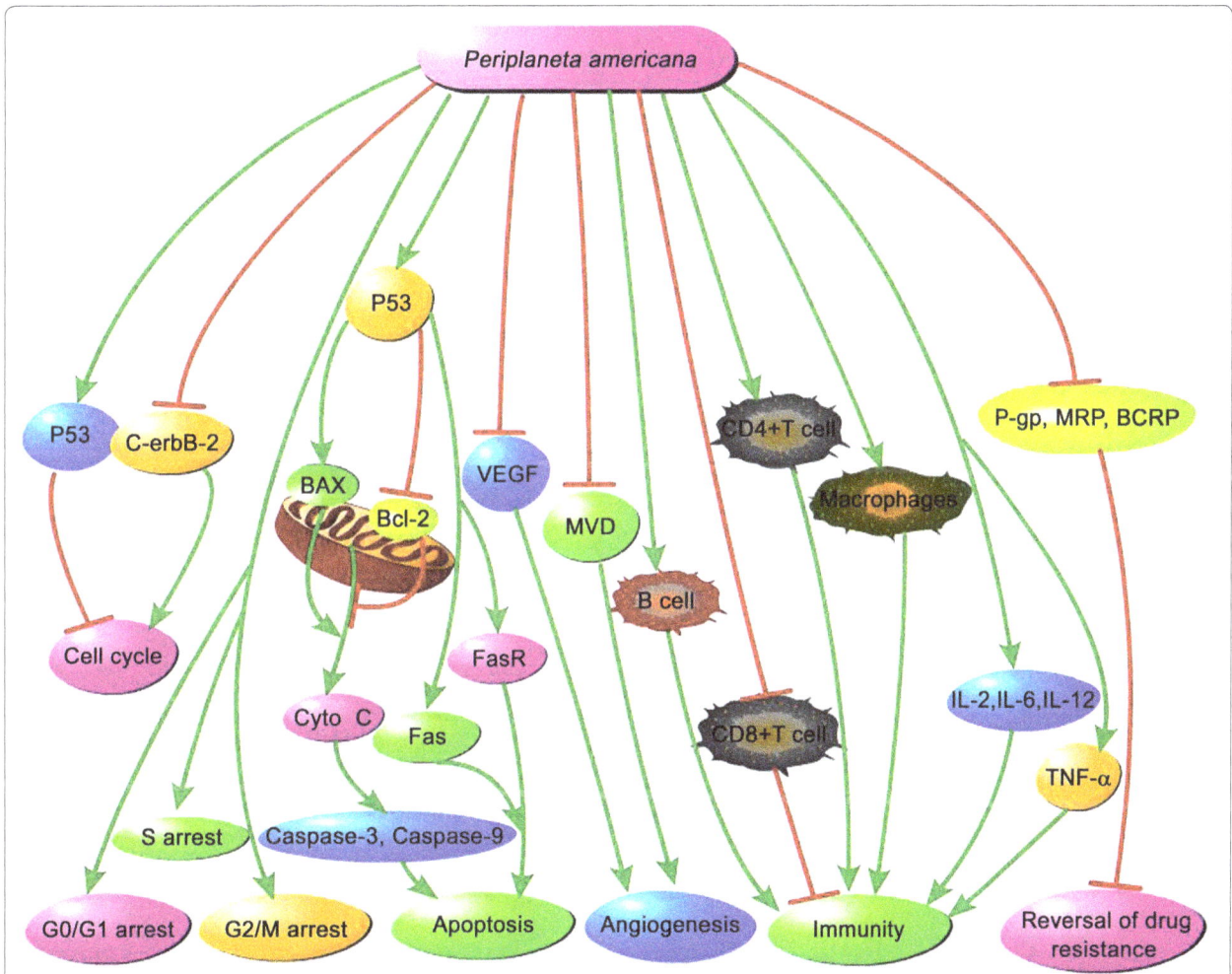

Fig. 1 Diagraphic illustration of mechanisms of anti-tumor effects of *P. americana*. *P. americana* extract inhibited cell proliferation via p53- and C-erbB-2-mediated cell-cycle arrest in progesterone-receptor negative endometrial cancer cells. *P. americana* extracts induced cell-cycle arrest of Lewis lung carcinoma (3LL) cells and human lung cancer cells H125 at G0/G1 phase and S phase, respectively. "Kangfuxin Liquid" induced cell-cycle arrest of human gastric cancer cells BGC-823 at G2/M phase. *P. americana* extract decreased the ratio of Bcl-2 to BAX by increasing p53 and upregulated Fas and FasR expression, which induced apoptosis of cancer cells. *P. americana* may depress angiogenesis by inhibiting VEGF expression and microvessel density (MVD). *P. americana* extract activated lymphocytes, increased the CD4/CD8 ratio of peripheral blood, prompted T- and B-lymphocytes proliferation, and modulated cytokines release, including TNF-α, IL-2, IL-6, and IL-12. In addition, the extract effectively reversed the drug resistance of human hepatoma cells (HepG2/ADM) by targeting P-gp, MRP, and BCRP

Abbreviations

TCM: traditional Chinese medicine; VEGF: vascular endothelial growth factor; TNF-α: tumor necrosis factor-α; *P. americana*: *Periplaneta americana*; MVD: microvessel density; HBV: hepatitis B virus; PAE60: 60% ethanol fraction of *Periplaneta americana* organic extracts; FasR: Fas receptor; MRP: multidrug resistance protein; BCRP: breast cancer resistance protein; P-gp: P-glycoprotein.

Authors' contributions

YZ, PT, and ZH conceived and designed the review. YZ, AY, PT, and ZH wrote the manuscript . All authors read and approved the final manuscript.

Acknowledgements

Not applicable.

Competing interests

The authors declare that they have no competing interests.

Consent for publication

All of authors consent to publication of this work in *Chinese Medicine*.

Funding

This work was supported by the Excellent Young Scientist Foundation of Beijing University of Chinese Medicine (2015-JYB-XYQ-004).

References

1. Siegel RL, Miller KD, Jemal A. Cancer statistics, 2016. CA Cancer J Clin. 2016;66:7–30.
2. Jemal A, Bray F, Center MM, Ferlay J, Ward E, Forman D. Global cancer statistics. CA Cancer J Clin. 2011;61:69–90.
3. Chen W, Zheng R, Baade PD, Zhang S, Zeng H, Bray F, Jemal A, Yu XQ, He J. Cancer statistics in China, 2015. CA Cancer J Clin. 2016;66:115–32.
4. He G, Liu J, Wang J, Xie S. The anti-tumor mechanism research status of traditional Chinese medicine. J Sichuan Tradit Chin Med. 2008;26:47–9.
5. Liweber M. Targeting apoptosis pathways in cancer by Chinese medicine. Cancer Lett. 2013;332:304–12.
6. Xia Q, Mao W. Anti-tumor effects of traditional Chinese medicine give a promising perspective. J Cancer Res Ther. 2014;10(Suppl 1):1–2.
7. Nie J, Zhao C, Deng LI, Chen J, Yu B, Wu X, Pang P, Chen X. Efficacy of traditional Chinese medicine in treating cancer. Biomed Rep. 2016;4:3–14.
8. Tan W, Lu J, Huang M, Li Y, Chen M, Wu G, Gong J, Zhong Z, Xu Z, Dang Y, et al. Anti-cancer natural products isolated from chinese medicinal herbs. Chin Med. 2011;6:27.
9. Efferth T, Li PC, Konkimalla VS, Kaina B. From traditional Chinese medicine to rational cancer therapy. Trends Mol Med. 2007;13:353–61.
10. Parekh HS, Liu G, Wei MQ. A new dawn for the use of traditional Chinese medicine in cancer therapy. Mol Cancer. 2009;8:21.
11. Li X, Yang G, Zhang Y, Yang J, Chang J, Sun X, Zhou X, Guo Y, Xu Y, Liu J, Bensoussan A. Traditional Chinese medicine in cancer care: a review of controlled clinical studies published in Chinese. PLoS ONE. 2013;8:e60338.
12. Ye L, Jia Y, Ji KE, Sanders AJ, Xue K, Ji J, Mason MD, Jiang WG. Traditional Chinese medicine in the prevention and treatment of cancer and cancer metastasis. Oncol Lett. 2015;10:1240–50.
13. Carmady B, Smith CA. Use of Chinese medicine by cancer patients: a review of surveys. Chin Med. 2011;6:22.
14. Shi W. The medical research advanced on *Periplaneta americana*. Chin J Ethnomed Ethnopharm. 2012;21:50–1.
15. Yu S, Zhang H, Zhang T, Liu J. Research advances in pharmacological action and clinical application of *Periplaneta americana*. J Liaoning Coll Tradit Chin Med. 2016;18:228–30.
16. He Z, Peng F, Song L, Wang X, Hu M, Zhao Y, Liu G. Advances in chemical constituents and pharmacological effects of *Periplaneta americana*. Chin J Chin Mater Med. 2007;32:2326–30.
17. Dai Y, Zeng M, Xiang P. The medicinal value of cockroaches. Chin Med Mat. 2005;28:848–9.
18. Ou W, Zhu C, Lin W. Observation of the clinical curative effects of Xiao zheng Yi gan Pian on chronic hepatitis B. Chin J Integr Tradit West Med Liver Dis. 1995;5:12–3.
19. Chen L. Observation of the curative effect of 66 cases with primary liver cancer treated with Xiao zheng Yi gan Pian. Fujian J Tradit Chin Med. 1986;6:16–7.
20. Zhang H, Geng F, Shen Y, Liu H, Zhao Y, Zhang C. Research progress of Kangfuxin Ye in pharmacological action and clinical application. Chin J Ethnomed Ethnopharm. 2017;26:57–60.
21. Du Y, Chen H, Li S, Li Z, Li X, Zhang H, Fang C. The hepatic pharmacological effects of Gan long capsules in vivo. Lishizhen Med Mater Med Res. 2006;17:1369–71.
22. Zhang L. Pharmacological effect and clinical curative effect of Xinmailong injection. Herald Med. 2001;20:250.
23. Wang XY, He ZC, Song LY, Spencer S, Yang LX, Peng F, Liu GM, Hu MH, Li HB, Wu XM, et al. Chemotherapeutic effects of bioassay-guided extracts of the American cockroach, *Periplaneta americana*. Integr Cancer Ther. 2011;10:NP12–23.
24. Jiang L, Li X, Xia C, Chen K, He S, Liu G. Research advance on chemical constituents and anti-tumor effects of *Periplaneta americana*. Med Plant. 2012;3:95–102.
25. Jiang W, Luo S, Wang Y, Wang L, Zhang X, Ye W. Chemical constituents of *Periplaneta americana*. J Jinan Univ. 2015;36:294–301.
26. Yu X, Xu L, Chen S, Sun Q, Zhang D. Analysis of supercritical carbon dioxide extraction of *Periplaneta americana* by GC-MS. J Luzhou Med Coll. 2016;39:344–6.
27. Li Y, Wang F, Zhang P, Yang M. Studies on chemical constituents of *Periplaneta american*. Chin Med Mat. 2015;38:2038–41.
28. Luo J, Xiao H, Dong G, Liu G. Analysis of the fat-soluble components in *Periplaneta americana* by GC-MS. Chin J Ethnomed Ethnopharm. 2009;18:26–7.
29. Meng S, Xiao X, Wang S, Luo C, Liu X. Liposoluble chemical constituents of *periplaneta americana* by GC-MS. Cent South Pharm. 2008;6:23–5.
30. Yao L. Study on the chemical ingredients of cockroach-preliminary analysis of amino acid composition. Tianjin Pharm. 1994;6:26–8.
31. He Z, Liu G, Wang X, Yang L, Zhao Y. Research advance on neuropeptides from *Periplaneta americana*. Nat Prod Res Dev. 2008;20:180–6.
32. Hu Y, Lu X, Wang Y, Peng F. Advances in medicinal value of *Periplaneta americana*. Med Rev. 2008;14:2822–4.
33. Xu J, Song Z, Guo Q, Li J. Synergistic effect and molecular mechanisms of traditional Chinese medicine on regulating tumor microenvironment and cancer cells. Biomed Res Int. 2016;2016:1490738.
34. Mu J, Liu T, Jiang L, Wu X, Cao Y, Li M, Dong Q, Liu Y, Xu H. The traditional Chinese medicine baicalein potently inhibits gastric cancer cells. J Cancer. 2016;7:453–61.
35. Cheng Y, Zhang L. Study progress on drug research and anti-tumor mechanisms of Chinese medicine. Chin Pharm. 2013;22:103–4.
36. Hu Y, Lu X, Liu G, Li M, Peng F. Effect of *Periplaneta americana* extract on two human lung tumor cell lines. J Pharm Anal. 2011;37:1245–50.
37. He Z, Hu M, Wang X, Liu G. Toxicity studies of American cockroach extract on three cell strains of human reproductive system cancer cell. Yunnan J Tradit Chin Med Mat Med. 2009;30:56–7.
38. He Z, Wang X, Yang L, Zhao Y, Liu G. Study on systena genitale tumor cell cytotoxicity of extracts from *Periplaneta americana*. Northwest Pharm J. 2009;24:271–2.
39. He Z, Wang X, Hu M, Liu G. The extracts of *Periplaneta americana* were applied to three human and mouse leukemia cell lines to study the cytotoxicity. Chin J Mod Drug Appl. 2009;30:56–7.
40. Malumbres M, Barbacid M. Cell cycle, CDKs and cancer: a changing paradigm. Nat Rev Cancer. 2009;9:153–66.
41. McDonald ER 3rd, El-Deiry WS. Cell cycle control as a basis for cancer drug development (Review). Int J Oncol. 2000;16:871–86.

42. Otto T, Sicinski P. Cell cycle proteins as promising targets in cancer therapy. Nat Rev Cancer. 2017;17:93–115.

43. Zhang X, Zhu Y. Impact of Total Matrine and *Periplaneta americana* extract on progesterone-receptor negative endometrial cancer cells (JEC). Chin J Chin Mater Med. 2015;40:2210–3.

44. Wang J. Effect of *Periplaneta americana* extract on lung cancer cell H125. Chin J Public Health. 2014;30:1400–2.

45. Jiang Y, Wang X, Jin C, Yuan F, Liu G, Li S. An experimental study of traditional Chinese medicine Kangfuxin inducing apoptosis in vitro of peptic carcinoma cell line BGC-823. J Kunming Med Coll. 2006;27:5–9.

46. Jiang Y, Wang X, Jin C, Chen X, Wang Q, Liu G. The inhibitory effect of *Periplaneta americana* extract on Lewis lung cancer in Mice. J Kunming Med Coll. 2007;5:13–6.

47. Elmore S. Apoptosis: a review of programmed cell death. Toxicol Pathol. 2007;35:495–516.

48. Brown JM, Attardi LD. The role of apoptosis in cancer development and treatment response. Nat Rev Cancer. 2005;5:231–7.

49. Reed JC. Apoptosis-targeted therapies for cancer. Cancer Cell. 2003;3:17–22.

50. Ghobrial IM, Witzig TE, Adjei AA. Targeting apoptosis pathways in cancer therapy. CA Cancer J Clin. 2005;55:178–94.

51. Johnson MI, Hamdy FC. Apoptosis regulating genes in prostate cancer (review). Oncol Rep. 1998;5:553–7.

52. Safarzadeh E, Sandoghchian Shotorbani S, Baradaran B. Herbal medicine as inducers of apoptosis in cancer treatment. Adv Pharm Bull. 2014;4:421–7.

53. Wang J, Li X. Mechanism study of *Periplaneta americana* extract on human hepatoma cells Bel-7402. Chin J Mod Appl Pharm. 2012;29:876–80.

54. Jiang Y, Wang X, Jin C, Chen X, Li J, Wu Z, Liu G, Li S. Inhibitory effect and mechanism research of *Periplaneta americana* extract on 3LL lung cancer cell in mice. Chin J Lung Cancer. 2006;9:488–91.

55. Dong J, Wei Z, Wang J. Apoptosis and the related mechanisms that *Periplaneta americana* extract on human hepatocellular carcinoma SMMC-7721 cells. Shandong Med J. 2012;52:32–4.

56. Nishida N, Yano H, Nishida T, Kamura T, Kojiro M. Angiogenesis in cancer. Vasc Health Risk Manag. 2006;2:213–9.

57. Hanahan D, Weinberg RA. Hallmarks of cancer: the next generation. Cell. 2011;144:646–74.

58. Hoeben A, Landuyt B, Highley MS, Wildiers H, Van Oosterom AT, De Bruijn EA. Vascular endothelial growth factor and angiogenesis. Pharmacol Rev. 2004;56:549–80.

59. Ferrara N. VEGF and the quest for tumour angiogenesis factors. Nat Rev Cancer. 2002;2:795–803.

60. Liang G, Zhang D, Zhang H, Liu M. The inhibitory effect of *Periplaneta americana* polypeptide on tumor growth and angiogenesis in nude mice bearing human hepatocellular carcinoma Bel-7402 cells. Chin J New Drug. 2016;25:687–91.

61. Chen J, Geng L, Zhang X, Yang T, Li H, He X, Pu X, Peng F. Effect of *Periplaneta americana* Extract CII-3 on angiogenesis in H22 hepatoma-bearing mice. J Chin Oncol. 2012;18:274–6.

62. Vesely MD, Kershaw MH, Schreiber RD, Smyth MJ. Natural innate and adaptive immunity to cancer. Annu Rev Immunol. 2011;29:235–71.

63. Terabe M, Berzofsky JA. Immunoregulatory T cells in tumor immunity. Curr Opin Immunol. 2004;16:157–62.

64. Papaioannou NE, Beniata OV, Vitsos P, Tsitsilonis O, Samara P. Harnessing the immune system to improve cancer therapy. Ann Transl Med. 2016;4:261.

65. van Horssen R, Ten Hagen TL, Eggermont AM. TNF-alpha in cancer treatment: molecular insights, antitumor effects, and clinical utility. Oncologist. 2006;11:397–408.

66. Parameswaran N, Patial S. Tumor necrosis factor-alpha signaling in macrophages. Crit Rev Eukaryot Gene Expr. 2010;20:87–103.

67. Wajant H, Pfizenmaier K, Scheurich P. Tumor necrosis factor signaling. Cell Death Differ. 2003;10:45–65.

68. Zhang D, Sun Y, Li M, Sun Q, Liu M. Effects of *Periplaneta americana* polypeptide extracts on tumor growth and immune function in tumor-bearing mice. Chin J New Drug. 2015;24:681–6.

69. He X, Pu X, Li J, Peng F. Effect of extractive from *Periplaneta americana* on immune on and inhibitory tumor action in S180-bearing mice. Chin J Exp Tradit Med Form. 2012;18:179–81.

70. Zhou Q, Wu Z, Li Z, Liu J, Wang C. Effect of *Periplaneta americana* on immune function of mice with low immunity. J Fujian Agricul Forest Univ. 2008;37:519–22.

71. Gottesman MM. Mechanisms of cancer drug resistance. Annu Rev Med. 2002;53:615–27.

72. Huang Y, Cole SP, Cai T, Cai YU. Applications of nanoparticle drug delivery systems for the reversal of multidrug resistance in cancer. Oncol Lett. 2016;12:11–5.

73. Liu J, Xia M, Peng F. Experimental research of *Periplaneta americana* extract on human drug resistant hepatocellular carcinoma cell line. Chin J Biochem Pharm. 2015;4:19–23.

74. Qiao T, Niu C, Peng F. Study of *Periplaneta americana* L. reversing multidrug resistance of hepatocellular carcinoma. Chin J Biochem Pharm. 2015;4:35–8.

15

Anti-cancer effects of Rhizoma Curcumae against doxorubicin-resistant breast cancer cells

Zhangfeng Zhong[1,2†], Haibing Yu[3†], Shengpeng Wang[2], Yitao Wang[2*] and Liao Cui[1*]

Abstract

Background: Chemotherapy is a primary approach in cancer treatment after routine surgery. However, chemo-resistance tends to occur with chemotherapy in clinic, resulting in poor prognosis and recurrence. Nowadays, Chinese medicine may shed light on design of new therapeutic modes to overcome chemo-resistance. Although Rhizoma Curcumae possesses anti-cancer activities in various types of cancers, the effects and underlying mechanisms of its bioactive components against chemo-resistance are not clear. Therefore, the present study aims to explore the potential effects of Rhizoma Curcumae on doxorubicin-resistant breast cancer cells.

Methods: The expression and function of ABC transporters in doxorubicin-resistant MCF-7 breast cancer cells were measured by western blotting and flow cytometry. Cell viability was detected using MTT assay. The combination index was analyzed using the CalcuSyn program (Biosoft, Ferguson, MO), based on the Chou–Talalay method.

Results: In our present study, P-gp was overexpressed at protein level in doxorubicin-resistant MCF-7 cell line, but short of MRP1 and BCRP1. Essential oil of Rhizoma Curcumae and the main bioactive components were assessed on doxorubicin-resistant MCF-7 cell line. We found that the essential oil and furanodiene both display powerful inhibitory effects on cell viability, but neither of these is the specific inhibitor of ABC transporters. Moreover, furanodiene fails to enhance the efficacy of doxorubicin to improve multidrug resistance.

Conclusion: Overall, our findings fill the gaps of the researches on chemo-resistance improvement of Rhizoma Curcumae and are also beneficial for Rhizoma Curcumae being developed as a promising natural product for cancer adjuvant therapy in the future.

Keywords: Rhizoma Curcumae, Multidrug resistance, Breast cancer, ABC transporters, Furanodiene

Background

Chemotherapy is regarded as one of adjuvant therapy after a routine surgery and being the primary approach for various cancer types [1–3]. However, many obstacles, including low efficacy and side effects, especially for chemo-resistance, still exist in cancer patients undergoing chemotherapy. There are a lot of strategies overcoming chemo-resistance, such as targeting ATP-binding cassette (ABC) transporters [4, 5], inducing cell apoptosis [6], inhibiting DNA repair [7], regulating metabolic reprogramming [8, 9], or applying combination therapy [10]. The role of ABC transporters is found to be closely related with chemo-resistance, thereby leading to poor prognosis and tumor recurrence in clinic [11]. Because of the expressions of ABC transporters, efflux pump decreases intracellular accumulation of drugs, then therapeutic concentrations of effective agents are reduced [12]. A thorough mechanisms of ABC transporters in chemo-resistance are still ongoing, and some typical proteins have been hot topics for a long time, including P-glycoprotein 1 (P-gp, MDR1, or ABCB1) [13], multidrug resistance-associated protein 1 (MRP1) [14], and ATP-binding cassette sub-family G member 2 (ABCG2 or BCRP) [15, 16].

*Correspondence: ytwang@umac.mo; cuiliao@163.com
[†]Zhangfeng Zhong and Haibing Yu contributed equally to this work
[1] Guangdong Key Laboratory for Research and Development of Natural Drugs, Guangdong Medical University, Zhanjiang, Guangdong, China
[2] State Key Laboratory of Quality Research in Chinese Medicine, Institute of Chinese Medical Sciences, University of Macau, Macao, China
Full list of author information is available at the end of the article

Overcoming chemo-resistance is a big challenge to chemotherapy. Natural products are rich sources of bioactive constitutes reversing cancer multidrug resistance, enhancing efficacy of anti-cancer agents, and decreasing side effects [9, 17, 18]. Currently, growing evidence show that Rhizoma Curcumae exhibits therapeutic value in overcoming chemo-resistance. The fractionated extracts of Rhizoma Curcumae improve the sensitivity of doxorubicin-resistant MCF-7 breast cancer cells to doxorubicin by blocking P-gp activity and down-regulating P-gp expression [19]. Furthermore, the fraction of CH_2Cl_2 extract is much more effective than that of EtOAc extract to restore the sensitivity of chemo-resistant MCF-7 cells to anti-neoplastic agents [20]. Meanwhile, several pure compounds (as shown in Fig. 1) isolated from Rhizoma Curcumae also have been reported to possess anti-cancer activities in multidrug resistant cancer cells. In detailly, curcumin inhibits viability of chemo-resistant breast cancer cells in an ER-independent manner and reverses multidrug resistance through ABC transporters [21]. β-elemene enhances cytotoxic effect of doxorubicin on doxorubicin-resistant MCF-7 breast cancer cells, which is related to increased doxorubicin accumulation and decreased Bcl-2 expression [22]. Germacrone reverses multidrug resistance through inducing cell apoptosis by down-regulation of Bcl-2 and up-regulation of p53 and Bax. In addition, germacrone significantly reduces P-gp expression in multidrug resistant breast cancer cells [23].

Combination therapy is a treatment combining two or more therapeutic agents, aiming to improve disease-specific symptoms and overall survival. During and after cancer treatment, combination therapy potentially reduces chemo-resistance and provide therapeutic anti-cancer benefits simultaneously [24, 25]. Meanwhile, a variety of components derived from Chinese medicinal herbs are undergoing extensive researches of combination treatments in overcoming multidrug resistance to enhance efficacy [26, 27]. Therefore, it is urgent to develop an integrative approach to cancer care, when combination therapy meets Chinese medicinal herbs [28, 29]. To the best of our knowledge, there is no report of furanodiene or essential oil from Rhizoma Curcumae exhibiting anti-cancer effects in chemo-resistant cancer cells by means of ABC transporters regulation. Therefore, our present study identified anti-cancer effects of those bioactive constituents from Rhizoma Curcumae initially and explored the related mechanisms in doxorubicin-resistant MCF-7 breast cancer cells.

Methods

The Minimum Standards of Reporting Checklist contains details of the experimental design, and statistics, and resources used in this study (Additional file 1).

Chemical and reagents

The Roswell Park Memorial Institute-1640 (RPMI-1640) culture medium were purchased from Gibco (Maryland, USA). Fetal bovine serum (FBS), phosphate-buffered saline (PBS), penicillin-streptomycin (PS), and 0.25% (w/v) trypsin/1 mM EDTA were obtained from

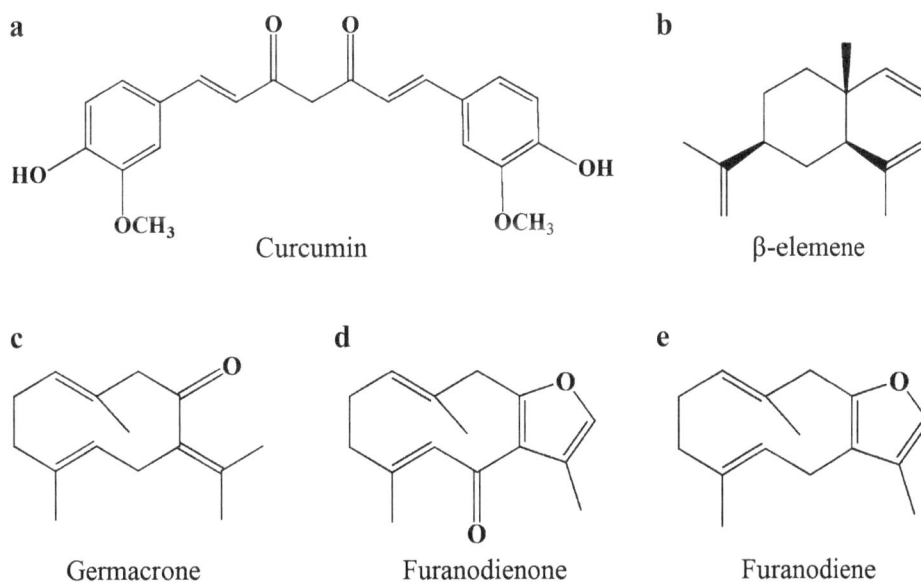

Fig. 1 Chemical structures of the main compounds derived from Rhizoma Curcumae. **a** Curcumin. **b** β-elemene. **c** Germacrone. **d** Furanodienone. **e** Furanodiene

Invitrogen (Carlsbad, USA). 3-[4, 5-Dimethyl-2-thia-zolyl]-2, 5-diphenyltetrazolium bromide (MTT) and Calcein AM were obtained from Molecular Probes (Eugene, USA). Doxorubicin (DOX) and Rhodamine 123 were supplied by Sigma-Aldrich (St. Louis, USA). Furanodiene and furanodienone were purchased from National Institutes for Food and Drug Control. Essential oil was obtained as our previous report [30]. Radioimmuno-precipitation assay (RIPA) lysis buffer and primary antibodies against P-gp, MRP1, and BCRP1 were obtained from Santa Cruz (Santa Cruz, USA). Primary antibodies against β-actin, as well as the secondary antibodies were purchased from Cell Signaling (Danvers, USA).

Cell culture and drug treatment
MCF-7 cell line was obtained from the ATCC (Manassas, USA) and was cultured as previously reported [31]. To induce doxorubicin-resistant cancer cell line, MCF-7 cells were cultured with RPMI1640 medium containing fetal bovine serum (10%), penicillin (100 units per mL), and streptomycin (100 µg/mL), at 37 °C in a humidified atmosphere of 5% CO_2 in air. Doxorubicin-resistance was established by stepwise exposure to increased concentrations of doxorubicin as described previously [32]. The stock solutions of essential oil (100 mg/mL), furanodiene (100 mM), furanodienone (100 mM), and doxorubicin (2 and 100 mM) dissolved in DMSO were diluted to different concentrations as required.

Cell viability assay
Cell viability was performed using MTT assay as described previously [33]. Briefly, exponentially growing cells were seeded in 96-well plates at a density of 2×10^4/well and allowed to attach overnight. Following the required incubation period, cell viability was determined by adding MTT working solution (100 µL/well, 1 mg/mL). The absorbance values at 570 nm were recorded using SpectraMax M5 microplate reader (Molecular Devices, Silicon Valley, USA).

Western blotting assay
Western blotting assay was performed according to previous studies [34]. Briefly, exponentially growing cells were seeded in culture dish (100 mm) at a density of 2×10^6/dish and allowed to attach overnight. After the required treatments, cells were harvested, and the total proteins were extracted with RIPA lysis buffer. Equal amounts of total proteins were separated by appropriate SDS-PAGE followed by transferring onto a PVDF membrane. After blocking with 5% non-fat milk, the membrane was incubated with specific primary antibodies (1:1000 v/v) and the corresponding second antibodies (1:2000 v/v), respectively. The specific protein bands were visualized with an Amersham™ ECL™ advanced western blotting detection kit (GE Healthcare Life Sciences, UK).

P-gp expression assay
P-gp expression was evaluated using the antibody of P-glycoprotein conjugated FITC (BD Biosciences, San Jose, USA) as described previously [35]. Cells were seeded into 6-well plates at a density of 2×10^5/well, followed by the required drug treatments. The cells were harvested and incubated with 100 µL of P-gp-FITC antibody dye-loading buffer at 37 °C for 30 min protected from light. The mean fluorescence intensity of FITC was detected using a flow cytometry (BD FACS Canto™, BD Biosciences, San Jose, USA). And the results were analyzed by FlowJo software (TreeStar, Ashland, OR, USA).

P-gp function assay
Rhodamine 123 and Calcein AM were applied to determine the activity of P-gp as described previously [35]. Cells were seeded into 6-well plates at a density of 2×10^5/well, followed by the required drug treatments. 100 µL of Rhodamine 123 or Calcein AM dye-loading solutions were added to each well and incubated at 37 °C for 30 min protected from light. The cells were harvested, and intracellular fluorescence was detected using a flow cytometry and analyzed by FlowJo software.

Doxorubicin uptake assay
Cells were seeded in 6-well plates at a density of 2×10^5/well and were treated with different concentrations of test agents in the presence of doxorubicin. Following a 2-h incubation, the cells were washed and re-suspended in dye-free culture medium. The doxorubicin uptake was assessed using flow cytometry and the results were also analyzed by FlowJo software.

Statistical analysis
All data represent the mean of three independently performed experiments, plus or minus standard deviation or standard error of the mean. The significance of inter-group differences was evaluated by one-way ANOVA using the GraphPad Prism software (GraphPad Software, USA). Newman–Keuls multiple comparison tests were performed for *post hoc* pairwise comparisons. *p*-values less than 0.05 were considered as significant.

Results
Establishment and characterization of doxorubicin-resistant MCF-7 breast cancer cell line
Doxorubicin-resistant MCF-7 breast cancer cell line was established by a stepwise exposure of MCF-7 cells to increasing concentrations of doxorubicin. Cell viability was tested by MTT assay after a 48-h treatment of

doxorubicin. Our results show that doxorubicin-resistant MCF-7 cells are resistant to doxorubicin with an IC50 value of 73.45 μM. And MCF-7 cells are sensitive to doxorubicin with an IC50 value of 2.87 μM (Fig. 2a). The drug resistance index (RI) is 25.60, calculated by the ratio of IC50 of doxorubicin-resistant MCF-7 cells and IC50 of MCF-7 cells. A chemo-resistant model with RI of 3 or more is considered a successful establishment. Then ABC transporters proteins were detected by western blotting. Results show that P-gp expression of doxorubicin-resistant MCF-7 cells is different from that of MCF-7 cells despite of absence or presence of doxorubicin. However, the protein expression levels of MRP1 and BCRP1 are not apparent both in MCF-7 cell line and doxorubicin-resistant MCF-7 cell line, even in the presence of doxorubicin (Fig. 2b). Furthermore, flow cytometry results confirm that the P-gp expression level of doxorubicin-resistant MCF-7

cells is much higher than that of MCF-7 cells, even in the presence of doxorubicin (Fig. 2c).

Effects of bioactive constituents of Rhizoma Curcumae on P-gp protein expression in doxorubicin-resistant MCF-7 breast cancer cells

Protein expression was assessed with western blotting, accompanied by FITC-P-gp staining assays. Different concentrations of essential oil (E30, E60, and E120 are 30, 60, and 120 μg/mL of essential oil, respectively) or furanodiene (F25, F50, and F100 are 25, 50, and 100 μM of furanodiene, respectively) do not show any inhibitory effects on P-gp expression, as shown in Fig. 3a, b. Meanwhile, FITC-P-gp staining assay using flow cytometry show that when compared with the red histogram of isotype control IgG, there are no any significant alterations in P-gp expression after treatment of essential oil or furanodiene at the indicated concentrations. That means

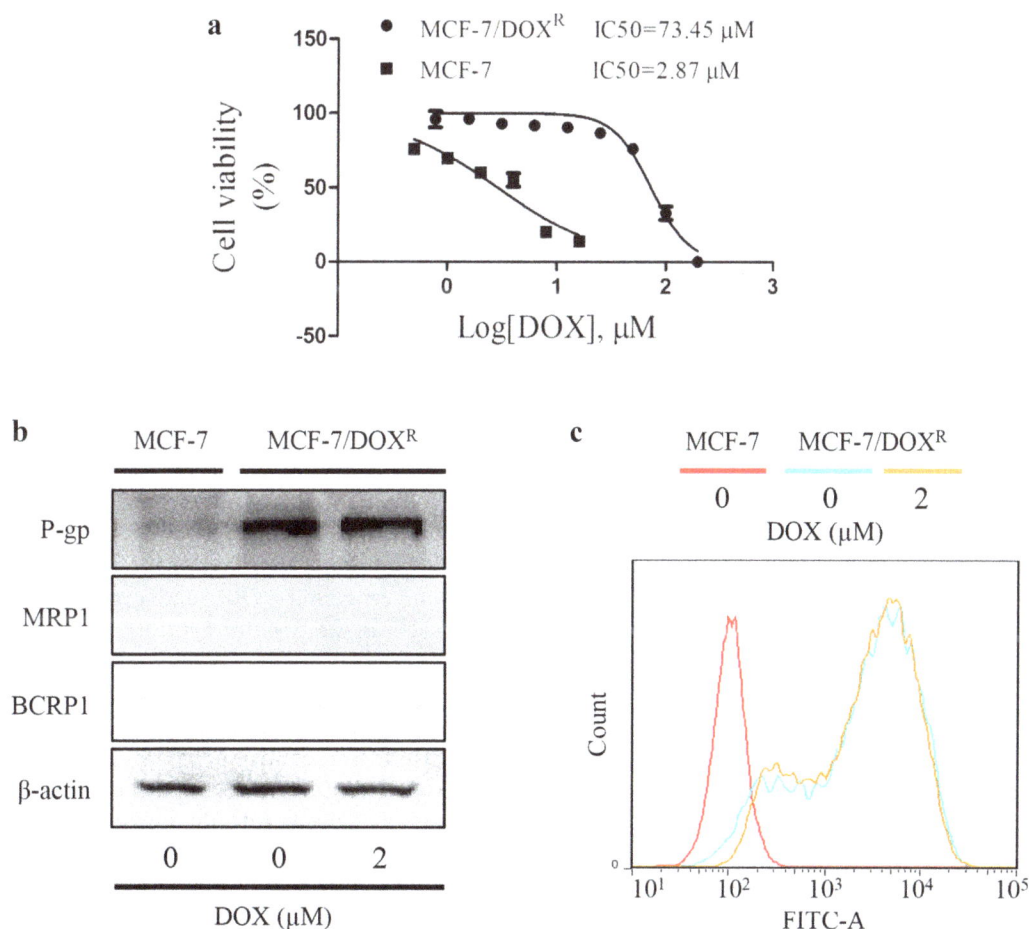

Fig. 2 Establishment and characterization of the doxorubicin (DOX)-resistant MCF-7 breast cancer cell line. Doxorubicin-resistant MCF-7 breast cancer cell line (MCF-7/DOX^R) was established by a stepwise exposure of MCF-7 cells to increasing concentrations of doxorubicin (DOX). Cells were treated with DOX for 48 h. **a** Cell viability was tested using MTT assay, represented by percentage of control. **b** Protein expression was evaluated using western blotting assay. **c** The expression alterations of P-gp were confirmed by FITC-P-gp antibody staining using flow cytometry

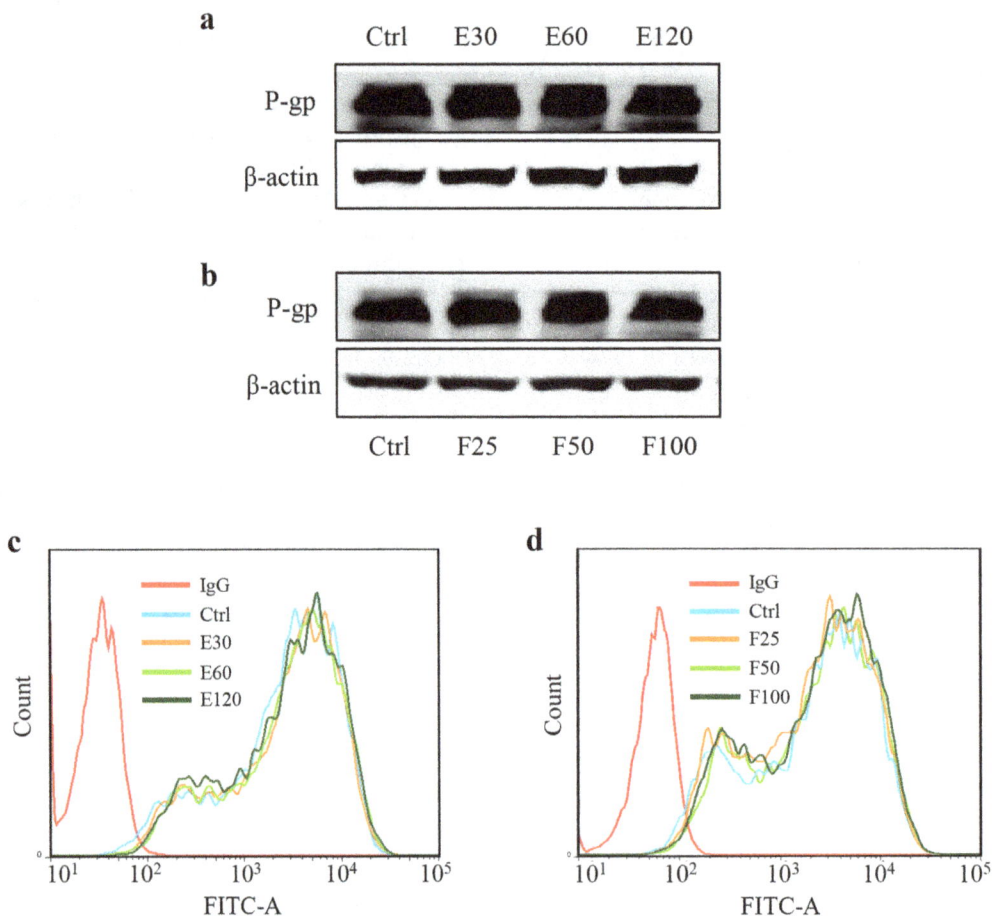

Fig. 3 Effects of bioactive constituents of Rhizoma Curcumae on P-gp protein expression in doxorubicin-resistant MCF-7 cells. Cells were treated with different concentrations of essential oil (E; µg/mL) and furanodiene (F; µM) for 24 h, compared with the control (Ctrl). **a, b** Protein expression was evaluated using western blotting assay. **c, d** Alterations of P-gp expression were confirmed by FITC-P-gp antibody staining using flow cytometry. Data were representative of at least three independent experiments

P-gp protein expression cannot be affected by essential oil or furanodiene in doxorubicin-resistant MCF-7 cells, as shown in Fig. 3c, d.

Effects of bioactive constituents of Rhizoma Curcumae on P-gp function in doxorubicin-resistant MCF-7 breast cancer cells

To further investigate influence of bioactive constituents on P-gp function, Rhodamine 123 and Calcein AM uptake assay were employed. After 1-h pre-treatment of essential oil or furanodiene, 30-min incubation with Rhodamine 123 or Calcein AM, fluorescence alterations were determined. Results show that 120 µg/mL of essential oil induces minor enhancements with mean fluorescence intensity (MFI) of 1359 and 2203, represented by P-gp-transported Rhodamine 123 (Fig. 4a) and the intracellular Calcein (Fig. 4b). It indicates that essential oil exerts a slight inhibitory effect on P-gp function in doxorubicin-resistant MCF-7 cells.

Regarding the potential effect of furanodiene on P-gp function, verapamil (VRP) and cyclosporine A (CYA) were used as the positive controls, both in Rhodamine 123 uptake assay and Calcein AM assay. In Rhodamine 123 uptake assay, compared with the remarkable increases (13.26-fold VRP and 37.28-fold CYA) induced by the positive controls, 1.47-fold increasement was observed after 100-µM furanodiene treatment (Fig. 5a, b). Similarly, in Calcein AM assay, compared with the remarkable increases (7.52-fold VRP and 7.16-fold CYA) induced by the positive controls, 1.77-fold increasement was observed after 100-µM furanodiene treatment (Fig. 5c, d).

Collectively, essential oil and furanodiene, both exert a mild inhibitory effect on efflux activity of P-gp in doxorubicin-resistant MCF-7 cells.

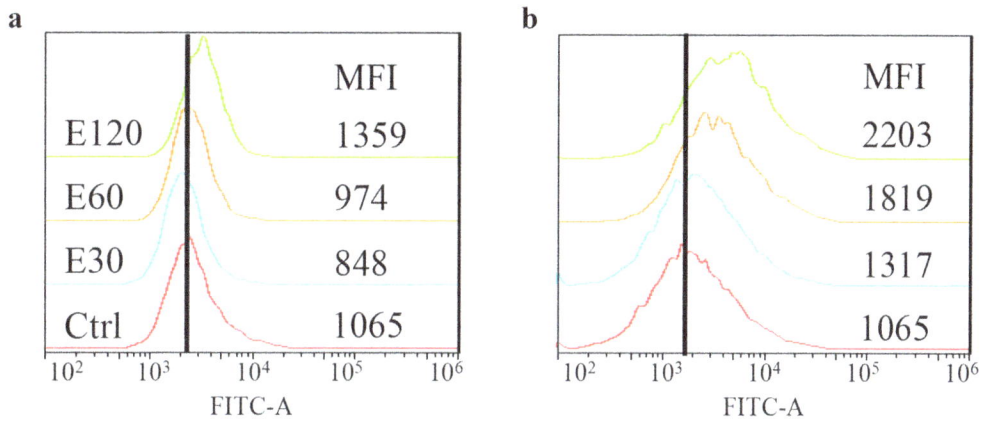

Fig. 4 Effect of essential oil on P-gp function in doxorubicin-resistant MCF-7 cells. P-gp function evaluation was performed by a 30-min incubation of **a** Rhodamine 123 and **b** Calcein AM using flow cytometry after 1-h treatment of essential oil (E; μg/mL). Ctrl stands for control. Data were representative mean fluorescence intensity (MFI) of at least three independent experiments

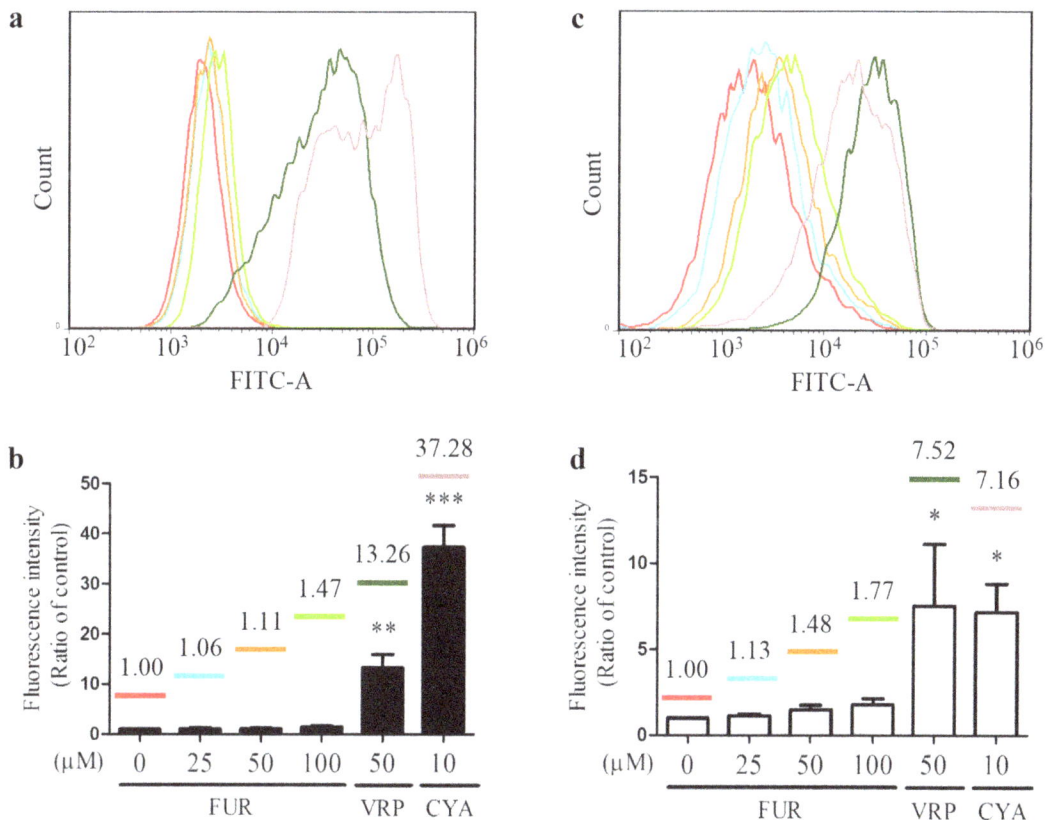

Fig. 5 Effect of furanodiene (FUR) on P-gp function in doxorubicin-resistant MCF-7 cells. P-gp function evaluation was performed by a 30-min incubation of Rhodamine 123 (**a**) and Calcein AM (**c**) using flow cytometry after 1-h treatments with furanodiene (FUR), verapamil (VRP), and cyclosporine A (CYA). The corresponding statistical result (**b, d**) was shown with VRP and CYA as positive controls. Data were expressed as mean ± S.E.M. *$P < 0.05$, **$P < 0.01$, and ***$P < 0.001$ vs. negative control

The enhancement of furanodiene on doxorubicin uptake in doxorubicin-resistant MCF-7 breast cancer cells

Doxorubicin uptake assay was performed to further confirm the regulatory effect of furanodiene on P-gp function. Results show that the positive drug verapamil (50 μM) can significantly increase doxorubicin uptake, represented by 19.06-fold fluorescence intensity compared with control. Meanwhile, furanodiene at the indicated concentrations slightly increases doxorubicin uptake without significance (Fig. 6a, b), which indicates that furanodiene may not be a specific inhibitor of ABC transporter protein as verapamil.

Effects of bioactive constituents of Rhizoma Curcumae on viability of doxorubicin-resistant MCF-7 breast cancer cells

To investigate the effect of Rhizoma Curcumae on viability of chemo-resistant cancer cells, doxorubicin-resistant MCF-7 cells were exposed to essential oil, furanodienone, and furanodiene. Cell viability was tested by MTT assay after a 48-h treatment. Results show that essential oil, furanodienone, and furanodiene display powerful inhibitory effects on viability of doxorubicin-resistant MCF-7 cells, with IC50 values of 76.98 μg/mL (Fig. 7a), 52.14 μM (Fig. 7b), and 69.63 μM (Fig. 7c), respectively.

Combined effects of furanodiene and doxorubicin on viability of doxorubicin-resistant MCF-7 breast cancer cells

Combined effects of furanodiene and doxorubicin on the viability of doxorubicin-resistant MCF-7 cells were determined after 24 h of treatment. Figure 8a, b show that the drug treatment alone (furanodiene or doxorubicin at concentrations of 25, 50, and 100 μM) dose-dependently inhibits the viability of doxorubicin-resistant MCF-7 cells. Doxorubicin (2 μM) and furanodiene (25 μM) are selected in subsequent experiments on account of non-toxic concentrations, as shown in Fig. 8a, b. However, there is no enhancement on sensitivity observed for furanodiene (Fig. 8a) or doxorubicin (Fig. 8b), no significance even at the highest concentration (100 μM of furanodiene or doxorubicin). To further assess the interaction of furanodiene and doxorubicin, cell viability results were analyzed using CalcuSyn program (Biosoft, Ferguson, MO), based on Chou–Talalay method. The combination index (CI) less than one is defined as synergism, while the CI greater than one is defined as antagonism. As shown in Fig. 8c, a synergistic inhibitory effect on the viability of doxorubicin-resistant MCF-7 cells is found when high concentrations of furanodiene combined with low concentrations of doxorubicin; On the contrary, drug antagonism occurs when low concentrations of furanodiene combined with high concentrations of doxorubicin.

Discussion

Growing evidence claim that Rhizoma Curcumae possesses anti-cancer activity mainly due largely in part to the essential oil and the bioactive components as well, containing curcumin, β-elemene, germacrone, furanodiene, furanodienone, and so on. However, the anti-cancer activities of Rhizoma Curcumae against chemo-resistant cancer cells are not clear yet. Therefore, we reviewed the anti-cancer effects of bioactive constituents of Rhizoma Curcumae against chemo-resistant cancer cells. Collectively, some reports demonstrated that Rhizoma

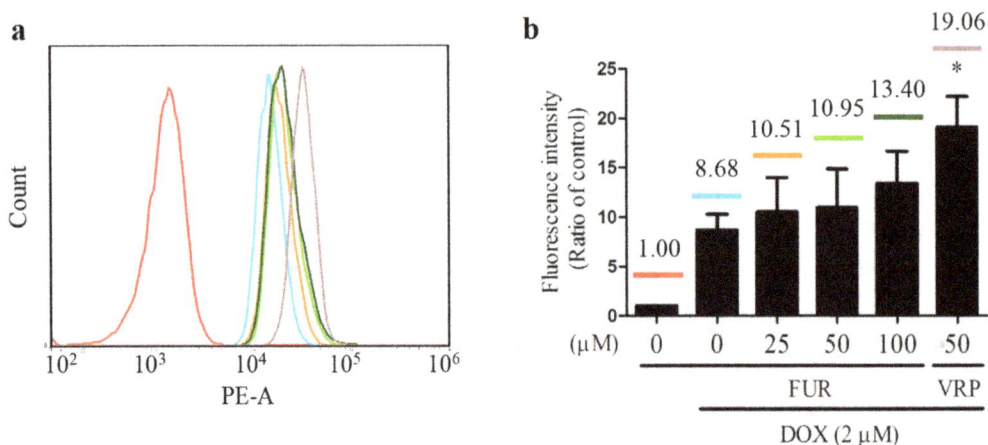

Fig. 6 Effect of furanodiene (FUR) on cellular uptake of doxorubicin in doxorubicin (DOX)-resistant MCF-7 cells. **a** After explosion to furanodiene (FUR) or verapamil (VRP) in the presence of doxorubicin (DOX) for 2 h, doxorubicin uptake was analyzed using flow cytometry. **b** Statistical result of **a**. Data shown were expressed as mean ± S.E.M. *$P < 0.05$ vs. negative control

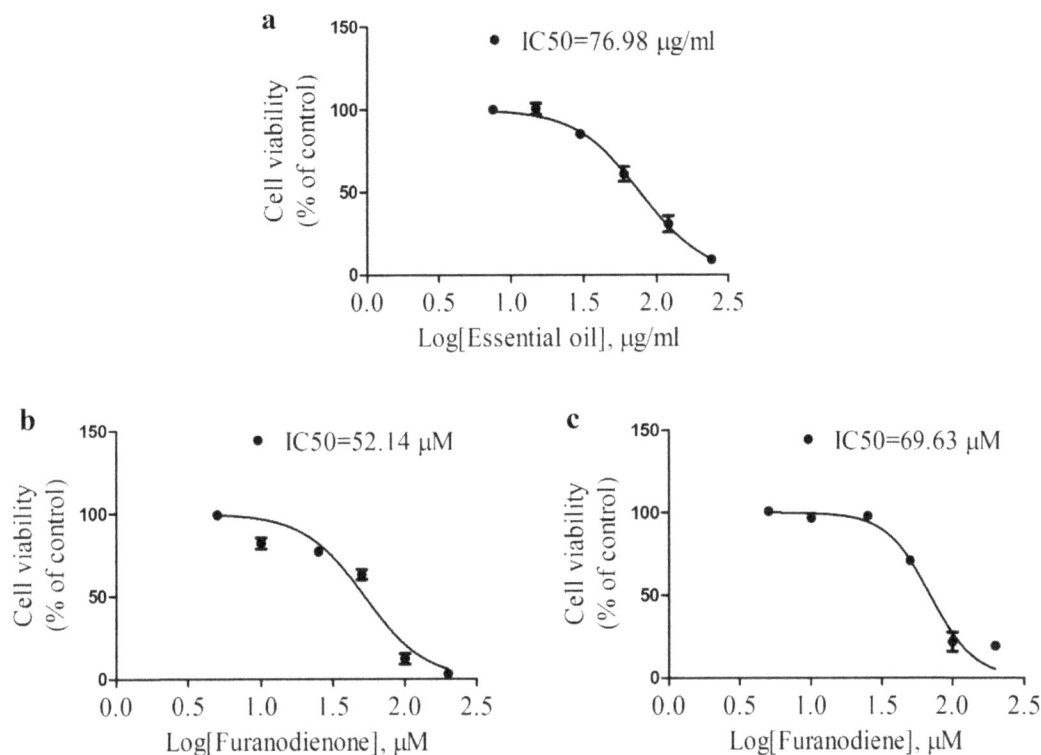

Fig. 7 Effects of bioactive constituents of Rhizoma Curcumae on viability of doxorubicin-resistant MCF-7 cells. Cells were treated with different concentrations of **a** essential oil, **b** furanodienone, and **c** furanodiene for 48 h. Cell viability was tested using MTT assay. Data shown were expressed as mean ± S.E.M

Curcumae extract [19], curcumin [36], β-elemene [37], and germacrone [23] exhibit anti-cancer activities in chemo-resistant cancer cells. However, to the best of our knowledge, there are still research gaps in the exact mechanisms of essential oil, furanodiene, and furanodienone on chemo-resistance. Therefore, our present study was designed to investigate the detailed anti-cancer effects of essential oil, furanodiene, and furanodienone against doxorubicin-resistant MCF-7 breast cancer cells.

Firstly, we identified whether these ingredients are specific inhibitors of ABC transporters or not. Unexpectedly, essential oil and furanodiene cannot affect P-gp expression and slightly inhibit P-gp activity. Accordingly, the underlying mechanisms of Rhizoma Curcumae on chemo-resistance improvement may not be limited to the ABC transporters. Afterwards, our findings show that essential oil, furanodienone, and furanodiene display powerful inhibitory effects on viability of doxorubicin-resistant MCF-7 cells. The results clarified that these ingredients also have anti-cancer activities in chemo-resistant cancer cells. Meanwhile, furanodiene, the potential bioactive compound, was confirmed to induce extrinsic and intrinsic apoptosis through altering mitochondrial function via AMPK-dependent and

NF-κB-independent pathways in doxorubicin-resistant MCF-7 cells [32, 38].

According to our previous study, ERα-negative MDA-MB-231 cells are much more sensitive to furanodiene than ERα-positive MCF-7 cells. Therefore, we concluded that furanodiene could significantly increase the efficacy of tamoxifen in ERα-positive breast cancer cells [31]. Therefore, we make an inference from these results that furanodiene may enhance the efficacy of non-steroidal agents in ERα-negative breast cancer cells, instead of in ERα-positive breast cancer cells. Considering these findings mentioned above, we presumed that furanodiene could significantly enhance the efficacy of doxorubicin in ERα-negative and ERα-low expression breast cancer cells [39]. That is why we proposed the subsequent study evaluating the anti-breast cancer activities of furanodiene in combined with doxorubicin on doxorubicin-resistant breast cancer cells. Interestingly, it is actually observed that high concentrations of furanodiene combined low concentrations of doxorubicin exhibit synergistic inhibitory effects on the viability of doxorubicin-resistant MCF-7 cells, and low concentrations of furanodiene combined with high concentrations of doxorubicin exhibit antagonism.

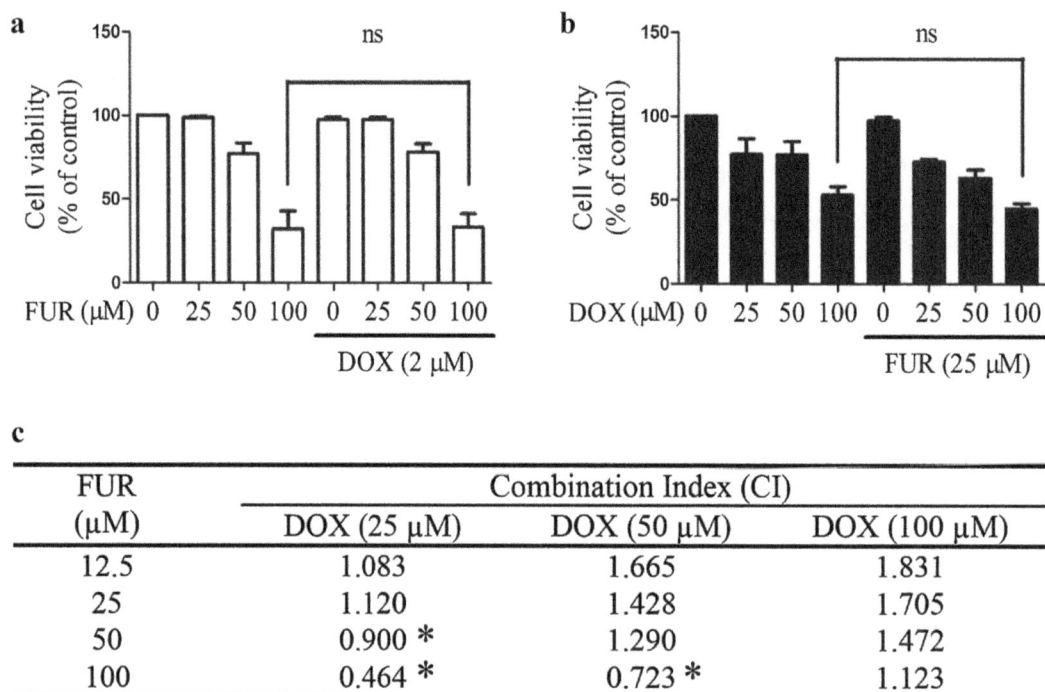

Fig. 8 Combined effects of furanodiene (FUR) and doxorubicin (DOX) on viability of DOX-resistant MCF-7 cells. **a** Cells were treated with different concentrations of furanodiene (FUR; 0–100 μM) in the presence or absence of doxorubicin (DOX; 2 μM) for 24 h. **b** Cells were treated with different concentrations of DOX (0–100 μM) in the presence or absence of FUR (25 μM) for 24 h. Cell viability was assessed using MTT assay. **c** The results were analyzed using CalcuSyn program (Biosoft), based on Chou–Talalay method. Data shown were expressed as mean ± S.E.M. ns stands for not significant. *, synergism

Conclusions

Overall, even though essential oil and furanodiene are not the specific inhibitors of ABC transporters, these ingredients still display powerful inhibitory effects on viability of doxorubicin-resistant breast cancer cells. The present study not only indicated Rhizoma Curcumae being a promising natural agent for cancer adjuvant therapy in the future, but also filled the gap of the researches on anti-cancer activities and corresponding mechanisms of Rhizoma Curcumae in chemo-resistant cancer cells.

Abbreviations
DOX: doxorubicin; FUR: furanodiene; VRP: verapamil; CYA: cyclosporine A; MTT: 3-[4, 5-Dimethyl-2-thiazolyl]-2, 5-diphenyltetrazolium bromide; CI: combination index; ABC transporters: ATP-binding cassette transporters; P-gp: P-glycoprotein 1; MRP1: multidrug resistance-associated protein 1; ABCG2: ATP-binding cassette sub-family G member 2; FBS: fetal bovine serum; PBS: phosphate-buffered saline; PS: penicillin–streptomycin; RIPA: radioimmunoprecipitation assay.

Authors' contributions
ZZ designed and performed the study. HY analyzed the data and revised the manuscript. SW participated in data analysis. YW and LC organized and supervised the study. All authors read and approved the final manuscript.

Author details
[1] Guangdong Key Laboratory for Research and Development of Natural Drugs, Guangdong Medical University, Zhanjiang, Guangdong, China. [2] State Key Laboratory of Quality Research in Chinese Medicine, Institute of Chinese Medical Sciences, University of Macau, Macao, China. [3] School of Public Health, Guangdong Medical University, Dongguan, Guangdong, China.

Acknowledgements
Not applicable.

Competing interests
The authors declare that they have no competing interests.

Consent for publication
Not applicable.

Funding
This study was supported by the Macao Science and Technology Development Fund (071/2017/A2), the Research Fund of University of Macau (CPG2014-00012-ICMS), the China Postdoctoral Science Foundation Funded Project (2017M622811), the Natural Science Foundation of Guangdong Province (2018A030310226), and the Features Innovative Projects of General Colleges and Universities of Guangdong Province (4SG18126G).

References

1. Kumagai K, Rouvelas I, Tsai JA, Mariosa D, Klevebro F, Lindblad M, et al. Meta-analysis of postoperative morbidity and perioperative mortality in patients receiving neoadjuvant chemotherapy or chemoradiotherapy for resectable oesophageal and gastro-oesophageal junctional cancers. Br J Surg. 2014;101(4):321–38.

2. Petrelli F, Borgonovo K, Cabiddu M, Lonati V, Barni S. Mortality, leukemic risk, and cardiovascular toxicity of adjuvant anthracycline and taxane chemotherapy in breast cancer: a meta-analysis. Breast Cancer Res Treat. 2012;135(2):335–46.

3. Ashraf N, Hoffe S, Kim R. Adjuvant treatment for gastric cancer: chemotherapy versus radiation. Oncologist. 2013;18(9):1013–21.

4. Schinkel AH, Jonker JW. Mammalian drug efflux transporters of the ATP binding cassette (ABC) family: an overview. Adv Drug Deliv Rev. 2003;55(1):3–29.

5. Chen Z, Shi T, Zhang L, Zhu P, Deng M, Huang C, et al. Mammalian drug efflux transporters of the ATP binding cassette (ABC) family in multidrug resistance: a review of the past decade. Cancer Lett. 2016;370(1):153–64.

6. Krishna R, Mayer LD. Multidrug resistance (MDR) in cancer. Mechanisms, reversal using modulators of MDR and the role of MDR modulators in influencing the pharmacokinetics of anticancer drugs. Eur J Pharm Sci. 2000;11(4):265–83.

7. Ding J, Miao ZH, Meng LH, Geng MY. Emerging cancer therapeutic opportunities target DNA-repair systems. Trends Pharmacol Sci. 2006;27(6):338–44.

8. Zhao Y, Butler EB, Tan M. Targeting cellular metabolism to improve cancer therapeutics. Cell Death Dis. 2013;4:e532.

9. Tan W, Zhong Z, Wang S, Liu H, Yu H, Tan R, et al. The typical metabolic modifiers conferring improvement in cancer resistance. Curr Med Chem. 2017;24(34):3698–710.

10. Al-Lazikani B, Banerji U, Workman P. Combinatorial drug therapy for cancer in the post-genomic era. Nat Biotechnol. 2012;30(7):679–92.

11. Lage H. ABC-transporters: implications on drug resistance from microorganisms to human cancers. Int J Antimicrob Agents. 2003;22(3):188–99.

12. Borowski E, Bontemps-Gracz MM, Piwkowska A. Strategies for overcoming ABC-transporters-mediated multidrug resistance (MDR) of tumor cells. Acta Biochim Pol. 2005;52(3):609–27.

13. Thomas H, Coley HM. Overcoming multidrug resistance in cancer: an update on the clinical strategy of inhibiting p-glycoprotein. Cancer Control. 2003;10(2):159–65.

14. Liang Z, Wu H, Xia J, Li Y, Zhang Y, Huang K, et al. Involvement of miR-326 in chemotherapy resistance of breast cancer through modulating expression of multidrug resistance-associated protein 1. Biochem Pharmacol. 2010;79(6):817–24.

15. Bisson C, Adams NBP, Stevenson B, Brindley AA, Polyviou D, Bibby TS, et al. The molecular basis of phosphite and hypophosphite recognition by ABC-transporters. Nat Commun. 2017;8(1):1746.

16. Natarajan K, Xie Y, Baer MR, Ross DD. Role of breast cancer resistance protein (BCRP/ABCG2) in cancer drug resistance. Biochem Pharmacol. 2012;83(8):1084–103.

17. Cao YJ, Pu ZJ, Tang YP, Shen J, Chen YY, Kang A, et al. Advances in bioactive constituents, pharmacology and clinical applications of rhubarb. Chin Med. 2017;12:36.

18. Zhang Y, Liang Y, He C. Anticancer activities and mechanisms of heat-clearing and detoxicating traditional Chinese herbal medicine. Chin Med. 2017;12:20.

19. Yang L, Wei DD, Chen Z, Wang JS, Kong LY. Reversal of multidrug resistance in human breast cancer cells by *Curcuma wenyujin* and *Chrysanthemum indicum*. Phytomedicine. 2011;18(8–9):710–8.

20. Yang L, Wei DD, Chen Z, Wang JS, Kong LY. Reversal effects of traditional Chinese herbs on multidrug resistance in cancer cells. Nat Prod Res. 2011;25(19):1885–9.

21. Labbozzetta M, Notarbartolo M, Poma P, Maurici A, Inguglia L, Marchetti P, et al. Curcumin as a possible lead compound against hormone-independent, multidrug-resistant breast cancer. Ann N Y Acad Sci. 2009;1155:278–83.

22. Hu J, Jin W, Yang PM. Reversal of resistance to adriamycin in human breast cancer cell line MCF-7/ADM by β-elemene. Zhonghua Zhong Liu Za Zhi. 2004;26(5):268–70.

23. Xie XH, Zhao H, Hu YY, Gu XD. Germacrone reverses Adriamycin resistance through cell apoptosis in multidrug-resistant breast cancer cells. Exp Ther Med. 2014;8(5):1611–5.

24. Bayat Mokhtari R, Homayouni TS, Baluch N, Morgatskaya E, Kumar S, Das B, et al. Combination therapy in combating cancer. Oncotarget. 2017;8(23):38022–43.

25. Rationalizing combination therapies. Nat Med. 2017;23(10):1113.

26. Wang S, Wang L, Shi Z, Zhong Z, Chen M, Wang Y. Evodiamine synergizes with doxorubicin in the treatment of chemoresistant human breast cancer without inhibiting P-glycoprotein. PLoS ONE. 2014;9(5):e97512.

27. Zhao Y, Yang A, Tu P, Hu Z. Anti-tumor effects of the American cockroach, *Periplaneta americana*. Chin Med. 2017;12:26.

28. Wang Z, Qi F, Cui Y, Zhao L, Sun X, Tang W, et al. An update on Chinese herbal medicines as adjuvant treatment of anticancer therapeutics. Biosci Trends. 2018;12(3):220–39.

29. Weerapreeyakul N, Machana S, Barusrux S. Synergistic effects of melphalan and *Pinus kesiya* Royle ex Gordon (*Simaosong*) extracts on apoptosis induction in human cancer cells. Chin Med. 2016;11:29.

30. Yang FQ, Li SP, Zhao J, Lao SC, Wang YT. Optimization of GC-MS conditions based on resolution and stability of analytes for simultaneous determination of nine sesquiterpenoids in three species of *Curcuma rhizomes*. J Pharm Biomed Anal. 2007;43(1):73–82.

31. Zhong ZF, Li YB, Wang SP, Tan W, Chen XP, Chen MW, et al. Furanodiene enhances tamoxifen-induced growth inhibitory activity of ERα-positive breast cancer cells in a PPARγ independent manner. J Cell Biochem. 2012;113(8):2643–51.

32. Zhong ZF, Tan W, Qiang WW, Scofield VL, Tian K, Wang CM, et al. Furanodiene alters mitochondrial function in doxorubicin-resistant MCF-7 human breast cancer cells in an AMPK-dependent manner. Mol BioSyst. 2016;12(5):1626–37.

33. Pauzi AZ, Yeap SK, Abu N, Lim KL, Omar AR, Aziz SA, et al. Combination of cisplatin and bromelain exerts synergistic cytotoxic effects against breast cancer cell line MDA-MB-231 in vitro. Chin Med. 2016;11:46.

34. Lai IC, Lai GM, Chow JM, Lee HL, Yeh CF, Li CH, et al. Active fraction (HS7) from *Taiwanofungus camphoratus* inhibits AKT-mTOR, ERK and STAT3 pathways and induces CDK inhibitors in CL1-0 human lung cancer cells. Chin Med. 2017;12:33.

35. Zhong ZF, Tan W, Wang SP, Qiang WA, Wang YT. Anti-proliferative activity and cell cycle arrest induced by evodiamine on paclitaxel-sensitive and -resistant human ovarian cancer cells. Sci Rep. 2015;5:16415.

36. Anuchapreeda S, Leechanachai P, Smith MM, Ambudkar SV, Limtrakul PN. Modulation of P-glycoprotein expression and function by curcumin in multidrug-resistant human KB cells. Biochem Pharmacol. 2002;64(4):573–82.

37. Xu HB, Li L, Fu J, Mao XP, Xu LZ. Reversion of multidrug resistance in a chemoresistant human breast cancer cell line by β-elemene. Pharmacology. 2012;89(5–6):303–12.

38. Zhong ZF, Yu HB, Wang CM, Qiang WA, Wang SP, Zhang JM, et al. Furanodiene induces extrinsic and intrinsic apoptosis in doxorubicin-resistant MCF-7 breast cancer cells via NF-κB-independent mechanism. Front Pharmacol. 2017;8:648.

39. Zhong ZF, Qiang WA, Wang CM, Tan W, Wang YT. Furanodiene enhances the anti-cancer effects of doxorubicin on ERα-negative breast cancer cells in vitro. Eur J Pharmacol. 2016;774:10–9.

16

Metabolic regulations of a decoction of *Hedyotis diffusa* in acute liver injury of mouse models

Min Dai[†], Fenglin Wang[†], Zengcheng Zou, Gemin Xiao, Hongjie Chen and Hongzhi Yang[*]

Abstract

Background: Dysfunctional metabolisms are contributed to LPS/GALN-induced hepatitis. However, whether *Hedyotis diffusa* (HD) employs metabolic strategies against hepatitis is unknown.

Methods: We use the cytokines expression, levels of serum alanine transaminase and aspartate transaminase, survival and histological analysis to measure the effect of decoction of HD on acute severe hepatitis of mouse induced by LPS/GALN. Meanwhile, we utilize GC/MS-based metabolomics to characterize the variation of metabolomes.

Results: The present study shows the relieving liver damage in HD decoction-treated mice. Metabolic category using differential metabolites indicates the lower percentage of carbohydrates in LPS/GALN + HD group than LPS/GALN group, revealing the value of carbohydrate metabolism in HD decoction-administrated mouse liver. Further pathway enrichment analysis proposes that citrate cycle, galactose metabolism, and starch and sucrose metabolism are three important carbohydrate metabolisms that involve in the protective effect of decoction of HD during acute hepatitis. Furthermore, other important enrichment pathways are biosynthesis of unsaturated fatty acids, alanine, aspartate and glutamate metabolism, and arginine and proline metabolism. Fatty acids or amino acids involved in above-mentioned pathways are also detected in high loading distribution on IC01 and IC02, thereby manifesting the significance of these metabolites. Other key metabolites detect in ICA analysis were cholesterol, lactic acid and tryptophan.

Conclusions: The variation tendency of above-mentioned metabolites is totally consistent with the protective nature of decoction of HD. These findings give a viewpoint that HD decoction-effected metabolic strategies are linked to underlying mechanisms of decoction of HD and highlight the importance of metabolic mechanisms against hepatitis.

Keywords: *Hedyotis diffusa*, Metabolomics, Carbohydrate metabolism, Hepatitis, Mouse

Background

The worldwide incidence of hepatocellular carcinoma (HCC), a major cause of human cancer death, has enhanced in recent years [1]. Hepatocyte death that drives liver disease progression from hepatitis associated with a number of liver insults, including steatosis, hepatotoxins, viral infection, and autoimmune disease, are responsible for the development of HCC [2, 3]. These liver insults are related to the subsequent development of inflammation, fibrosis, and cirrhosis. Actually, inflammation, a syndrome responsive to pathogen infection or injury, is a hallmark of liver disease that may represent a cause of HCC development [3, 4]. Therefore, it is an urgent clinical challenge to develop new therapeutic interventions through targeting hepatic inflammation, which may ultimately provide therapeutic benefit for the treatment of HCC [3].

Hedyotis diffusa, a traditional Chinese herbal medicine that belongs to the Rubiaceae family and also known as *Oldenlandia diffusa* and Bai Hua She She Cao [5], is widely spread in South of China and other Asian countries. *H. diffusa* has been largely employed

*Correspondence: Hongzhiyang1960@163.com
[†]Min Dai and Fenglin Wang contributed equally to this work
Traditional Chinese Medicine Department, The Third Affiliated Hospital of Sun Yat-sen University, Guangzhou 510630, China

in the treatments of inflammation-involved diseases, such as bronchitis, arthritis, rheumatism, appendicitis, sore throat, urethral infection, contusions, and ulcerations [6]. Accumulating evidence also proposes that *H. diffusa* is capable of controlling the liver, breast, lung, colon, brain and pancreatic cancers through promoting apoptosis of cancer cell and inhibiting tumor angiogenesis [7–11]. Moreover, the isolated splenocytes from *H. diffusa* extract-administrated leukemic mice manifest an improvement of T- and B- cell proliferation in vivo [12]. Also, *H. diffusa* addition affects the levels of cell markers (CD3, CD11b, and CD19) in white blood cell, enhances macrophage phagocytosis, and increases the cytotoxic activities of NK cells in normal Balb/c mice [13]. All above-mentioned studies show that *H. diffusa* has anti-inflammatory, anti-cancer and immunomodulatory activities. Actually, recent papers coincidentally demonstrate that inflammatory process, cancer development and progression, and immune response have strong inter-relationship with metabolism happened in host cells [14–17]. Currently, only one paper focuses on metabolic alterations of *H. diffusa* in tumor-bearing rat [18]. The underlying metabolic mechanisms related to *H. diffusa*-involved activities need to be elaborated further, and the metabolic activities of this herb in liver inflammation is unknown.

Metabolomics is a powerful new technology studying metabolic processes, identifying crucial biomarkers responsible for metabolic characteristics, and revealing metabolic mechanisms. Analysis of the key metabolites in various samples has become a meaningful part of improving the diagnosis, prognosis, and therapy of diseases [19]. Gas chromatography/mass spectrometry (GC–MS), liquid chromatography–mass spectrometry (LC–MS) and nuclear magnetic resonance (NMR) are three most common analytical technologies in metabolomics investigation [20]. While each technology has its own unique advantages and disadvantages, GC–MS is specifically becoming for the analyses of volatile compounds and thus is widely applied [21–23]. Here, we report the use of GC–MS combined with multivariate statistical tools to exploit, among the differential metabolites, key metabolites and important pathways as biomarkers capable of differentiating LPS/GALN treatment from the treatment of decoction of *H. diffusa* plus LPS/GALN in the liver metabolome.

Methods
Animals and experimental design
Adult female mice (C57BL/6, pathogen-free), weighing 24 ± 2 g from the same litters, were reared in an environmentally controlled breeding room (temperature: 20 ± 2 °C, humidity: $60 \pm 5\%$, 12 h dark/light cycle), and in cages fed with sterile water and dry pellet diets.

They were maintained in accordance with internationally accepted principles for laboratory animal use. All work was conducted in strict accordance with the recommendations in the Guide for the Care and Use of Laboratory Animals of the National Institutes of Health. The protocol was approved by the Institutional Animal Care (Animal Welfare Assurance Number: IS06). The Minimum Standards of Reporting Checklist (Additional file 1) contained details of the experimental design, and statistics, and resources used in this study.

According to the previous study [24], murine model of acute hepatitis was induced by combined injection of LPS (50 g/kg) and D-GALN (1.2 g/kg). Mice were randomly separated into 3 groups ($n = 26$ per group). The control and model groups were injected intraperitoneally with 200 μL of saline twice a day [6]; the treatment group received the 200 μL of decoction of *H. diffusa* (5 g/kg) twice a day [6]. Three days after injection, the mice in both model and treatment groups were challenged intraperitoneally by LPS/GALN. Twelve hours later, six mice in each group were euthanized by decapitation, and blood and livers were collected for following studies. The remaining 20 mice in each group were observed for 20 days to examine their survival.

Preparation of a decoction of *H. diffusa*
According the previous procedure [5], 100 g of dried *H. diffusa* were cut into 1–1.5 mm pieces and crushed using a mortar and pestle, and then boiled with 1 L of deionised water for 1 h. After cooling, the decoction was centrifuged at 3000 rpm for 20 min, and filtered through a 0.45 μm filter. The filtrate was evaporated in vacuum (EYELA N-1001, Tokyo, Japan) and a dry residue was recovered. Finally, the total residue was reconstituted in saline and the final volume of extract is 100 mL (equal to 1.0 g raw material/mL).

Histology analysis
The liver sample was fixed in 4% paraformaldehyde overnight at room temperature, then embedded in paraffin, sliced into 5-μm sections. For histological analysis, paraffin sections were stained with hematoxylin and eosin (H&E). The morphologic criteria used to determine the degree of necrosis included portal inflammation, hepatocellular necrosis, inflammatory cell infiltration, and loss of cell architecture. The pathological changes were evaluated in nonconsecutive, randomly chosen 200× histological fields.

Quantitative RT-PCR assay
For quantitative RT-PCR assay, RNA was isolated from mouse livers using the TRIzol reagent according to the manufacturer's instructions. 2 μg of total RNA was

provided to generate the first-strand cDNAs by using commercially available kits (Applied Biosystems). All subsequent PCR reactions were carried out using the 7 Universal PCR Master Mix (Applied Biosystems). PCR primers of mouse CXCL1 were 5′-TCGTCTTTCAT-ATTGTATGGTCAAC-3′ and 5′-CGAGACGAGAC-CAGGAGAAA C-3′. The primers for mouse TNFα were 5′-CATCTTCTAAAATTCGAGTGACAA-3′ and 5′-TGGGAGTAGACAAGGTACAACCC-3′. The real-time PCR primers for mouse IL-1β were 5′-ACA-GATGAAGTGCTCCTTCCA-3′ and 5′-GTCGGAGA-TTCGTAGCTGGAT-3′. The real-time PCR primers for mouse MIP-2 were 5′-CCCCCTGGTTCAGAAAAT-CATC-3′ and 5′-AACTCTCAGACAGCGAGGCA-CATC-3′. The primers for the mouse housekeeping gene GAPDH were 5′-TTCACCACCATGGAGAAGGC-3′ and 5′-GGCATGGACTGTGGTCATGA-3′ and were used as a control.

Measurement of cytokines in liver
Concentrations of TNF-α, IL-1β, IL-6, and MCP-1 in liver were measured through mouse-specific enzyme-linked immunosorbent assay (ELISA) kits (NeoBioscience, Shenzhen, China). Each analysis was carried out according to the manufacturer's instruction, and the concentrations of cytokines were determined according to the standard curves.

Measurement of serum alanine transaminase and aspartate transaminase activities
Blood samples were centrifuged at 1500g for 20 min at 4 °C, and alanine transaminase (ALT) and aspartate transaminase (AST) activities in serum were measured by commercial kits from Randox Laboratories (UK).

Extraction of metabolites in mouse liver
For the metabolomics investigation, the extraction of total metabolites in mouse liver was performed according a procedure described previously [25]. Briefly, 1 g of liver tissue was homogenized and dissolved for 1 min in 1 mL of methanol at 4 °C. The homogenates were centrifuged at 12,000×g for 10 min at 4 °C. 300 μL of supernatant was transferred to a GC sampling vial containing ribitol (10 μL, 0.1 mg/mL), an internal standard, and then dried in a vacuum centrifuge concentrator before the subsequent derivatization.

Derivatization and GC–MS analysis
Prior to GC–MS analysis, deriving liver samples was required. After drying samples, 80 μL of methoxamine/pyridine hydrochloride (20 mg/mL) was added to induce oximation for 1.5 h at 37 °C and then 80 μL of MSTFA, a derivatization reagent (Sigma), was mixed and reacted

with the liver sample for additional 0.5 h at 37 °C. By centrifuging, 1 μL of supernatant derivative was added to a tube and analyzed using GC–MS (Trace DSQ II, Thermo Scientific). The separation conditions of GC–MS consisted of an initial temperature of 70 °C (5 min) with a uniform increase to 270 °C at a speed of 2 °C/min (5 min); 0.5 μL sample volume, splitless injection; injection temperature, 270 °C; interface temperature, 270 °C; ion source (EI) temperature, 30 °C; ionization voltage, 70 eV; quadrupole temperature, 150 °C; carrier gas, highly pure helium; velocity, 1.0 mL/min; and full scan way, 60–600 m/z.

Statistical and bioinformatics analysis
The data of liver metabolome were collected using Thermo Foundation 1.0.1. The sum abundance value was employed for normalizing the resulting data matrix, and then the computed abundance of metabolites was centered for each tissue sample on their median value and scaled by their inter-quartile range (IQR) to decline between-sample variation [25, 26]. The significant analysis of microarray (SAM), a permutation-based hypothesis testing method for the analysis of proteomic and metabolomic data [27, 28], was applied to analyze the differential metabolites. Independent component analysis (ICA) was chosen as the pattern recognition method [29]. Statistical significance between groups was determined with the unpaired two-tailed Student t test. All data were analyzed by Prism (GraphPad Software, Inc.), and P values less than 0.05 and 0.01 were deemed as two significant levels.

Results
Decoction of *H. diffusa* (HD) attenuates the acute inflammation in hepatitis mouse
Normally, the most important criterion in evaluating a potential drug against hepatitis is its efficacy in vivo. Thus, we employed a hepatitis mouse model reported previously and revealed the potential effect of decoction of *H. diffusa* (HD) on acute inflammation. In brief, decoction of HD or saline control was injected into C57BL/6 mice 3 days and LPS/GALN was applied subsequently to induce the liver damage. Firstly, the mRNA levels of CXCL1, TNFα, IL-1β and MIP-2 gene, and productions of vital cytokines in liver were measured (Fig. 1a, b). Injection of LPS/GALN caused a significant elevation in the mRNA levels of CXCL1, TNFα, IL-1β and MIP-2 gene, and increased the secretions of TNFα, IL-1β, IL-6 and MCP-1 in mouse liver. The administration of decoction of HD (5 g/kg) had an ability to decrease the mRNA levels of these genes and production of these cytokines. Furthermore, the levels of alanine transaminase and aspartate transaminase were also reduced in serum of HD decoction-treated mice (Fig. 1c, d). By using survival

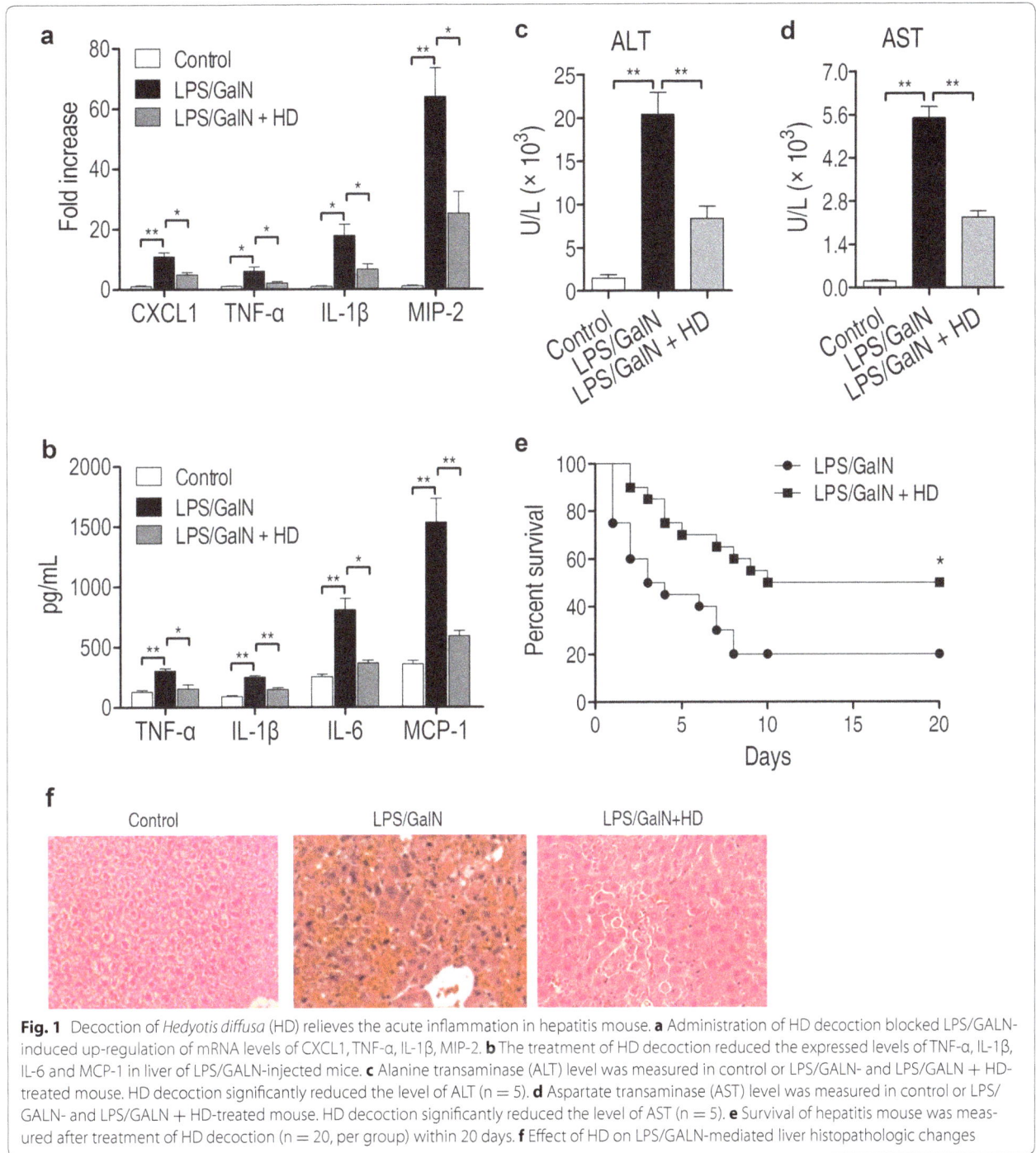

Fig. 1 Decoction of *Hedyotis diffusa* (HD) relieves the acute inflammation in hepatitis mouse. **a** Administration of HD decoction blocked LPS/GALN-induced up-regulation of mRNA levels of CXCL1, TNF-α, IL-1β, MIP-2. **b** The treatment of HD decoction reduced the expressed levels of TNF-α, IL-1β, IL-6 and MCP-1 in liver of LPS/GALN-injected mice. **c** Alanine transaminase (ALT) level was measured in control or LPS/GALN- and LPS/GALN + HD-treated mouse. HD decoction significantly reduced the level of ALT (n = 5). **d** Aspartate transaminase (AST) level was measured in control or LPS/GALN- and LPS/GALN + HD-treated mouse. HD decoction significantly reduced the level of AST (n = 5). **e** Survival of hepatitis mouse was measured after treatment of HD decoction (n = 20, per group) within 20 days. **f** Effect of HD on LPS/GALN-mediated liver histopathologic changes

analysis, we found that LPS/GALN led to rapid death of animals as early as 24 h after injection (Fig. 1e). Importantly, the application of decoction of HD delayed the incidence of death and increased the survival rate by two-folds, when compared with the saline control (Fig. 1e). The histological analysis of mouse liver in the control group indicated normal liver lobular architecture and

cell structure (Fig. 1f). However, livers exposed to GalN/LPS presented numerous and extensive areas of portal inflammation and cellular necrosis and a significant increase in inflammatory cell infiltration. These changes were rescued by the application of decoction of HD (5 g/kg). Taken together, these data suggest that decoction of

HD is an efficient Chinese Medicine that attenuates LPS/GALN-induced liver inflammation in vivo.

Metabolomic profiling of mouse liver

To identify the vital metabolic pathways and important metabolites that acted the helpful effect of decoction of HD on mouse hepatitis, GC–MS was employed to quantitatively evaluate the level of known metabolites in mouse livers which were obtained from six individuals each group. Typical total ion current chromatograms (TIC) were presented in Fig. 2a. 73 metabolites with dependable signal were found each sample. The correlation coefficient of two technical repeats revealed the reliability of the detection technology (Fig. 2b). The category showed that 49.32, 17.81, 31.51 and 1.37% of metabolites belonged to carbon sources, amino acids, lipids and

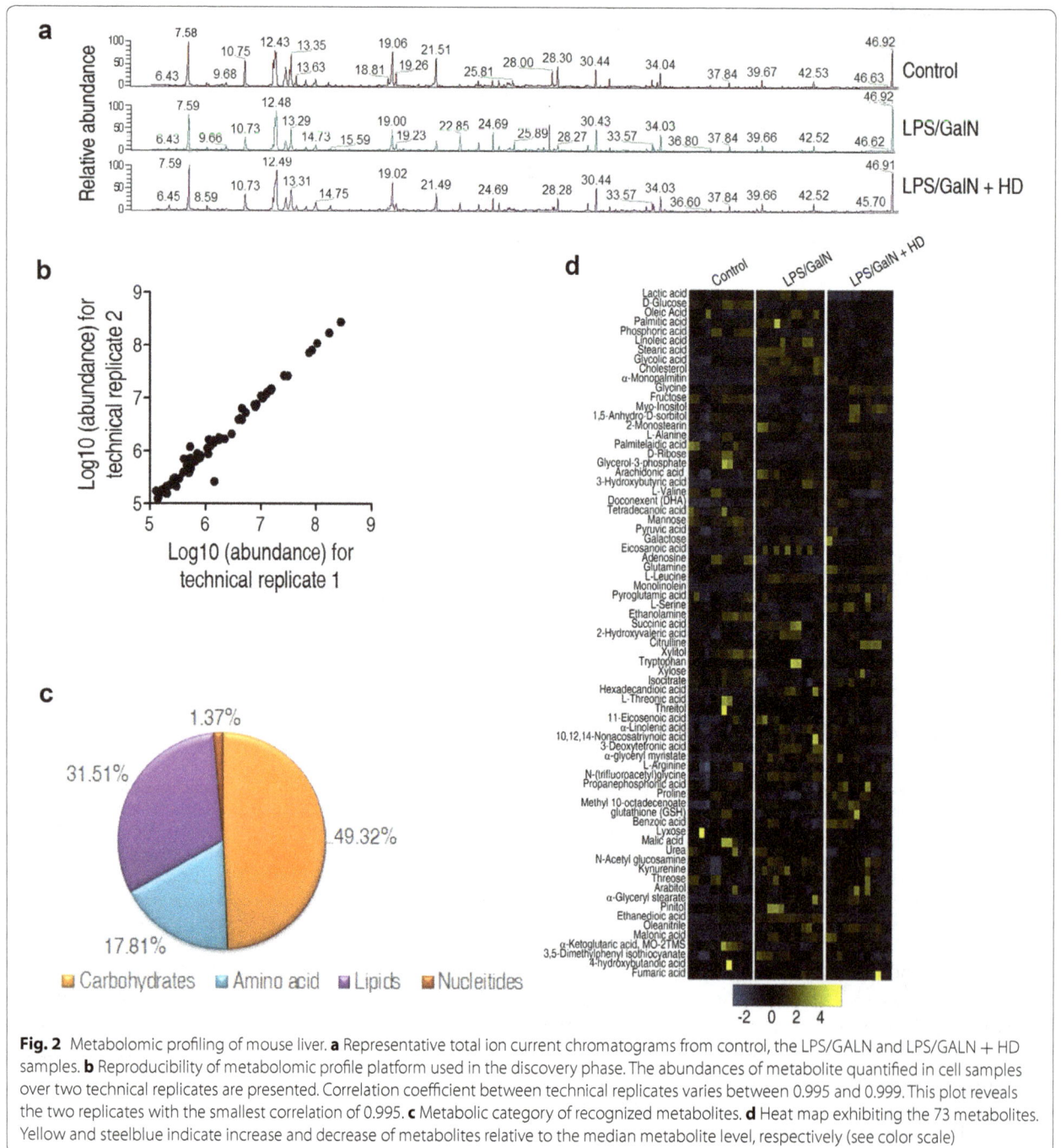

Fig. 2 Metabolomic profiling of mouse liver. **a** Representative total ion current chromatograms from control, the LPS/GALN and LPS/GALN + HD samples. **b** Reproducibility of metabolomic profile platform used in the discovery phase. The abundances of metabolite quantified in cell samples over two technical replicates are presented. Correlation coefficient between technical replicates varies between 0.995 and 0.999. This plot reveals the two replicates with the smallest correlation of 0.995. **c** Metabolic category of recognized metabolites. **d** Heat map exhibiting the 73 metabolites. Yellow and steelblue indicate increase and decrease of metabolites relative to the median metabolite level, respectively (see color scale)

nucleotides, respectively (Fig. 2c). Heat map showed the abundance of the metabolites, which came from the three groups (Fig. 2d). These data indicated that a carbohydrates-, amino acids- and lipids-dominant metabolome of mouse liver is developed. The metabolome varied among the three groups, suggesting an association between the metabolomics responses and degree of liver damage.

Decoction of HD varied the metabolomic profiling of liver in LPS/GALN-injected mice

To further investigate a changed metabolome identifying the LPS/GALN + HD group from the LPS/GALN group, a two-sided Wilcoxon rank-sum test coupled with a permutation test was applied to detect differential metabolites. Fifty-four (73.97%) and forty (54.79%) metabolites out of the 73 metabolites were differential at $P < 0.05$ in LPS/GALN and LPS/GALN + HD group (Fig. 3a),

respectively. Z value based on the control group was calculated for comparative study. Z score plot showed that it spanned from -25.41 to 66.78 in LPS/GALN group and from -15.61 to 55.21 in LPS/GALN + HD group (Fig. 3b). Higher varied abundances of metabolites were found in the LPS/GALN group than in the LPS/GALN + HD group. Notably, 20 metabolites down-regulated and 34 metabolites were up-regulated in the LPS/GALN group, while 14 were metabolites decreased and 26 metabolites increased in the LPS/GALN + HD group (Additional file 2).

Metabolic categories of these differential metabolites in abundance were explored further. They presented analogous varying percentage in the two groups, ranking lipids > carbohydrates > amino acids > nucleotides, but relative higher percentage of lipids and amino acid, and lower carbohydrates were discovered in the LPS/GALN + HD than the LPS/GALN groups (Fig. 3c).

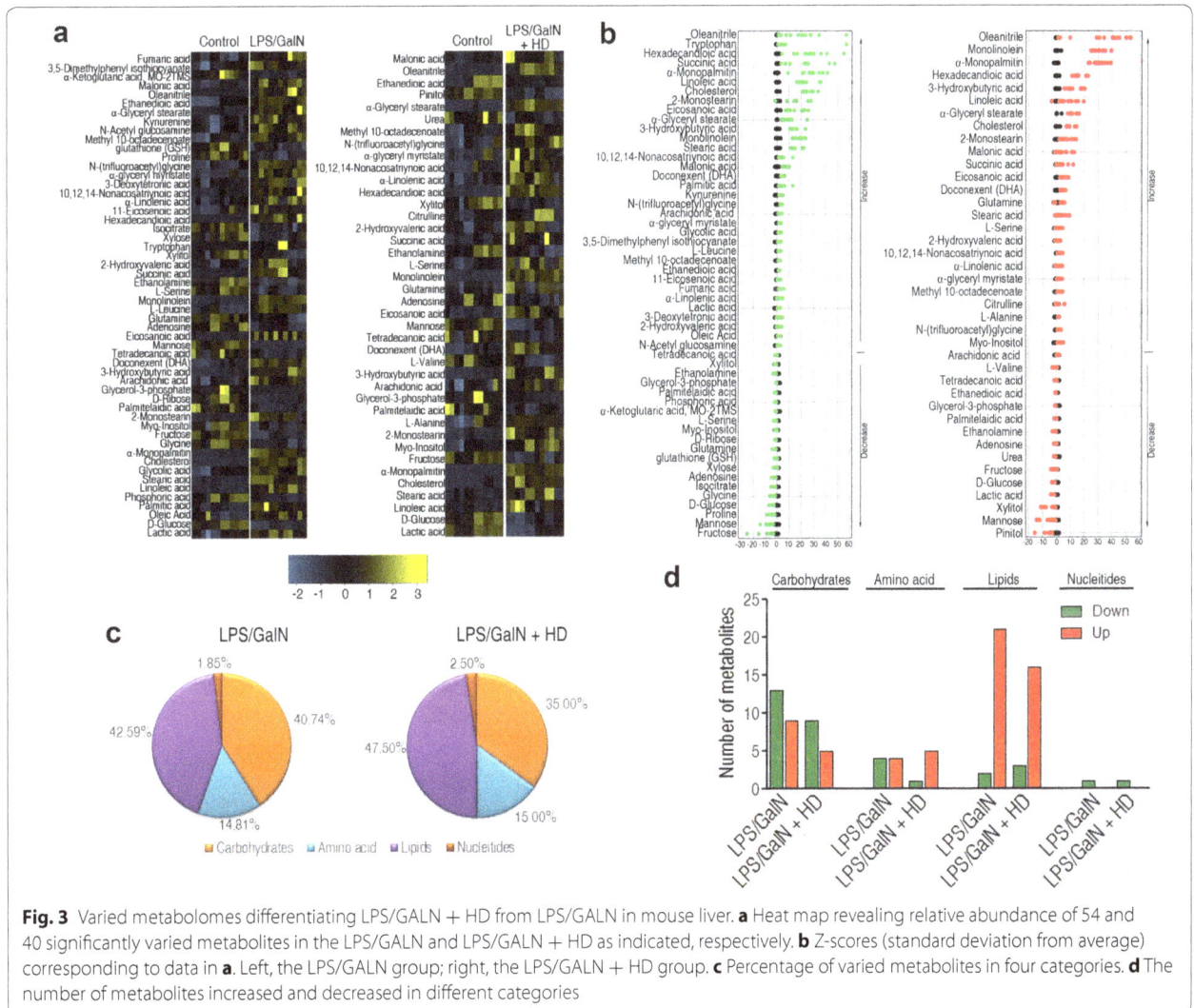

Fig. 3 Varied metabolomes differentiating LPS/GALN + HD from LPS/GALN in mouse liver. **a** Heat map revealing relative abundance of 54 and 40 significantly varied metabolites in the LPS/GALN and LPS/GALN + HD as indicated, respectively. **b** Z-scores (standard deviation from average) corresponding to data in **a**. Left, the LPS/GALN group; right, the LPS/GALN + HD group. **c** Percentage of varied metabolites in four categories. **d** The number of metabolites increased and decreased in different categories

Figure 3d visualized the numbers of up-regulated and down-regulated metabolites in these categories. HD reduced the numbers of up-regulated and down-regulated carbohydrates caused by LPS/GALN, and up-regulated lipids and down-regulated amino acid in LPS/GALN group were declined after HD administration. These data reveal that decoction of HD might provide a helpful response through a change in metabolome.

Differential enriched pathways responsible for the helpful response induced by HD

To further investigate which pathways were enriched and what difference of the enriched pathways were detected between LPS/GALN and LPS/GALN + HD groups, an online tool, Metaboanalyst 3.0 was utilized. Shared and differential enriched pathways between them were showed in Fig. 4a. Three shared pathways were biosynthesis of unsaturated fatty acids, alanine, aspartate and glutamate metabolism, and galactose metabolism. Specifically, biosynthesis of unsaturated fatty acids was a pathway that had the lowest *P* value in both LPS/GALN and LPS/GALN + HD groups. Besides that, arginine and proline metabolism, and starch and sucrose metabolism were enriched only in LPS/GALN + HD group, and cyanoamino acid metabolism, citrate cycle and, nitrogen metabolism, and fatty acid biosynthesis were enriched only in LPS/GALN group.

Among these pathway, two were uniquely related to the relief of liver damage, which were arginine and proline metabolism, and starch and sucrose metabolism (Fig. 4b). Metabolites enriched in the starch and sucrose metabolism were all decreased. Although all metabolites enriched in biosynthesis of unsaturated fatty acids had higher abundance in LPS/GALN and LPS/GALN + HD groups in contrast to control group, abundance of most metabolites in LPS/GALN + HD group were lower than LPS/GALN group. In other words, HD was capable of reducing the abundance of these up-regulated metabolites enriched in biosynthesis of unsaturated fatty acids in LPS/GALN-treated liver. These metabolites included

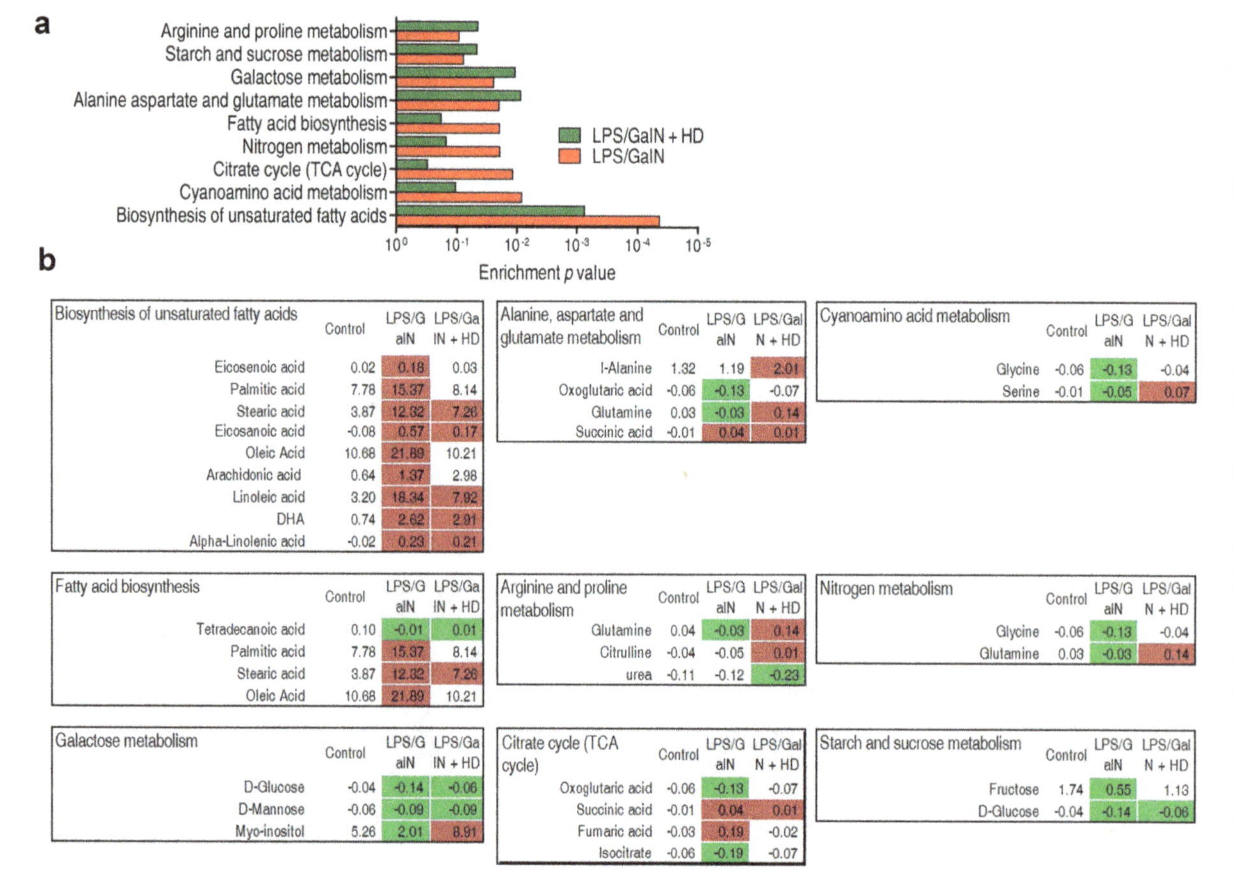

Fig. 4 Pathway analysis and integrative analysis. **a** Pathway enrichment analysis of differential metabolites form LPS/GALN and LPS/GALN + HD using an online tool, Metaboanalyst 3.0 (http://www.metaboanalyst.ca/). Significantly enriched pathways are selected to plot. **b** Integrative analysis of metabolites in significantly enriched pathways. Up-regulation and down-regulation of metabolites are indicated as red and green, respectively. The number reveals the ratio of differential metabolites

eicosenoic acid, palmitic acid, stearic acid, eicosanoic acid, oleic acid, arachidonic acid and linoleic acid. More importantly, some of metabolites in alanine, aspartate and glutamate metabolism, arginine and proline metabolism, and galactose metabolism were reversal between LPS/GALN and LPS/GALN + HD groups. These metabolites included glutamine and myo-inositol, and were all declined in LPS/GALN group and augmented in LPS/ GALN + HD group. Besides, L-alanine enriched in alanine, aspartate and glutamate metabolism and citrulline enriched in arginine and proline metabolism was only boosted, and urea enriched in arginine and proline metabolism was only reduced in LPS/GALN + HD group. Moreover, three of four metabolites (oxoglutaric acid, fumaric acid and isocitrate), which were enriched in citrate cycle and showed higher abundance in LPS/GALN group, had the similar metabolic levels between control and LPS/GALN + HD groups. Meanwhile, remaining metabolite, succinic acid, had a lower abundance in LPS/ GALN + HD group, when compared to the LPS/GALN group. Collectively, these results indicated that biosynthesis of unsaturated fatty acids, alanine, aspartate and glutamate metabolism, arginine and proline metabolism and citrate cycle might be significantly related to the HD decoction-induced benefit for hepatitis mouse.

Identification of crucial metabolites using ICA analysis

ICA was an available and alternative application to be designed to recognize the sample pattern. As shown in Fig. 5a, control group and LPS/GALN group was separated obviously on IC01, and IC02 depicted the obvious differentiation between LPS/GALN and LPS/ GALN + HD groups. Because of a clear sample discrimination by ICA in Fig. 5a, it was possible to detect the significant metabolites differentiating LPS/GALN and LPS/ GALN + HD. In Fig. 5b, the loadings of different independent component IC01 and IC02 were visualized in a heat map. Ranking of the varied metabolites displayed that 25 metabolites (blue boxes in Fig. 5b) have the largest loading in IC01 and IC02.

Out of these metabolites, D-glucose, fructose, palmitic acid, stearic acid, oleic acid, glycine, L-alanine, myo-inositol, succinic acid, arachidonic acid, eicosanoic acid, DHA, 3-hydroxybutyric acid and linoleic acid were the shared significant metabolites found in above pathway enrichment analysis, while others were the new crucial metabolites detected in ICA analysis. More interestingly, only tryptophan, lactic acid and cholesterol were differentiated significantly between control and LPS/ GALN group, as well as between LPS/GALN and LPS/ GALN + HD group (Fig. 5c).

Discussion

The latest new in anticancer study suggests that *H. diffusa* treatment is capable of reducing the injury caused by Walker 256 tumor and maintaining a metabolic balance [18]. In addition, recent evidence reveals that the dysfunctional metabolisms are responsible for LPS/D/ GALN-induced acute hepatitis [30, 31]. However, it is unknown that whether HD may protect host against LPS/D/GALN-induced liver damage through mounting metabolic strategy. Therefore, in the present study, we focus on the examination of metabolic response of HD decoction-pretreated acute hepatitis through using GC/MS-based metabolomic. Our study not only reveals that metabolic response is likely linked to the degree of LPS/D/GALN-induced acute hepatitis through overall understanding the metabolomes among control, LPS/D/ GALN and LPS/D/GALN + HD groups, but also detects some crucial pathways and key metabolites (Fig. 6).

The finding of current metabolic category shows that LPS/D/GALN + HD have a lower percentage of carbohydrates than LPS/GALN group (Fig. 3c, d), subsequent pathway enrichment analysis further make clear that citrate cycle, galactose metabolism, and starch and sucrose metabolism are able to be involved in the metabolic activities of HD. Among these, citrate cycle is more striking because two metabolites (oxoglutaric acid and isocitrate) are down-regulated but others (succinic acid and fumaric acid) are up-regulated after LPS/GALN treatment (Fig. 6). Consistent with this, previous study show the down-regulation of isocitrate, and up-regulation of succinic acid and fumaric acid in LPS-treated mice [32]. In fact, recent papers demonstrate that LPS stimulates a profound metabolic transition to aerobic glycolysis through phosphatidyl inositol 3′-kinase/Akt pathway and inhibits mitochondrial oxidative phosphorylation, an action that have an indispensable connection with citrate cycle [33, 34]. Succinic acid is an inflammatory signal that activate IL-1β through stabilizing the hypoxia-inducible factor-1α (HIF-1α) [32]. Similarly, fumaric acid also have a function in HIF stability and fumaric acid up-regulation can be recognized as a tumor-promoting event [35]. Given that the lower abundance of succinic acid and fumaric acid are found in LPS/D/GALN + HD group than that in LPS/D/GALN group, thus a becoming possibility is that modulation of succinic acid and fumaric acid concentrations and following HIF-dependent cytokine production partly explains how decoction of HD possesses strong host protection in liver damage. Other interesting carbohydrates are D-glucose and myo-inositol enriched by pathway analysis (Fig. 4b), and lactic acid detected by ICA analysis (Fig. 5c). In patients, glucose metabolism is abnormal when the liver cell damage occurs [36], and the higher level of lactic acid

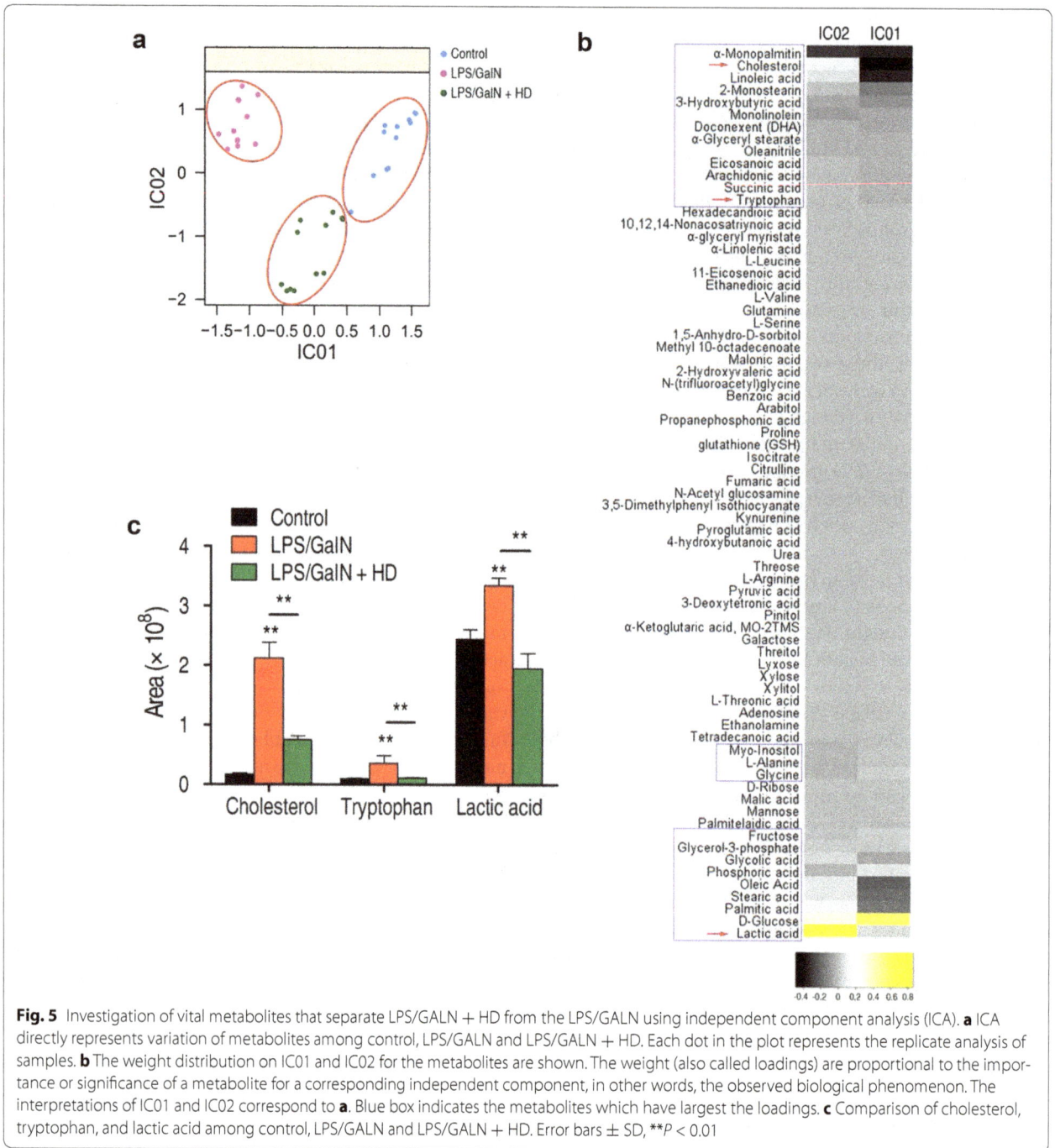

Fig. 5 Investigation of vital metabolites that separate LPS/GALN + HD from the LPS/GALN using independent component analysis (ICA). **a** ICA directly represents variation of metabolites among control, LPS/GALN and LPS/GALN + HD. Each dot in the plot represents the replicate analysis of samples. **b** The weight distribution on IC01 and IC02 for the metabolites are shown. The weight (also called loadings) are proportional to the importance or significance of a metabolite for a corresponding independent component, in other words, the observed biological phenomenon. The interpretations of IC01 and IC02 correspond to **a**. Blue box indicates the metabolites which have largest the loadings. **c** Comparison of cholesterol, tryptophan, and lactic acid among control, LPS/GALN and LPS/GALN + HD. Error bars ± SD, **$P < 0.01$

in LPS/GALN group can be explained by the acceleration of aerobic glycolysis [33, 34]. After HD decoction treatment, the abundance of D-glucose and lactic acid is almost equal to the control group, indicating that maintaining the normal glucose metabolism and glycolysis is the potential metabolic mechanisms to relieve the acute hepatitis. It has been reported that myo-inositol plays an important role in immunity system [25, 37]. However, the

detailed meaning of myo-inositol elevated by decoction of HD still needs to be studied in future.

Combining current pathway enrichment analysis with ICA analysis, the shared lipid-related metabolites are palmitic acid (PA), stearic acid (SA), oleic acid (OA), linoleic acid (LA), eicosanoic acid (EA) and arachidonic acid (AA). We know that PA (16:0), stearic acid (18:0), OA (18:1) and LA (18:2) are capable of stimulating TLR4

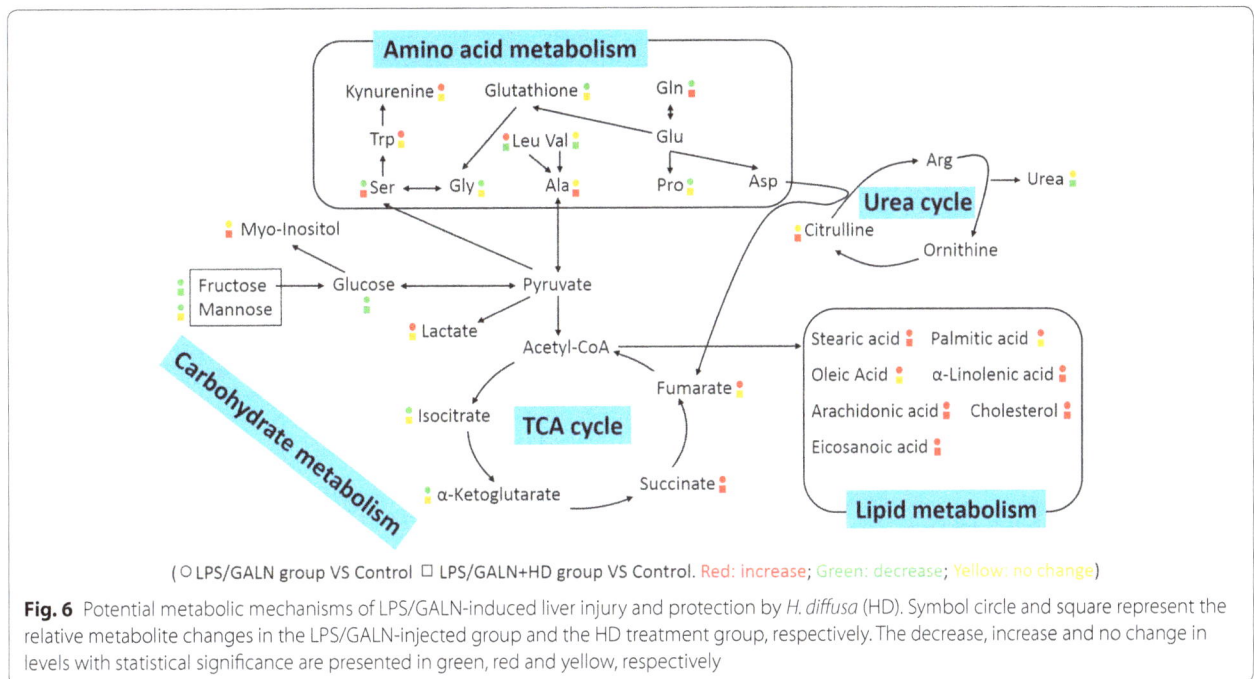

Fig. 6 Potential metabolic mechanisms of LPS/GALN-induced liver injury and protection by *H. diffusa* (HD). Symbol circle and square represent the relative metabolite changes in the LPS/GALN-injected group and the HD treatment group, respectively. The decrease, increase and no change in levels with statistical significance are presented in green, red and yellow, respectively

signaling to produce an inflammatory response [38], which may eventually contribute to acute severe hepatitis [39]. Other lipid-related metabolites are AA and cholesterol, which also have an excellent action in inducing the severe inflammation [40]. These metabolites were up-regulated by LPS/GALN treatment but decoction of HD down-regulated these metabolites, indicating that decoction of HD has an anti-inflammatory action through declining the abundance of lipids including PA, SA, OA, LA, AA and cholesterol (Fig. 6).

For amino acid metabolisms, alanine, aspartate and glutamate metabolism, and arginine and proline metabolism, cyanoamino acid metabolism, and nitrogen metabolism are enriched by pathway analysis. In these pathway, L-alanine, L-glutamine, citrulline, glycine and serine are involved (Fig. 6). L-Alanine, a significant energy substrate for cell, is beneficial for supporting gluconeogensis and leucocyte metabolism through unknown mechanism [41]. L-Glutamine is known to support the anti-inflammatory response through various signal pathways [42–44]. Serine and glycine are two potent antioxidants that scavenge free radicals, thereby playing an essential role in anti-oxidative defense of liver cell [45, 46]. There is also in vivo evidence that glycine blunts the production of TNFα and reduces inflammatory reactions [47, 48]. When compared to the LPS/GALN group, the boosted level of L-alanine, L-glutamine, glycine and serine found in LPS/GALN + HD group indicates that the high level of these amino acids is benefit for the alleviation of acute severe hepatitis. Citrulline and nitric oxide (NO)

are produced by the metabolic response of L-arginine through NO synthase (NOS) and L-arginine also can generate urea and ornithine through arginase [23, 49]. The boosted citrulline and declined urea in LPS/GALN + HD revealed that NO may be involved in the protective effect of HD decoction on acute severe hepatitis, which certainly requires to be determined in further investigation. In addition, tryptophan is a high loading in differentiating LPS/GALN + HD from LPS/GALN. Tryptophan metabolism is increased during inflammation or stimulation by LPS or certain cytokines [50]. Most of tryptophan in mammals is oxidized along kynurenine pathway and kynurenine promotes carcinogenesis by acting on the aryl hydrocarbon receptor [51]. Thus inhibiting tryptophan metabolism is a possible metabolic mechanisms for HD decoction-induced protection.

Conclusions

The current study uses GC/MS-based metabolomics to characterize variation of metabolomes in response to LPS/GALN and HD decoction treatment before LPS/GALN. Metabolic category using differential metabolites showed the lower percentage of carbohydrate in LPS/GALN + HD group than LPS/GALN group, revealing that carbohydrates metabolism may play an important role in HD-treated mice to combat liver damage. Subsequent pathway enrichment analysis further find out that citrate cycle, galactose metabolism, and starch and sucrose metabolism are three important carbohydrate metabolisms that involve in the protective effect of decoction of HD during acute severe hepatitis. Thus, these findings provide a viewpoint that underlying mechanisms of decoction of HD are connected to the metabolic strategies and highlight the value of metabolic strategies against hepatitis.

Authors' contributions
Designed the experiments: HZY, MD, FLW. Performed the experiments: MD, FLW, ZCZ, GMX. Analyzed the data: MD, FLW, ZCZ, HJC. Wrote the paper: MD, FLW, HZY. All authors read and approved the final manuscript.

Acknowledgements
Not applicable.

Competing interests
The authors declare that they have no competing interests

Consent for publication
Not applicable.

Funding
This work was sponsored by Grants from State Administration of Traditional Chinese Medicine (JDZX2015173).

References
1. Fitzmorris P, Shoreibah M, Anand B, Singal A. Management of hepatocellular carcinoma. J Cancer Res Clin Oncol. 2015;141:861.
2. Luedde T, Kaplowitz N, Schwabe RF. Cell death and cell death responses in liver disease: mechanisms and clinical relevance. Gastroenterology. 2014;147(765–83):e4.
3. Han MS, Barrett T, Brehm MA, Davis RJ. Inflammation mediated by JNK in myeloid cells promotes the development of hepatitis and hepatocellular carcinoma. Cell Rep. 2016;15:19–26.
4. Sun B, Karin M. Inflammation and liver tumorigenesis. Front Med. 2013;7:242–54.
5. Ganbold M, Barker J, Ma R, Jones L, Carew M. Cytotoxicity and bioavailability studies on a decoction of *Oldenlandia diffusa* and its fractions separated by HPLC. J Ethnopharmacol. 2010;131:396–403.
6. Ye JH, Liu MH, Zhang XL, He JY. Chemical profiles and protective effect of *Hedyotis diffusa* Willd in lipopolysaccharide-induced renal inflammation mice. Int J Mol Sci. 2015;16:27252–69.
7. Niu Y, Meng QX. Chemical and preclinical studies on *Hedyotis diffusa* with anticancer potential. J Asian Nat Prod Res. 2013;15:550–65.
8. Ahmad R, Shaari K, Lajis NH, Hamzah AS, Ismail NH, Kitajima M. Anthraquinones from *Hedyotis capitellata*. Phytochemistry. 2005;66:1141–7.
9. Li C, Xue X, Zhou D, Zhang F, Xu Q, Ren L, et al. Analysis of iridoid glucosides in *Hedyotis diffusa* by high-performance liquid chromatography/electrospray ionization tandem mass spectrometry. J Pharm Biomed Anal. 2008;48:205–11.
10. Lin J, Chen Y, Wei L, Chen X, Xu W, Hong Z, et al. *Hedyotis diffusa* Willd extract induces apoptosis via activation of the mitochondrion-dependent pathway in human colon carcinoma cells. Int J Oncol. 2010;37:1331–8.
11. Lin J, Wei L, Xu W, Hong Z, Liu X, Peng J. Effect of *Hedyotis diffusa* Willd extract on tumor angiogenesis. Mol Med Rep. 2011;4:1283–8.
12. Lin CC, Kuo CL, Lee MH, Hsu SC, Huang AC, Tang NY, et al. Extract of *Hedyotis diffusa* Willd influences murine leukemia WEHI-3 cells in vivo as well as promoting T-and B-cell proliferation in leukemic mice. In Vivo. 2011;25:633–40.
13. Kuo YJ, Lin JP, Hsiao YT, Chou GL, Tsai YH, Chiang SY, et al. Ethanol extract of *Hedyotis diffusa* Willd affects immune responses in normal Balb/c mice in vivo. In Vivo. 2015;29:453–60.
14. Hotamisligil GS. Inflammation and metabolic disorders. Nature. 2006;444:860–7.
15. Chawla A, Nguyen KD, Goh YS. Macrophage-mediated inflammation in metabolic disease. Nat Rev Immunol. 2011;11:738–49.
16. Cairns RA, Harris IS, Mak TW. Regulation of cancer cell metabolism. Nat Rev Cancer. 2011;11:85–95.
17. Pearce EL, Poffenberger MC, Chang C-H, Jones RG. Fueling immunity: insights into metabolism and lymphocyte function. Science. 2013;342:1242454.
18. Wang Z, Gao K, Xu C, Gao J, Yan Y, Wang Y, et al. Metabolic effects of *Hedyotis diffusa* on rats bearing Walker 256 tumor revealed by NMR-based metabolomics. Magn Reson Chem. 2017;56:5–17.
19. Sun H, Zhang A, Yan G, Piao C, Li W, Sun C, et al. Metabolomic analysis of key regulatory metabolites in hepatitis C virus–infected tree shrews. Mol Cell Proteom. 2013;12:710–9.
20. Kuehnbaum NL, Britz-McKibbin P. New advances in separation science for metabolomics: resolving chemical diversity in a post-genomic era. Chem Rev. 2013;113:2437–68.
21. Besada C, Sanchez G, Salvador A, Granell A. Volatile compounds associated to the loss of astringency in persimmon fruit revealed by untargeted GC–MS analysis. Metabolomics. 2013;9:157–72.
22. Fiehn O. Extending the breadth of metabolite profiling by gas chromatography coupled to mass spectrometry. Trends Analyt Chem. 2008;27:261–9.
23. Chen XH, Liu SR, Peng B, Li D, Cheng ZX, Zhu JX, et al. Exogenous L-valine promotes phagocytosis to kill multidrug-resistant bacterial pathogens. Front Immunol. 2017;8:207.
24. Ma L, Gong H, Zhu H, Ji Q, Su P, Liu P, et al. A novel small-molecule tumor necrosis factor α inhibitor attenuates inflammation in a hepatitis mouse model. J Biol Chem. 2014;289:12457–66.
25. Chen XH, Zhang BW, Li H, Peng XX. Myo-inositol improves the host's ability to eliminate balofloxacin-resistant *Escherichia coli*. Sci Rep. 2015;5:10720.
26. Sreekumar A, Poisson LM, Rajendiran TM, Khan AP, Cao Q, Yu J, et al. Metabolomic profiles delineate potential role for sarcosine in prostate cancer progression. Nature. 2009;457:910–4.
27. Amathieu R, Nahon P, Triba M, Bouchemal N, Trinchet JC, Beaugrand M, et al. Metabolomic approach by 1H NMR spectroscopy of serum for the assessment of chronic liver failure in patients with cirrhosis. J Proteome Res. 2011;10:3239–45.
28. Naccarato WF, Ray RE, Wells WW. Biosynthesis of myo-inositol in rat mammary gland. Isolation and properties of the enzymes. Arch Biochem Biophys. 1974;164:194–201.
29. Wienkoop S, Morgenthal K, Wolschin F, Scholz M, Selbig J, Weckwerth W. Integration of metabolomic and proteomic phenotypes analysis of data covariance dissects starch and RFO metabolism from low and high temperature compensation response in *Arabidopsis thaliana*. Mol Cell Proteom. 2008;7:1725–36.
30. Kim SJ, Chung WS, Kim SS, Ko SG, Um JY. Antiinflammatory effect of *Oldenlandia diffusa* and its constituent, hentriacontane, through suppression of caspase-1 activation in mouse peritoneal macrophages. Phytother Res. 2011;25:1537–46.
31. Chou TW, Feng JH, Huang CC, Cheng YW, Chien SC, Wang SY, et al. A plant kavalactone desmethoxyyangonin prevents inflammation and fulminant hepatitis in mice. PLoS ONE. 2013;8:e77626.
32. Tannahill GM, Curtis AM, Adamik J, Palsson-McDermott EM, McGettrick AF, Goel G, et al. Succinate is an inflammatory signal that induces IL-1β through HIF-1α. Nature. 2013;496:238–42.
33. Krawczyk CM, Holowka T, Sun J, Blagih J, Amiel E, DeBerardinis RJ, et al. Toll-like receptor–induced changes in glycolytic metabolism regulate dendritic cell activation. Blood. 2010;115:4742–9.

34. Cheng SC, Joosten LA, Netea MG. The interplay between central metabolism and innate immune responses. Cytokine Growth Factor Rev. 2014;25:707–13.

35. Isaacs JS, Jung YJ, Mole DR, Lee S, Torres-Cabala C, Chung YL, et al. HIF overexpression correlates with biallelic loss of fumarate hydratase in renal cancer: novel role of fumarate in regulation of HIF stability. Cancer Cell. 2005;8:143–53.

36. Guo CH, Sun TT, Weng XD, Zhang JC, Chen JX, Deng GJ. The investigation of glucose metabolism and insulin secretion in subjects of chronic hepatitis B with cirrhosis. Int J Clin Exp Pathol. 2015;8:13381.

37. Jiang WD, Hu K, Liu Y, Jiang J, Wu P, Zhao J, et al. Dietary myo-inositol modulates immunity through antioxidant activity and the Nrf2 and E2F4/cyclin signalling factors in the head kidney and spleen following infection of juvenile fish with *Aeromonas hydrophila*. Fish Shellfish Immunol. 2016;49:374–86.

38. Shi H, Kokoeva MV, Inouye K, Tzameli I, Yin H, Flier JS. TLR4 links innate immunity and fatty acid—induced insulin resistance. J Clin Invest. 2006;116:3015–25.

39. Eguchi K, Manabe I, Oishi-Tanaka Y, Ohsugi M, Kono N, Ogata F, et al. Saturated fatty acid and TLR signaling link β cell dysfunction and islet inflammation. Cell Metab. 2012;15:518–33.

40. Tall AR, Yvan-Charvet L. Cholesterol, inflammation and innate immunity. Nat Rev Immunol. 2015;15:104–16.

41. Calder P, Yaqoob P. Glutamine and the immune system. Amino Acids. 1999;17:227–41.

42. Singleton KD, Beckey VE, Wischmeyer PE. Glutamine prevents activation of NF-κB and stress kinase pathways, attenuates inflammatory cytokine release, and prevents acute respiratory distress syndrome (ARDS) following sepsis. Shock. 2005;24:583–9.

43. Hou YC, Liu JJ, Pai MH, Tsou SS, Yeh SL. Alanyl-glutamine administration suppresses Th17 and reduces inflammatory reaction in dextran sulfate sodium-induced acute colitis. Int Immunopharmacol. 2013;17:1–8.

44. Hou YC, Wu JM, Wang MY, Wu MH, Chen KY, Yeh SL, et al. Glutamine supplementation attenuates expressions of adhesion molecules and chemokine receptors on T cells in a murine model of acute colitis. Mediators Inflamm. 2014;2014:837107.

45. Fang YZ, Yang S, Wu G. Free radicals, antioxidants, and nutrition. Nutrition. 2002;18:872–9.

46. Li P, Yin YL, Li D, Kim SW, Wu G. Amino acids and immune function. Br J Nutr. 2007;98:237–52.

47. Wheeler MD, Thurman RG. Production of superoxide and TNF-α from alveolar macrophages is blunted by glycine. Am J Physiol. 1999;277:L952–9.

48. Konashi S, Takahashi K, Akiba Y. Effects of dietary essential amino acid deficiencies on immunological variables in broiler chickens. Br J Nutr. 2000;83:449–56.

49. Morris SM Jr. Arginine: master and commander in innate immune responses. Sci Signal. 2010;3:e27.

50. Platten M, Ho PP, Youssef S, Fontoura P, Garren H, Hur EM, et al. Treatment of autoimmune neuroinflammation with a synthetic tryptophan metabolite. Science. 2005;310:850–5.

51. Stone TW, Stoy N, Darlington LG. An expanding range of targets for kynurenine metabolites of tryptophan. Trends Pharmacol Sci. 2013;34:136–43.

Permissions

All chapters in this book were first published in CM, by BioMed Central; hereby published with permission under the Creative Commons Attribution License or equivalent. Every chapter published in this book has been scrutinized by our experts. Their significance has been extensively debated. The topics covered herein carry significant findings which will fuel the growth of the discipline. They may even be implemented as practical applications or may be referred to as a beginning point for another development.

The contributors of this book come from diverse backgrounds, making this book a truly international effort. This book will bring forth new frontiers with its revolutionizing research information and detailed analysis of the nascent developments around the world.

We would like to thank all the contributing authors for lending their expertise to make the book truly unique. They have played a crucial role in the development of this book. Without their invaluable contributions this book wouldn't have been possible. They have made vital efforts to compile up to date information on the varied aspects of this subject to make this book a valuable addition to the collection of many professionals and students.

This book was conceptualized with the vision of imparting up-to-date information and advanced data in this field. To ensure the same, a matchless editorial board was set up. Every individual on the board went through rigorous rounds of assessment to prove their worth. After which they invested a large part of their time researching and compiling the most relevant data for our readers.

The editorial board has been involved in producing this book since its inception. They have spent rigorous hours researching and exploring the diverse topics which have resulted in the successful publishing of this book. They have passed on their knowledge of decades through this book. To expedite this challenging task, the publisher supported the team at every step. A small team of assistant editors was also appointed to further simplify the editing procedure and attain best results for the readers.

Apart from the editorial board, the designing team has also invested a significant amount of their time in understanding the subject and creating the most relevant covers. They scrutinized every image to scout for the most suitable representation of the subject and create an appropriate cover for the book.

The publishing team has been an ardent support to the editorial, designing and production team. Their endless efforts to recruit the best for this project, has resulted in the accomplishment of this book. They are a veteran in the field of academics and their pool of knowledge is as vast as their experience in printing. Their expertise and guidance has proved useful at every step. Their uncompromising quality standards have made this book an exceptional effort. Their encouragement from time to time has been an inspiration for everyone.

The publisher and the editorial board hope that this book will prove to be a valuable piece of knowledge for researchers, students, practitioners and scholars across the globe.

List of Contributors

H. P. Cheung, S. W. Wang, Y. B. Zhang, L. X. Lao, Z. J. Zhang, Y. Tong, F. W. S. Chung and S. C. W. Sze
School of Chinese Medicine, Li Ka Shing Faculty of Medicine, The University of Hong Kong, 10 Sassoon Road, Pokfulam, Hong Kong, SAR, China

T. B. Ng
School of Biomedical Science, Faculty of Medicine, The Chinese University of Hong Kong, Shatin, N.T., Hong Kong, SAR, China

Yan Yan, Zhenyu Li, Jinping Jia, Aiping Li and Xuemei Qin
Modern Research Center for Traditional Chinese Medicine of Shanxi University, No. 92, Wucheng Road, Taiyuan 030006, Shanxi, China

Min Zhang
Modern Research Center for Traditional Chinese Medicine of Shanxi University, No. 92, Wucheng Road, Taiyuan 030006, Shanxi, China
College of Chemistry and Chemical Engineering of Shanxi University, No. 92, Wucheng Road, Taiyuan 030006, Shanxi, China

Chenhui Du, Jin Li and Qiang Song
School of Traditional Chinese Materia Medica, Shanxi University of Chinese Medicine, No. 121, Daxue Street, Taiyuan 030619, Shanxi, China

Wenlong Huang and Li Liu
China Pharmaceutical University, Longmian Road 639, Nanjing 211198, China

Haitao Tang
China Pharmaceutical University, Longmian Road 639, Nanjing 211198, China
Jiangsu Suzhong Pharmaceutical Group Co., Ltd., No. 1, Suzhong Road, Jiangyan District, Taizhou 225500, Jiangsu, China

Jimei Ma
Jiangsu Suzhong Pharmaceutical Group Co., Ltd., No. 1, Suzhong Road, Jiangyan District, Taizhou 225500, Jiangsu, China

Yue Yan, Chun-Lei Li, Qi Shi, Yan-Hua Kong, Ting Yao and You-Lin Li
The 2nd Department of Pulmonary Disease in TCM, The Key Unit of SATCM Pneumonopathy Chronic Cough and Dyspnea, Beijing Key Laboratory of Prevention and Treatment of Allergic Diseases With TCM (No. BZ0321), Center of Respiratory Medicine, China-Japan Friendship Hospital, National Clinical Research Center for Respiratory Diseases, Beijing 100029, China

Hai-Peng Bao
Beijing University of Chinese Medicine, Beijing 100029, China

Chuen Heung Yau, Cheuk Long Ip and Yuk Yin Chau
School of Chinese Medicine, Hong Kong Baptist University, Kowloon Tong, Hong Kong

Jin-Ni Hong, Wei-Wei Li, Lin-Lin Wang and Xue-Mei Wang
Integrated Laboratory of Traditional Chinese Medicine and Western Medicine, Peking University First Hospital, Beijing, People's Republic of China

Hao Guo
Institute of Basic Medical Sciences, Xiyuan Hospital, China Academy of Chinese Medical Sciences, Beijing, People's Republic of China

Yong Jiang, Yun-Jia Gao and Peng-Fei Tu
School of Pharmaceutical Science, Peking University, Beijing, People's Republic of China

Jiatong Li, Jianfan Zhu, Hao Hu and Ging Chan
State Key Laboratory of Quality Research in Chinese Medicine, Institute of Chinese Medical Sciences, University of Macau, Taipa, Macao

Carolina Oi Lam Ung
State Key Laboratory of Quality Research in Chinese Medicine, Institute of Chinese Medical Sciences, University of Macau, Taipa, Macao
The University of Sydney School of Pharmacy, Faculty of Medicine and Health, The University of Sydney, Sydney, Australia
Pharmaceutical Society of Macau, Taipa, Macau

Joanna E. Harnett
The University of Sydney School of Pharmacy, Faculty of Medicine and Health, The University of Sydney, Sydney, Australia

Chi Ieong Lei
Pharmaceutical Society of Macau, Taipa, Macau

Ka Yin Chau
City University of Macau, Taipa, Macau

Ying Yang and Yijia Chen
State Key Laboratory of Quality Research in Chinese Medicine, Institute of Chinese Medical Sciences, University of Macau, Taipa, Macao, China

Ru Yan
State Key Laboratory of Quality Research in Chinese Medicine, Institute of Chinese Medical Sciences, University of Macau, Taipa, Macao, China
Zhuhai UM Science & Technology Research Institute, Zhuhai 519080, China

Liang Shen, Jiang Xu, Lu Luo, Haoyu Hu, Xiangxiao Meng, Xiwen Li and Shilin Chen
Institute of Chinese Materia Medica, China Academy of Chinese Medical Sciences, Beijing 100700, China

Zhongzhen Zhao, Ping Guo and Eric Brand
School of Chinese Medicine, Hong Kong Baptist University, Kowloon Tong, Hong Kong, China

Ling-Wei Hsu, Meng-Che Yu, Ting-Lin Yen and Thanasekaran Jayakumar
Graduate Institute of Medical Sciences, College of Medicine, Taipei Medical University, Taipei, Taiwan

Wei-Cheng Shiao
Graduate Institute of Medical Sciences, College of Medicine, Taipei Medical University, Taipei, Taiwan
Department of Internal Medicine, Yuan's General Hospital, Kaohsiung, Taiwan

Joen-Rong Sheu
Graduate Institute of Medical Sciences, College of Medicine, Taipei Medical University, Taipei, Taiwan
Department of Pharmacology, School of Medicine, Taipei Medical University, Taipei, Taiwan

Nen-Chung Chang
Department of Internal Medicine, School of Medicine, Taipei Medical University, Taipei, Taiwan

Philip Aloysius Thomas
Department of Microbiology, Institute of Ophthalmology, Joseph Eye Hospital, Tiruchirappalli, Tamil Nadu 620 001, India

Xiaomei Wang and Huangan Wu
Shanghai Research Institute of Acupuncture and Meridian, Shanghai University of Traditional Chinese Medicine, 650 South Wanping Road, Xuhui District, Shanghai 200030, China
Key Laboratory of Acupuncture and Immunological Effects, Shanghai University of Traditional Chinese Medicine, Shanghai 200030, China

Qin Qi, Yuanyuan Wang, Duiyin Jin, Yanan Liu and Cun Wang
Yueyang Clinical Medical College, Shanghai University of Traditional Chinese Medicine, Shanghai 200437, China

Xiaoming Jin
Stark Neurosciences Research Institute & Department of Anatomy and Cell Biology, Indiana University School of Medicine, Indianapolis, IN 46202, USA

Huan Yao
Department of Radiation Oncology, Indiana University School of Medicine, Indianapolis, IN 46202, USA

Qing-Wen Zhang and Li-Gen Lin
State Key Laboratory of Quality Research in Chinese Medicine, Institute of Chinese Medical Sciences, University of Macau, Macao, People's Republic of China

Wen-Cai Ye
Institute of Traditional Chinese Medicine & Natural Products, and Guangdong Provincial Engineering Research Center for Modernization of TCM, College of Pharmacy, Jinan University, Guangzhou 510632, People's Republic of China

Yanan Zhao, Ailin Yang, Pengfei Tu and Zhongdong Hu
Modern Research Center for Traditional Chinese Medicine, School of Chinese Materia Medica, Beijing University of Chinese Medicine, No.11 North Third Ring Road, Chaoyang District, Beijing 100029, China

Liao Cui
Guangdong Key Laboratory for Research and Development of Natural Drugs, Guangdong Medical University, Zhanjiang, Guangdong, China

Zhangfeng Zhong
Guangdong Key Laboratory for Research and Development of Natural Drugs, Guangdong Medical University, Zhanjiang, Guangdong, China State Key Laboratory of Quality Research in Chinese Medicine, Institute of Chinese Medical Sciences, University of Macau, Macao, China

Shengpeng Wang and Yitao Wang
State Key Laboratory of Quality Research in Chinese Medicine, Institute of Chinese Medical Sciences, University of Macau, Macao, China

Haibing Yu
School of Public Health, Guangdong Medical University, Dongguan, Guangdong, China

Min Dai, Fenglin Wang, Zengcheng Zou, Gemin Xiao, Hongjie Chen and Hongzhi Yang
Traditional Chinese Medicine Department, The Third Affiliated Hospital of Sun Yat-sen University, Guangzhou 510630, China

Index